CW00516469

# The Eighteenth-Century Origins of Angina Pectoris

(*Medical History*, Supplement No. 21)

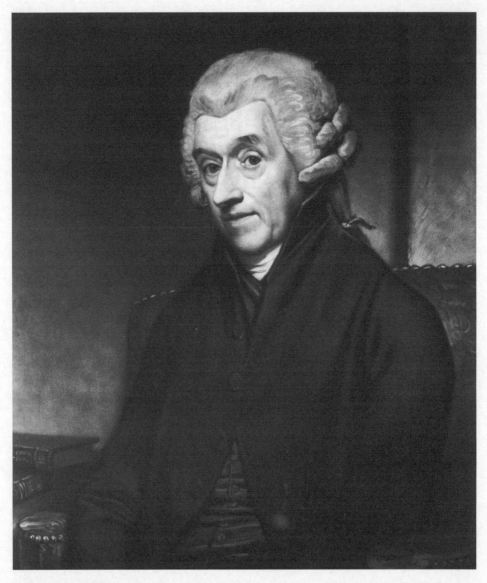

*Frontispiece:* William Heberden (1710–1801). Mezzotint by J Ward after Sir W Beechey (Wellcome Library, London).

# The Eighteenth-Century Origins of Angina Pectoris: Predisposing Causes, Recognition and Aftermath

by

## LEON MICHAELS

(*Medical History*, Supplement No. 21)

London
The Wellcome Trust Centre for the History of Medicine at UCL
2001

ISBN 0-85484-073-7

Supplements to *Medical History* may be obtained by post from Professional & Scientific Publications, BMA House, Tavistock Square, London WC1H 9JR, UK; and The Wellcome Library, Wellcome Building, 183 Euston Road, London NW1 1BE, UK.

# Contents

## Contents

# List of Illustrations, Tables, and Figures

*Tables*

## Illustrations, Tables and Figures

### Figures

# Acknowledgements

Help has been received from innumerable sources, always given with great kindness and consideration. My grateful thanks go to those who so generously gave of their time, facilities and expertise.

At what is now the Wellcome Trust for the History of Medicine at UCL, Sir Christopher Booth provided useful insights concerning the early descriptions of angina pectoris. The text was enhanced by inclusion of supplementary topics suggested by Professor W F Bynum. Professor R Porter furnished valuable general information about life in Georgian England, Dr S R Johanssen provided material from her PhD thesis concerning eighteenth-century medicine in general, and Mr Ernest Heberden, biographer of William Heberden, supplied uniquely helpful background information about his distinguished forebear.

Professor Margaret Visser of the University of Toronto and Miss C Mullins, Clinical Dietician, Health Sciences Centre, Winnipeg, gave advice about relevant eighteenth- and twentieth-century dietary matters respectively. Professors R Gold and I McDougall of the Department of Classics at the University of Winnipeg helped with English translations of medical writings from the original Latin. Professor E A Wrigley of the Cambridge Group for the History of Population and Social Structure furnished demographic data additional to that available in his published works. Professor J Wortley, Department of History, University of Manitoba, reviewed the section on eighteenth-century religious history for its relevance to dietary changes at that time. Dr J Wood of the Division of Food and Animal Science of the University of Bristol directed me to source material dealing with the connections between farming practice and the fat characteristics of animals raised for food. In the latter respect I am also indebted to Professor M Eskins of the Department of Food and Nutrition and to Professors R J Parker and R Ingalls of the Department of Animal Science and the Faculty of Agricultural and Food Sciences, all of the University of Manitoba. They were initially somewhat nonplussed by requests for information about past research into feeding techniques that were designed to *increase* the fat content and the proportion of saturated fats in animals raised for human consumption. It was the exact opposite of their own and their departments' current endeavours and indeed of their life work. However, once my purpose was clarified, they were extremely helpful in providing information and source material dealing with animal husbandry as practised in the mid-twentieth century, a period that antedated current concerns about fats in general and cholesterol in particular. Professor R A Hegele of the University of Toronto introduced me to genetics as related to ischaemic heart disease.

Considerable help was provided by my colleagues who are members of the Medical Faculty of the University of Manitoba. Dr C Greenberg lent her expertise to the chapter on heredity. Dr P Bolli gave specialist advice with respect to the relationships between dietary fat, lipid biochemistry and their epidemiological significance. Dr I Carr, lecturer in Medical History, read a draft of the completed manuscript. His criticisms were constructive and much appreciated. Mr R Tate, consultant at the Biostatistical Unit, provided assistance with statistical material and presentation of numerical data. The librarians of the Wellcome Library, the British Museum and London Guildhall Libraries, and the Elizabeth Dafoe and Neil John Maclean Libraries of the University of Manitoba gave generous help, notwithstanding a penchant for shelving almost all of the materials that I needed at either floor or ceiling level. They were endlessly patient with provision of source material and provided help when my own computer skills proved less than adequate for some literature searches. The London staff of Messrs Berry and Rudd were most considerate in making available their records of the weights of their eighteenth-century clients. The resources of the Manitoba Clinic, Winnipeg, Canada, were put freely at my disposal, and Mrs April Borgford and Ms Lelia Beaufoy provided unstinting and thoughtful secretarial help from the earliest draft to the final manuscript, coping tirelessly with the necessary revisions. My wife Joan Michaels edited the manuscript, effecting improvements in style and lucidity. I am deeply indebted to everyone concerned and wish to express to them my most sincere thanks.

# Abbreviations

| | |
|---|---|
| ACE | Angiotensin Converting Enzyme. Involved in a cascade of reactions leading ultimately to elevation of blood pressure. |
| AP | Angina Pectoris. Also referred to simply as "angina". |
| APO | Apolipoprotein. A protein in the blood concerned with lipid (i.e. fat) transport. High levels of type A are desirable; raised concentrations of type B undesirable and predispose to CHD. |
| BMI | Body Mass Index. Derived from height and weight, and an indicator of obesity when elevated. |
| C | Carbon |
| CCF | Congestive Cardiac Failure |
| CHD | Coronary Heart Disease |
| CL | Confidence Limits |
| cwt | Hundredweight (112 pounds) |
| dl | Decilitre |
| g | Grams |
| HDL | High Density Lipoprotein—elevation of blood levels is associated with reduced liability to develop CHD; low levels with increased risk. Sometimes referred to as the "good cholesterol". |
| LDL | Low Density Lipoprotein. Predisposes to CHD when blood levels are excessive. It is sometimes referred to as the "bad cholesterol". |
| Lipid Profile | An overview of fats in the blood, including serum triglycerides, total cholesterol, HDL and LDL. |
| Lipoproteins | Serum proteins which act as carriers for fats in the blood. |
| Lp(a) | Lipoprotein (a). A variant of the above. High blood levels are associated with increased CHD incidence. |
| METS | Metabolic equivalents. A measure of exercise intensity. |
| mg | Milligrams |
| mg/dl | Milligrams per decilitre |
| mg/g | Milligrams per gram |
| mg/L | Milligrams per litre |
| MI | Myocardial Infarction |
| mmHg | Millimetres of Mercury |
| mmol | Millimoles |
| MRFIT | Multiple Risk Factor Intervention Trial |
| MUFA | Monounsaturated Fatty Acids |
| P | Probability. $<0.05$ conventionally implies (statistical) significance. |
| P/S ratio | Ratio of polyunsaturated to saturated fats (or fatty acids). |
| PUFA | Polyunsaturated Fatty Acids. The commonest is linoleic acid. |
| RF | Risk Factor. One which predisposes to development of CHD. |
| RR | Relative Risk |

*Abbreviations*

SD          Standard Deviation
SE          Standard Error
SFA         Saturated Fatty Acids
TC          Total Serum Cholesterol
TFA         Trans-fatty Acids
VLDL        Very Low Density Lipoprotein
μg/L        Micrograms per Litre
μU/L        Microunits per Litre

# Terminology and Definitions

"When I use a word, it means just what I choose it to mean, neither more nor less."[1]

*Agricultural Revolution:* this term is used to describe the developments in animal husbandry and crop management that took place during the eighteenth century. Although in their ultimate effects the changes over many decades were revolutionary, nothing cataclysmic is implied by this expression.

*Aristocracy* or *nobility:* describe members of the peerage, both spiritual and temporal, together with their spouses, children and any of their parents who had not themselves been ennobled.

*Cis-* and *trans-fatty acids:* these are formulaically identical unsaturated fatty acids, the former occurring more commonly in natural fats, the latter in margarines. They differ in the spacial arrangements of hydrogen atoms attached to double bonded carbon atoms and function differently in vivo.

*Coronary heart disease:* this refers to the common atherosclerotic disease of the coronary arteries unless otherwise specified, for example in reference to coronary ostial narrowing of syphilitic origin. When epidemiological data concerning unstable angina, myocardial infarction or sudden death are mentioned, the definitions used by the investigators being quoted have been accepted.

*England:* the name is never used in the Continental sense as synonymous with the United Kingdom. It refers strictly to England, excluding Wales and Monmouthshire. When these *are* included, the term England and Wales is employed. Prior to the Act of Union with Scotland of 1707, England and Wales was a distinct political entity. Even after the Union, demographic, economic and sociological data for either England alone or for England and Wales continued to be compiled separately from Scotland. From 1707 until 1800 the term Great Britain applied strictly to the geographical description of the island. Politically, the country created by the union of England and Wales with Scotland became "the United Kingdom of Great Britain". The term United Kingdom of Great Britain and Ireland was included after the union of 1800. In 1922 the name was finally modified to "The United Kingdom of Great Britain and Northern Ireland".[2]

---

[1] Humpty Dumpty in Lewis Carroll, *Through the looking glass and what Alice found there* (first published 1872), London, Macmillan, 1968, p. 130.

[2] Frank O'Gorman, *The long eighteenth century: British political and social history 1688–1832*, London, Arnold, 1997, p. 124.

## Terminology and Definitions

*Gentry:* includes baronets, knights and large-scale landowners together with their immediate families.

*Georgian era:* has been used on occasion in place of "eighteenth century", although not quite identical with it. The consecutive reigns of the four monarchs named George extended from 1714 to 1830. However, as the changes in cardiac risk factors to be described were gradual and continuous and did not fit neatly into the years 1700 to 1800, no serious inaccuracy results from the substitution and needless repetition is thereby avoided.

*Middle aged* and *elderly:* unless stated otherwise, both these terms indicate all persons aged 45 or more. A little arbitrary, but includes almost all people susceptible to coronary heart disease. A frequent division in demographic tabulations.

*Middle class:* although this term was not used before the late eighteenth century and many of the more affluent members of society would have considered themselves demeaned by being so classified, the term has sociological value. Here it is used to include families whose heads were in offices, places, liberal arts and sciences, clergymen below the rank of bishop, naval and military officers (unless members of the nobility), merchants, professional persons, freeholders and small landowners not engaged personally in farm work. Towards the end of the eighteenth century, manufacturers and providers of financial services became important additions to this group. Eighteenth-century writers sometimes referred to "the middling sort" or "the middling orders".[3]

*Monounsaturated fats* or *monounsaturates:* triglycerides in which fatty acids bound by glycerol have one double bond linkage in the carbon chain.

*Polyunsaturated fats* or *polyunsaturates:* As above, except for two or more double bonds linking the carbon chain.

*Saturated fats or saturates:* triglycerides in which all bonds in the carbon chains are single.

*Secondary study*: one designed to observe the effect of an intervention on the recurrence rate of cardiac events in a population whose members had already suffered a CHD episode.

*South Asian*: this term is used to describe migrants from the Indian subcontinent whose forebears had lived there for very many generations. The adjective Indian would have applied prior to 1947, Indian or Pakistani after independence and Indian, Pakistani or Bangladeshi after 1971. A further complication is introduced because migrants from India to the United Kingdom during the late 1940s

[3] Ibid., p. 108.

consisted very largely of people of British origin leaving the subcontinent when imperial rule ended. The term South Asian circumvents these complexities, providing it is understood that it excludes both British returnees from the subcontinent *and* migrants to the UK from any other parts of Asia.

*Traditional risk factors:* include age, male sex, abnormalities of lipid profile, diabetes mellitus, high blood pressure, smoking, stress and physical inactivity. Any other risk factors, of which some 246 were listed at a recent count,[4] are specified when alluded to. Examples of the latter include elevation of serum homocysteine, Lp(a) levels and coagulation or clotting factors. On occasion, the term "nontraditional risk factor" is used as a generalization.

*Traditional societies:* communities in developing countries whose farming practices had not been affected appreciably by the types of change introduced into Western Europe and North America during the past three centuries.

*Victorian era:* strictly from 1837 to 1901. It has been used in practice to denote the middle and late nineteenth century.

*1768:* this date is used at times without explanation in order to denote the year of Heberden's first description of angina pectoris.

[4] Paul N Hopkins and Roger R Williams, 'A survey of 246 reputed coronary risk factors', *Atherosclerosis*, 1981, **40**: 1–52, pp. 2–8.

# I

# Introduction

Old diseases are passing away ... but new ones are continually taking their place.[1]

In 1768 William Heberden made a presentation to the Royal College of Physicians of London in which he described angina pectoris in a manner that is readily recognizable to the twentieth-century physician and patient. He reported on a score of individuals who clearly could be grouped together as having a symptom complex common to them all.[2] The number of similar patients that he saw subsequent to his initial presentation rose nearly fourfold in the next decade,[3] during which reports of angina by many other English medical writers appeared for the first time. This is in striking contrast to the paucity of earlier accounts and to the degree of uncertainty with which they could be identified as being descriptions of the characteristic pain.

There are two mutually exclusive explanations for these developments. The first is that angina pectoris had long afflicted humankind and not been uncommon, but had largely gone unrecognized. The second is that coronary heart disease was for all practical purposes a condition emerging *de novo*, its symptoms afflicting sufferers in the mid-eighteenth century for what was virtually the first time, and with its incidence increasing dramatically thereafter. The present work is devoted to the thesis that the second explanation is the correct one. Reasons why angina first made its appearance at that time have been sought among the many changes in living patterns that took place uniquely in England, during the eighteenth century in particular, and at a greater speed and extent than ever before. The subsequent relationships between risk factors new and old and the natural history of coronary heart disease during the succeeding 200 years have been outlined.

The history of clinical medicine consists not only of the record of the recognition of disease patterns and the evolution of ideas about causation of illnesses and their treatment, but also a record of the disease processes themselves. Some conditions have varied in their severity over the course of human history while others have changed in their presentation. Some have become more common and others more rare. Some illnesses have disappeared, others have emerged.

Human history and prehistory have been characterized by a succession of adverse events and forces, each capable of causing a great variety of diseases to which our progenitors had never been subject during human beginnings in the Olduvai Gorge. As migration took them into areas of desert, they became subject to extreme heat, dehydration and solar exposure, with all their consequences. Wandering further

---

[1] William Boyd, *A textbook of pathology*, 8th ed., Philadelphia, Lea and Febiger, 1970, pp. 10–11.

[2] William Heberden, 'Some account of a disorder in the breast', *Med Trans Coll Physns Lond*, 1772, **2**: 59–67, pp. 59–62.

[3] William Heberden, *Commentaries on the history and cure of diseases*, Boston, Wells and Lilly, 1818, p. 294.

northward into the temperate zones and beyond exposed them to the effects of wet, cold and lack of ultraviolet light. Ascent into mountain ranges brought hypoxia and its secondary effects and, more recently, the bends became manifest with descent into the depths of the sea for the first time. With the move from nomadic hunting and gathering to settlement in agricultural communities and the accompanying changes to diets that became excessively reliant on cereals, a variety of deficiency diseases became manifest. Development of animal husbandry brought in its train close and prolonged contact with animal pathogens that could be transmitted, with the resulting emergence of new human infections. The back-breaking work of cultivation resulted in orthopaedic problems. Increasing population density facilitated the spread of transmittable diseases in epidemic form. Examination of skeletal remains at archaeological sites has revealed the telltale evidence of bone thinning and inflammatory and osteoarthritis changes.[4] The beginning of communal living resulted in exposure to the stresses linked with crowding and disruption of earlier social patterns. A high incidence of fractures found at sites associated with early farming communities is a possible indicator of resulting violence.[5] More recently, illnesses attributable to excess have superseded those due to deficiency, at first among the privileged few but subsequently among widespread populations that had previously suffered deprivation.[6]

The long sea voyages of exploration beginning in the late fifteenth century led to a greatly increased prevalence of deficiency diseases such as scurvy and the spread of illnesses endemic in one part of the world to other regions previously spared.[7] A possible example in Europe is syphilis, first recorded after Columbus' crews returned from their first voyage to the New World and disseminated widely following a series of military campaigns in southern Italy in the early sixteenth century.[8] Sometimes migrants moved into areas inhabited by pathogens or their carriers, with neither of which there had been any previous contact;[9] at other times the pathogens became disseminated into areas of long-standing human habitation that had previously been spared, examples being malaria and yellow fever introduced into America after its original inhabitants' first contact with people from the Old World.[10]

In recent times, the increasing impact of human activity on the environment has brought new diseases in its train. The first industrial exposure probably came with inhalation of smoke from wood fires in caves. This was the forerunner of a myriad of toxic factors produced during farming, mining and manufacturing, and resulting in an increasingly polluted environment.[11] The resulting diseases were not necessarily

---

[4] Clark Spencer Larson, 'Biological changes in human populations with agriculture', *Annu Rev Anthropol*, 1995, **24**: 185–213, pp. 198–200.

[5] Ibid., p. 198.

[6] Ellen Ruppel Shell, 'New World Syndrome', *Atlantic Monthly*, 2001, **287**: 50–3.

[7] J Diamond, *Guns, germs and steel: the fates of human societies*, London, W W Norton, 1997, p. 210.

[8] Albert S Lyons and R Joseph Petricelli II, *Medicine: an illustrated history*, New York, Harry N Abrams, 1978, p. 376.

[9] Diamond, op. cit., note 7 above, p. 327.

[10] Ibid., p. 358.

[11] Bernardino Ramazzini, *Diseases of workers*, transl. from the Latin text, *De morbis artificum*, of 1713, by Wilmer Cave Wright, London, Hafner, 1964, pp. 15, 62, 337.

confined to the respiratory system. In 1817, James Parkinson described for the first time the "shaking palsy", the neurologic illness to which his name was later attached.[12] The absence of earlier clinical descriptions of this obvious and readily identifiable disability raises the possibility that Parkinsonism is a condition which only became manifest early in the nineteenth century. An association with manganese and carbon monoxide poisoning has since been recognized and exposure to industrial pollutants consequent to the industrial revolution proposed as a cause. Cerebral lesions resembling those of Parkinsonism have been produced in experimental animals by exposure to coal tar derivatives.[13] Environmental diseases have culminated in the late twentieth century in an array of illnesses associated with exposure to radiation.

Throughout the ages the endeavours of physicians have made their contribution to new diseases. Sometimes these were caused by medication. At other times they resulted from non-pharmacological forms of treatment, examples being the anaemia and complications of reduced blood volume that on occasion followed the frequent bloodletting of earlier times. Lately, the increased longevity which has resulted from the successes of medicine has brought in its train a rise in prevalence of the degenerative diseases of later life. Within the sphere of cardiology, an example of an apparently new disease is provided by Dressler's syndrome. Myocardial infarction with initial survival was described by W P Obrastzow and N D Straschesko in 1910,[14] and followed by James Herrick in 1912.[15] The auscultatory features of pericarditis had been reported by Joseph Skoda in the middle of the nineteenth century.[16] However, it was not until 1953 that L Faure and M Cazeilles described a patient with initial electrocardiographic evidence of acute myocardial infarction accompanied by a transient pericardial rub, a scratching sound heard with a stethoscope and associated with inflammation of the membranes covering the heart. In this individual, who was being treated with anticoagulants, initial improvement was followed after an interval by episodes of fever, lancinating chest pain and recurrence of the rub.[17] Three years later William Dressler, who had already described a similar course of events after heart valve surgery, reported ten similar patients. He described them as having a condition which did not "fit in any of the usual complications of myocardial infarction listed in the textbooks".[18] In these patients too, myocardial infarction was followed after an interval of comparative wellbeing by a succession of pleuritic and pericardial pains, fever and a pericardial rub.[19] The number of patients was sufficient to qualify the condition as a distinctly recognizable

[12] James Parkinson, 'An essay on the shaking palsy 1817', reprinted in Robert H Wilkins and Irwin A Brody, *Neurological classics*, New York, Johnson Reprint Corporation, 1973, pp. 88–92, 89–90.

[13] Carl Pinsky and R Bose, 'Pyridine and other coal tar constituents as free radical-generating environmental neurotoxicants', *Mol Cell Biochem*, 1988, **84**: 217–22, p. 219.

[14] W P Obrastzow and N D Straschesko, 'Zur Kenntnis der Thrombose der Koronarterien des Herzens', *Zschrf Klin Med*, 1910, **71**: 116–32, pp. 118–23.

[15] James B Herrick, 'Clinical features of sudden obstruction of the coronary arteries', *JAMA*, 1912, **59**: 2015–20, pp. 2017–18.

[16] L J Acierno, *The history of cardiology*, Camforth, Lancs, Parthenon, 1994, p. 466.

[17] L Faure and M Cazeilles, 'Pericardite aiguë récidivante et infarctus du myocarde', *Journal de Médecine de Bordeaux et du Sud Ouest*, 1953, **130**: 489–92, pp. 490–1.

[18] William Dressler, 'A post-myocardial-infarction syndrome', *JAMA*, 1956, **160**: 1379–83.

[19] Ibid., pp. 1379–83.

and eponymously named Dressler's syndrome. Speculation as to its causes included activation of a viral infection of the heart and, in some instances, an inflammatory response to bleeding into the pericardial sac as a consequence of the anticoagulant therapy which had recently been introduced for treatment of ischaemic heart disease.[20] In addition to the patient of Faure and Cazeilles, some of Dressler's patients were treated with anticoagulants, as were many others who were subsequently recognized as having the condition.

In some cases recognition followed the appearance of a disease that may never have been manifest previously. At other times a disease formerly extremely rare may have become significantly more common. In some instances the "newness" of a disease is speculative; in others it is definite. Certainly the spread of Acquired Immune Deficiency Syndrome (AIDS) over the past twenty years has shown in dramatic fashion that a completely new human ailment can become manifest.[21] L Garrett, writing in 1994, added nine other formerly unknown infectious diseases, and the list continues to grow.[22]

The emergence of new diseases continues and is not confined to physical complaints. Thus in 1979, Gerald Russell described thirty patients that he had seen during the previous six and a half years. In all cases periods of self-imposed near starvation were interrupted by uncontrollable binge eating followed by self-induced vomiting or purgation. The author, who named the condition "bulimia nervosa", noted that there were only three previous references in the literature, the earliest as recently as 1976. None had described the full-blown syndrome. No association with any endocrine disturbance was found and the condition had diagnostic criteria clearly distinguishable from anorexia nervosa.[23] It would be hard to imagine that a symptom complex so dramatic would have gone totally unnoticed before the 1970s, suggesting therefore that bulimia nervosa too is a new condition.

The present work is devoted to the thesis that the description of angina pectoris in 1768 by William Heberden marked not a first recognition of a syndrome formerly widespread although unrecognized, but rather the appearance and subsequent increase in frequency of a condition previously rare almost to the point of being non-existent. It is also suggested that such few earlier and questionable descriptions as are extant may, in some instances at least, have referred to angina pectoris caused by other than arteriosclerotic coronary arterial disease, the latter being a virtually "new" condition. This was my hypothesis, put forward over thirty years ago. I then suggested that increasing expectation of life could not alone explain the phenomenon and noted that even before the eighteenth century a privileged minority of the population of England had lived to late middle and old age and had access to adequate or even excessive amounts of animal foods. Reasons for the apparent appearance of angina pectoris on the medical scene *de novo* were not therefore

---

[20] George E Burch and H L Colcolough, 'Postcardiotomy and postinfarction syndromes—a theory', *Am Heart J*, 1970, **80**: 290–1, p. 290.

[21] Samuel Broder, T C Memgan Jr and D Bolognesi, *Textbook of AIDS medicine*, London, Williams and Wilkins, 1994, pp. 3–5.

[22] L Garrett, *The coming plague*, New York, Farrar, Straus and Giroux, 1994, p. ix.

[23] G Russell, 'Bulimia nervosa': an ominous variant of anorexia nervosa', *Psychol Med*, 1979, **9**: 429–48, p. 429.

adequately explained at that time.[24] My hypothesis received some attention, with a contrary view being expressed by Howard Sprague.[25] J O Leibowitz, in his classical history of coronary arterial disease, quoted the two opposing opinions without attempting to arbitrate between them.[26] Subsequent histories of cardiovascular disease have tended to record the late eighteenth-century descriptions of angina pectoris by Heberden without discussing possible reasons for its sudden widespread recognition. The present work reviews the evidence, necessarily in some measure negative, for angina pectoris being considered a condition that had been virtually non-existent before the mid-eighteenth century. The limitations of applying twentieth-century understanding to eighteenth-century conditions are acknowledged. Developments from the beginning of the eighteenth century and even somewhat earlier are con-sidered, as the onset and progression of coronary atherosclerotic changes usually precede the onset of symptoms by many years and the pain may be present for a long time before medical help is sought. One of Heberden's patients first developed angina pectoris as early as 1734, some thirty-four years before his ground-breaking oral report to a medical audience.

For several reasons, the emphasis is mainly on conditions in England, where the original classical description of angina pectoris was made and where Heberden's patients lived. As detailed later, the factors thought to have contributed to the emergence of overt coronary arterial disease developed both earlier and more rapidly in eighteenth-century England than elsewhere. The report by Samuel Black from Ireland may appear to be an exception as far as location is concerned. However, as he practised in Ulster and saw "none in the poor and laborious", it is probable that his patients were drawn from the Protestant minority with English middle-class lifestyles. Many English descriptions of angina pectoris followed closely upon that of Heberden, but almost half a century separated his description from any but the most scanty of written accounts emanating from either the Continent of Europe or from North America. As will become evident in the text, population records and other pertinent documentation were developed to a surprisingly advanced extent in England at that time. Furthermore, all its imports and exports of commodities such as coffee, sugar and tobacco were shipborne so that the amounts involved could be tallied the more readily at the ports and documented for posterity. Lastly, the study of trends extending for nearly a century is facilitated by the constancy of England's boundaries. Their political and economic significance remained unchanged from the 1707 union with Scotland until that with Ireland in 1800. In contrast, data for Austria, for example, would have had to take account of the loss of Silesia in the mid-eighteenth century; data for Prussia would have had to take note of its acquisition. The initial failure of physicians to report angina pectoris in countries other than England was the subject of comment by Samuel Black scarcely half a century after

[24] Leon Michaels, 'Aetiology of coronary heart disease: an historical approach', *Br Heart J*, 1966, **28**: 258–64, p. 263.

[25] Howard Sprague, 'Environment in relation to coronary artery disease', *Arch Environ Health*, 1966, **13**: 4–12, p. 11.

[26] J O Leibowitz, *The history of coronary heart disease*, London, Wellcome Institute of the History of Medicine, 1970, pp. 173–5.

*Table I.1*
Male manifestations of coronary heart disease.
Framingham Study: 10 year follow-up, age 50 to 59 at entry

|  | Cohort | |
| --- | --- | --- |
| Year | 1950 | 1970 |
| Number of subjects at entry | 485 | 512 |
| Myocardial infarction | 54 | 43 |
| Angina pectoris | 60 | 44 |
| Other (AP CCF & sudden death) | 26 | 22 |
| All CHD | 140 | 109 |

Adapted from data published by Pamela A Sytkowski, William B Kannel and Ralph B D'Agostino, 'Changes in risk factors and the decline in mortality from cardiovascular disease. The Framingham Heart Study', in *New Engl J Med*, 1990, **322**: 1635–41, pp. 1637–8.

Heberden's first presentation. Writing in 1819, he remarked on the failure of Baron Corvisart, Napoleon's physician, to make any mention of angina pectoris in a book devoted exclusively to diseases of the heart and great vessels. Black concluded that this failure reflected a real disparity between the United Kingdom and France with respect to the incidence of the complaint.[27]

Whilst angina pectoris was the subject of eighteenth-century descriptions, twentieth-century epidemiologic studies commonly use myocardial infarction, fatal or nonfatal, as additional end points, chosen because of their objective nature. Deductions from such investigations are here considered justified because in the eighteenth-century case reports already included worsening angina pectoris, onset of the pain at rest, prolonged episodes unrelieved by rest and ultimately death, instantaneous on occasion. It would therefore appear that the constellation of symptoms reported by Heberden and his contemporaries included not only classical stable angina of effort but other manifestations now recognizable as unstable angina, acute coronary insufficiency, myocardial infarction and death due to coronary heart disease. Its various presentations have pathological features in common making it probable that any risk factor relevant to one clinical variant would be similarly relevant to others. A number of large-scale studies have shown this to be the case. As examples, the Framingham study demonstrated a reduction in frequency of coronary heart disease between male cohorts enrolled in either 1950 or 1970, free of cardiovascular disease at baseline and followed for ten years. The incidence of angina pectoris and other clinical manifestations all lessened to about the same extent (Table I.1).[28] In a meta-analysis, Jesse A Berlin and Graham A Colditz found that the increase in relative risk of coronary heart disease associated with physical inactivity was about the same for cardiac deaths, angina pectoris and all clinical manifestations when considered

[27] Samuel Black, *Clinical and pathological reports*, Newry, Alexander Wilkinson, 1819, p. 31.
[28] Pamela A Sytkowski, William B Kannel and Ralph B D'Agostino, 'Changes in risk factors and the decline in mortality from cardiovascular disease. The Framingham Heart Study', *N Engl J Med*, 1990, **322**: 1635–41, pp. 1637–8.

*Table I.2*
Physical inactivity and risk of coronary heart disease

| Manifestation | Relative Risk* | Confidence Limits |
|---|---|---|
| CHD | 1.8 | 0.9–3.3 |
| CHD Death | 1.7 | 1.3–2.2 |
| Angina Pectoris | 2.2 | 1.3–3.9 |

* Physically active subjects: RR = 1.0.

Source: Jesse A Berlin and Graham A Colditz, 'A meta-analysis of physical activity in the prevention of coronary heart disease', *Am J Epidemiol*, 1990, **132**: 612–28, p. 623. (By permission of Oxford University Press.)

together (Table I.2).[29] The Whitehall II study of British government personnel included patients with new onset angina, prolonged chest pain suggestive of acute coronary insufficiency, proven myocardial infarction and any other coronary event as end points. They found, *inter alia*, that "the classic coronary risk factors were related to all four outcomes".[30] The Seven Countries study results showed that "except in the Netherlands the distribution of the several manifestations of the disease was similar in the several regions in the study" and "[f]or all diagnoses of coronary heart disease ... the same cohorts provided the extremes of incidence rates".[31]

This book is not directed solely to cardiologists but also to the general medical community and allied health professionals. The work gives the view of a clinical cardiologist enquiring into fields that include, amongst other disciplines, medical, general and economic history, sociology and demography, history of agriculture and current food chemistry. It is hoped therefore that it will interest persons working in any of these fields as well as the general reader. The text has been designed to be read independently of the tables which are inserted in order to provide supporting data for readers with a special interest in any particular topic. I trust that anyone properly concerned with women's rights will forgive the not infrequent use of masculine nouns and pronouns without accompanying feminine equivalents. This has been done, although only in part, for reasons of style. More importantly, the greater incidence of angina pectoris among men as compared to women seems to have been much more marked in the late eighteenth century than is now the case. Enquiry into possible reasons for its late eighteenth-century emergence can therefore legitimately include studies confined to men. The incidence of coronary heart disease is hardly something for which equality of the sexes is to be sought, even by the most ardent of feminists.

[29] Jesse A Berlin and Graham A Colditz, 'A meta-analysis of physical activity in the prevention of coronary heart disease', *Am J Epidemiol*, 1990, **132**: 612–28, p. 622.
[30] Hans Bosma *et al.*, 'Low job control and risk of coronary heart disease in Whitehall II (prospective cohort) study', *Br Med J*, 1997, **314**: 558–65, p. 563.
[31] Ancel Keys, *Seven countries: a multivariate analysis of death and coronary heart disease*, Cambridge, MA, and London, Harvard University Press, 1980, p. 319.

# II

# The Historical Evidence

1768 and all that.[1]

## The Impact of William Heberden

This chapter examines in a historical context the hypothesis that with exceedingly rare exceptions angina pectoris began to afflict patients only in the middle of the eighteenth century, after which its emergence was followed by a rapid increase in incidence, i.e. it had *not* been a symptom prevalent earlier but unrecognized.

An enquiry into the history of angina pectoris can do no better than begin with William Heberden's verbal but landmark description of 1768.[2] This was a time during which the ideas of the Enlightenment were spreading throughout Western Europe but the *anciens régimes* still managed to maintain their power: the French Revolution was nearly a quarter of a century away. Great Britain had just been victorious in the Seven Years' War and was about to obtain control of India. She ruled over the entire eastern seaboard of North America, Canada having been won and the American colonies not yet lost.[3] George III was on the throne and had yet to suffer his first bout of insanity.[4] The rural landscape was being transformed as enclosed fields replaced open scattered strips[5] and the urban scene was changing beyond recognition with the early stages of the Industrial Revolution.[6] Medical thought had become liberated from its former blind adherence to Galenic concepts and the four humours were no longer providing explanations for causation of disease. Instead, debate was raging between advocates of mechanistic theories of disease and those who considered disorders of the "anima" more significant.[7] Giovanni Battista Morgagni had recently expanded the scope of clinical-anatomical correlations with his 500 cases, usually followed to death and autopsy.[8] Daniel Gabriel Fahrenheit had developed a calibrated mercury thermometer and Herman Boerhaave applied it to the first instrumental assessment of illness at the bedside.[9] Leopold Auenbrugger had just widened the scope of physical examination by adding percussion to inspection

---

[1] With acknowledgments to W C Sellar and R J Yeatman, *1066 and all that*, London, Methuen, 1930.

[2] William Heberden, 'Some account of a disorder in the breast', *Med Trans Coll Physns*, London, 1772, **2**: 59–67, pp. 59–60, 63.

[3] Frank O'Gorman, *The long eighteenth century: British political and social history 1688–1832*, London, Arnold, 1997, p. 183.

[4] Ibid., p. 205.

[5] Ibid., p. 330.

[6] Ibid., pp. 113–15.

[7] Roy Porter, *The greatest benefit to mankind: a medical history of humanity from antiquity to the present*, London, HarperCollins, 1997, pp. 246–7.

[8] Giovanni Battista Morgagni, *The seats and causes of diseases*, vols. I–III, transl. B Alexander, London, A Miller and T Cadell, 1769.

[9] Porter, op. cit., note 7 above, p. 344.

and palpation.[10] In England the surgeons had recently become divorced from the barbers. The medical supremacy of Oxford and Cambridge was being challenged by physicians graduating from Edinburgh or Continental medical schools. John Hunter was transforming experimental medicine and surgery,[11] his brother William transforming obstetrics.[12] The management of heart disease was about to be advanced by introduction of the leaf of the foxglove for treating cardiac failure.[13]

Heberden first publicly described the symptoms of angina pectoris on 21 July 1768, in a presentation to the Royal College of Physicians of London, it being the first time that the term had ever been used. His description of the most salient features of the pain warrants reproduction *verbatim* as it appeared in 1772 when published in the *Transactions* of the Royal College of Physicians of London under the title of 'Some account of a disorder of the breast'.[14]

> There is a disorder of the breast marked with strong and peculiar symptoms, considerable for the kind of danger belonging to it, and not extremely rare, which deserves to be mentioned more at length and of which I do not recollect any mention among medical authors. The seat of it, and sense of strangling, and anxiety with which it is attended, may make it not improperly be called Angina pectoris.
>
> Those who are afflicted with it are seized, while they are walking and more particularly when they walk soon after eating with a painful and most disagreeable sensation in the breast, which seems as if it would take their life away if it were to increase or to continue; the moment they stand still, all this uneasiness vanishes. In all other respects, the patients are, at the beginning of this disorder perfectly well, and in particular have no shortness of breath, from which it is totally different.
>
> After it has continued for some months, it will not cease so instantaneously upon standing still; and it will come on not only when the persons are walking, but when they are lying down and oblige them to rise up out of their beds every night for many months together; and in one or two very inveterate cases it has been brought on by the motion of a horse, or a carriage, and even by swallowing, coughing, going to stool or speaking, or any disturbance of mind.
>
> The os sterni is usually pointed to as the seat of this malady, but it seems sometimes as if it was under the lower part of it, and at other times under the middle or upper part, but always inclining more to the left side, and sometimes there is joined with it a pain about the middle of the left arm.

In the *Commentaries* written subsequently and published some thirty years later, Heberden added some variants of the location of the pain, its natural history and some associated symptoms. These too warrant reproducing in his own words.[15]

> The pain sometimes reaches to the right arm, as well as to the left, and even down to the hands, but this is uncommon: in a very few instances the arm has at the same time been

---

[10] Ibid., p. 256.

[11] Ibid., p. 280.

[12] Ibid., p. 291.

[13] William Withering, *An account of the foxglove, and some of its medical uses: with practical remarks on dropsy, and other diseases*, Birmingham, M Swinney, 1785, pp. 2, 6, 11.

[14] Heberden, op. cit., note 2 above, pp. 59–64.

[15] W Heberden, *Commentaries on the history and cure of diseases*, Boston, Wells and Lilly, 1818, pp. 293–4.

numb and swelled. In one or two persons the pain has lasted some hours, or even days; but this has happened, when the complaint has been long lasting and thoroughly rooted in the constitution.

The descriptions are, of course, a composite based on nearly a hundred patients, but the individual case histories, many of which are now in the archives of the Royal College of Physicians of London, described the individual features which now clearly identify the presenting pain as anginal.[16] Although Heberden was initially unaware of any association with coronary arterial disease, his description of angina pectoris with its wealth of detail has never been bettered. It includes a clear-cut account of the distribution of the pain and its relation to exertion, other aggravating and some relieving factors, associated symptoms, and, in addition, the sense of impending dissolution or *angor animi*, and the natural history of the condition. William Heberden was one of the most learned physicians of his day and by 1768 a Fellow of the Royal College of Physicians of London of more than thirty years standing.[17] He had been chosen to give the Royal College Harveian oration and was a Gulstonian and Croonian lecturer. He was acquainted with the recent works of physicians on the Continent of Europe and was a classicist with a sound knowledge of Hebrew, Greek and Latin.[18] He was medically well read, yet even when his *Commentaries* were being written he had become acquainted with but one possible account, a two thousand year earlier observation by Erasistratus of Chios of a symptom complex that might conceivably be understood as being anginal. In his *Commentaries*, Heberden continued to describe angina pectoris as a condition which, "hitherto hardly had a place ... in medical books", the description of Erasistratus being the *only* earlier one to which he did make reference.[19] In 1772 he apparently knew of but one other physician who had seen any similar patients. John Fothergill, a prominent contemporary physician with wide general interests, writing in 1776, referred to angina pectoris specifically as, "the disease of that kind which is so fully and judiciously described by Dr. Heberden". Fothergill too was apparently unaware of any earlier descriptions.[20]

## The Earlier Years

The enquiry will continue with a review of the clinical records prior to 1768 that have been considered by some medical historians to be possible descriptions of the pain of angina pectoris, whether typical or otherwise. The first phrase that is relevant to the present investigation is that of Erasistratus. It has come down to us through

---

[16] W Heberden, case notes, *Index historiae morborum*, Royal College of Physicians of London, manuscript 342.

[17] Ernest Heberden, *William Heberden: physician of the age of reason*, London, Royal Society of Medicine Services, 1989, p. 13.

[18] Ibid., pp. 167, 111.

[19] Heberden, op. cit., note 15 above, p. 297, fn.

[20] John Fothergill, 'Case of an angina pectoris with remarks', *Medical Observations and Inquiries*, 1776, **5**: 233–51, p. 235.

a fifth-century Latin translation from the original Greek by Caelius Aurelianus.[21] "Erasistratus memorat paralyseos genus et paradoxon apellat quo ambulantes repente sistuntur et ambulare non possunt et tum rursum ambulare sinuntur." It may be translated as a report that Erasistratus of Chios had mentioned a kind of paralysis that he called a "paradoxon" which comes suddenly and repeatedly with walking so that subjects cannot walk, but after stopping it leaves and they can walk again. The Latin fragment has been quoted in full to highlight two points. First, the use of the plural forms *ambulantes* and *possunt* indicates that more than one patient was being described. It is not known whether the original Greek used the dual number or the plural, so whether there were only two patients or more than two is unknown, the text being available only in Latin translation. Secondly, the word *dolor* or an equivalent Latin term denoting pain does not appear. The description of the symptom as starting with effort and stopping with rest is compatible with exertional angina, and was considered as such by Heberden but must nevertheless be considered inconclusive. Erasistratus was not an unknown in the ancient world and although born on the Aegean Island of Chios he became a member of the Alexandrian School early in the third century before the Common Era. The School then flourished under the patronage of Ptolemy Soter, a general in the army of Alexander the Great who had become the first Hellenic King of Egypt. Erasistratus was a pupil of Theophrastus, himself a student of Aristotle. He achieved prominence in his own lifetime and was recognized as an authority in many aspects of medicine. Galen, through whom his writings have been preserved, acknowledged his influence, referring to his followers as "Erasistreans".[22] His teachings subsequently became known to a wide medical readership following Caelius Aurelianus' translation into Latin. Physicians in the Classical Era and subsequently were therefore alerted to there having once been patients with an exertionally related symptom that was sudden in onset and relieved by rest. Their silence on the subject is therefore all the more remarkable.

Seneca, in the first century of the Common Era, described a condition from which he himself suffered, and commented on his own symptoms. "The attack is very short and like a storm. It usually ends within an hour. To have any other abnormality is only to be sick, to have this is to be dying."[23] There was no mention of pain or relation to effort so that, apart from its episodic nature and the associated *angor animi*, there is nothing to suggest angina pectoris. Caleb Parry, writing at the end of the eighteenth century when the relationship of angina to coronary arterial disease was already known, thought that Seneca's symptoms were pulmonary in origin,[24] and in his twentieth-century history of coronary heart disease, J O Leibowitz described this as a view shared by modern medical historians.[25]

The next possible description is a thousand years later and had its origins in

[21] Caelius Aurelianus, *On acute diseases, and On chronic diseases*, transl. I E Drabkin, University of Chicago Press, 1950, p. 574–5.

[22] J F Dobson, 'Erasistratus', *Proc Royal Soc Med*, 1927, **20** (2): 825–32, p. 825.

[23] Clifford Allbutt, *Diseases of the arteries including angina pectoris*, London, Macmillan, 1915, p. 319.

[24] Caleb H Parry, *An inquiry into the symptoms and causes of the syncope anginosa, commonly called angina pectoris*, Bath, R Cruttwell, 1799, p. 36.

[25] J O Leibowitz, *The history of coronary disease*, London, Wellcome Institute of the History of Medicine, 1970, p. 97.

England. Mayr-Harting and Harris have suggested that Gervase, a twelfth-century Norman official of the Sheriff of Ely, a Cathedral City in the Fens district of England, suffered a myocardial infarct prior to his sudden death. He was reportedly a "craftsman of anger, an inventor of crime". The night before he was due to appear in a lawsuit, St Etheldreda, then dead some 500 years, appeared before him in a dream and rebuked him in a terrifying voice. She then pushed the point of her staff heavily on the place of his heart, as if to pierce him through, and her two accompanying sisters attacked him in similar fashion. The fearful groans and horrible cries of Gervase aroused his servants, to whom he described the episode. The pain returned, presumably after a short remission, and having cried out that he was dying, he did indeed expire. Mayr-Harting and Harris speculated that he had suffered a myocardial infarction precipitated by the acute emotional distress associated with a nightmare. There seems to have been an accompanying sense of pressure on his chest and *angor animi*.[26] However, there is no record of his having suffered any preceding pain on effort, and alternate explanations for chest pain in association with sudden death are possible.

The Chronicles of Sir John Froissart contain an account of the sudden death of the Comte de Foix in France in 1391. He had been hunting on a hot day and in the evening, while about to wash his hands, he changed colour from an oppression at his heart, fell back on his seat exclaiming, "I am a dead man", suffered great pain and died within half an hour. It is possible that he was having a myocardial infarct accompanied by *angor animi*, but the description is not detailed enough to warrant a definite diagnosis.[27] Certainly there is no recording of preceding chest pain, either with the exertion of hunting or with any other physical activity.

In the early seventeenth century, William Harvey engaged in correspondence with Jean Riolan, Professor of Anatomy and Botany at the University of Paris and committed to Galen's theories concerning the circulation, including belief in direct flow of blood between the ventricles. In one of his communications to Riolan, William Harvey described the case of Sir Robert Darcy who in middle life suffered frequent distressing pain in the chest, especially in the "night season" (*nocturno tempore*), accompanied by a dread of fainting or suffocation. He grew steadily worse, became cachectic, developed dropsy and finally died in a paroxysm. The autopsy showed a rupture of the left ventricle and therefore suggests a terminal acute myocardial infarction.[28] The earlier pains could have been anginal, but there is no record of any relation to exertion. This omission is particularly noteworthy because Harvey, although best known for his discovery of the circulation of the blood, was also a very observant and experienced clinician. Sir Robert almost certainly suffered a myocardial infarction, but the cause, as discussed in a later chapter, could have been other than coronary arteriosclerosis or thrombosis.

[26] H Mayr-Harting and P Harris, 'St. Etheldreda and the death of Gervase', *Int J Cardiol*, 1986, **12**: 369–71, p. 370.

[27] Sir John Froissart, *Chronicles*, transl. Thomas Johnes, London, H G Bohn, 1849, vol. 2, pp. 498–9, quoted in Leibowitz, op. cit., note 25 above, pp. 179–80.

[28] William Harvey, *Exercitatio anatomica, de motu cordis et sanguinis in animalibus*, Rotterdam, Arnold Leers, 1648, pp. 99–102.

The illness suffered by Henry Hyde in the years preceding his death in 1632 was chronicled by his son Edward Hyde, Earl of Clarendon, who described how his father suffered repeated episodes of left arm pain prior to the terminal event. These pains were very severe and associated with *angor animi,* or fear of dying. They were episodic with a sense of well-being between the paroxysms. Death came during one of his usual attacks.[29] This is a very perceptive recording by a man who was a statesman, a member of Charles II's Privy Council and Lord Chancellor, but who had no medical training. The description of episodic pain is certainly compatible with angina pectoris, notwithstanding the absence of any mention of relation to effort.

There are two descriptions of chest pain related to exertion in Giovanni Battista Morgagni's monumental 1761 work *De sedibus et causis morborum,* translated into English in 1769 by Benjamin Alexander as *The seats and causes of disease.* As the original description was in Latin, the *lingua franca* of the eighteenth-century medical world, its contents could have been read and understood by any physician in Europe. Morgagni, who could be considered one of the fathers of clinical pathology, recorded about 500 cases, brief clinical descriptions being followed in most instances by autopsy findings. Among them he described a nobleman of over fifty years of age about whom he had been consulted in 1730. The patient had by then suffered for some ten years from a sense of weight and constriction in the chest, as if something was wedged in his oesophagus. The sensation radiated to the lower sternum and was accompanied by some difficulty in breathing. At the onset the distress only occurred when he walked, especially if up a steep slope. Subsequently, it would come more often and when bending forward, especially after dinner and when going to bed, but it eased if he stood up. The final attack awoke him at night and lasted two or three hours. He collapsed after repeated venesections and died, but there was no autopsy. Some of the associated features described by Morgagni are suggestive of gastro-oesophageal reflux, which often coexists with ischaemic heart disease in patients over the age of fifty. However, the description of pain brought on by effort and relieved by rest but with progressive worsening suggests very strongly that, whatever else were his complaints, the nobleman from Padua did indeed suffer from angina pectoris.[30] A second patient of Morgagni was a woman of forty-two who had painful chest "crises" with physical effort accompanied by left arm numbness and respiratory "torture", but which were relieved when she rested. She died suddenly in 1707. At autopsy her heart was found to be voluminous. There were extensive irregularities and "ossified" plaques in the aorta and its main branches.[31] Although known since the late fifteenth century,[32] the coronary arteries were not mentioned in the postmortem report and there was no description of anything that could now be understood as a myocardial infarction. Nevertheless, the account of her symptoms stands out as the earliest ever description that is clear cut and highly suggestive of angina, occurring as it did repeatedly on effort and being relieved by rest.

[29] Leibowitz, op. cit., note 25 above, pp. 65–7.
[30] Morgagni, op. cit., note 8 above, vol. I, epistle xviii, p. 455.
[31] Ibid., epistle xxvi, p. 819.
[32] Leibowitz, op. cit., note 25 above, p. 47.

In 1748 another typical case was described by Friedrich Hoffmann, Professor of Medicine at the University of Halle. He recorded the history of a man in his seventies who had, over the space of years, a tight and severe pain in the region of the heart extending to the breastbone and radiating throughout his chest. This was accompanied by anxiety and difficulty in breathing that began to overcome him. The symptoms became more intense with any physical movement, and in particular they occurred if when unwell he walked up a slope or climbed some stairs. It even came with the effort of dressing himself. The severity was such that more often than not he had to desist from all activity in order to obtain relief from pain. Hoffmann made no mention of any other patient with similar symptoms, either in his practice or in the literature.[33]

Nicolas Rougnon described a patient with chest pain in 1768, five months before Heberden's presentation to the Royal College of Physicians of London. The patient, a retired captain and son of a professor of medicine in Besançon, was rather obese and had a history of difficulty in breathing brought on by slight physical exertion. This worsened and as his disease progressed the patient could not walk more than 100 steps quickly without feeling a kind of suffocation, especially when trying to speak. The attack would subside when he stopped walking for a few moments and he was rarely affected when he walked slowly. Six weeks before his death he complained of a strange discomfort over the whole anterior part of his breast, as if caused by a breastplate. During silence and rest he hardly experienced this disorder. Finally, after hurrying and then climbing two flights of stairs after a meal, he sat down and died on the instant.[34] Despite absence of pain, the symptoms might be considered an angina equivalent, but without any degree of certainty as a sense of suffocation and discomfort in the chest can accompany left heart failure of any cause. Other early descriptions of chest pain must be regarded as non-specific in character even when followed by sudden death, as the causes of this combination are legion. In particular, from about 1500 onwards, syphilis reached epidemic proportions in Europe[35] and many pre-terminal chest pains were associated with the aneurysms of the aorta with which the disease is associated and with death frequently following rupture of the artery.[36]

This review shows that between the immediate post-Hippocratic era in the ancient Hellenic world and the mid-eighteenth century, the occasion of Heberden's first presentation, it was possible to find just ten recorded clinical reports that have suggested to some medical historians the possibility that they were descriptions of angina pectoris. Of these, only eight were described as having episodic symptoms, a relationship of the dominant symptom to exertion was present in just six, but in three only was there any suggestion of pain brought on repeatedly by effort and relieved by rest. These three alone could be considered unequivocal descriptions of

[33] Friedrich Hoffmann, 'Consultationes medicae: casus lxxxiii', 1748, **1**: 385. Quoted in the original Latin in H Bogart, *An inaugural dissertation on angina pectoris*, New York, C S Van Winkle, 1813, pp. 19–20.
[34] N F Rougnon, *Journal de Sçavans*, July 1768, quoted in Leibowitz, op. cit., note 25 above, p. 99.
[35] Porter, op. cit., note 7 above, p. 167.
[36] Ibid., p. 361.

angina pectoris, the remaining seven accounts varying from possible to unlikely. With just two exceptions, no author described more than a single patient during the two millennia that linked the times of Erasistratus with those of Heberden. Certainly there are other descriptions in earlier writings of chest pain, sweating, shortness of breath, distress and ultimate death, but before 1768 there is, apart from those just listed, no other mention of the distinctive and characteristic features of angina of effort. This silence is of special note as the physicians responsible for the earlier descriptions were men of standing and their accounts appeared in books or journals that were widely available. They were therefore of easy access to the general medical community and would have sufficed to make angina pectoris a potentially recognizable entity were it anything but phenomenally rare.

Noteworthy among the absences in early medical writings is the failure of Pliny the Elder to describe anything remotely resembling the pain of angina pectoris in a work devoted exclusively to sudden death.[37] Even more remarkable is the omission of any such descriptions in the writings of Giovanni Maria Lancisi. He had been specifically asked by Pope Clement VII to review all aspects of sudden death as this had reached epidemic proportions in Rome in the year 1705. Lancisi's results were published in 1707 in considerable detail in a wide ranging book devoted exclusively to the topic. In this volume, *De subitaneis mortibus*, there is but one conceivable allusion to angina pectoris.[38] Lancisi reports, "interni pectoris dolores, qui modo spirandi difficultatem, praesertim per acclivia modo cordis angorum, saepe pulses inaequalitatem". This can be rendered into English as, "there are pains of the interior of the chest which are accompanied sometimes by difficulty in breathing, especially on going uphill; sometimes by distress of the heart and often by irregularity of the pulse". Critical examination of the Latin text shows that it is indeed, as in the above translation, not the pain but the difficulty in breathing that is related to going uphill. This distinction was noted by J Iain McDougall when publishing with me an English rendering of the sections of Lancisi's book dealing with the cardiovascular causes of sudden death.[39] A similar conclusion was reached by Paul Dudley White and Alfred Boursy in their translation. Although they considered that the pain might have been anginal, they listed left ventricular failure or mitral valve disease with pulmonary congestion as possible causes. These conditions are typically associated with painless shortness of breath that occurs not only with effort but typically when the patient is recumbent, as instanced by Lancisi.[40]

Morgagni was not alone in documenting case histories and this practice was not confined to teachers in the great universities. As an example, Doctor William Brownrigg, who practised in the remote northwestern Cumberland port of White-haven in the early part of the eighteenth century, kept case histories of 127 patients, none of whom had any symptoms that could be remotely associated with angina

[37] Pliny the Elder, 'Sudden death' in *Natural history*, transl. H Rackham, 10 vols., Cambridge, MA, Harvard University Press, 1942, vol. 2, book 7.

[38] Giovanni Maria Lancisi, *De subitaneis mortibus Liber I*, Rome, F Bagni, 1707, p. 66.

[39] J Iain McDougall and Leon Michaels, 'Cardiovascular causes of sudden death in "De subitaneis mortibus" by Giovanni Maria Lancisi', *Bull Hist Med*, 1972, **45**: 486–94, p. 489.

[40] Giovanni Maria Lancisi, *De subitaneis mortibus*, transl. Paul D White and A V Boursy, New York, St John's University Press, 1971, p. 52.

pectoris.[41] Apart from the exceptions already noted, there was none in any other case record collections from before the late eighteenth century.

The possibility of severe, recurrent, disabling and eventually life-threatening chest pain going unnoticed must be viewed in the light of our understanding of the art and science of medicine as it existed 200 and more years ago. Knowledge of anatomy was limited and that of physiology in its infancy. There was no understanding of the causes of disease as perceived nowadays, and there was in consequence a tendency to confuse illnesses with similar clinical presentations but different causes. Symptoms were sometimes described as if they were disease entities and disease entities were categorized primarily by their symptoms. Examination of the patient was very limited and largely confined to inspection and palpation, notably of the pulse. As physicians were invariably men, concern for the proprieties as then conceived often prevented any physical examination of female patients. Consultations could even be based on accounts of symptoms given by third parties, the patient not being seen at all by the physician rendering an opinion. However, these limitations should not obscure the fact that many physicians who lived before the mid-eighteenth century were very astute observers and possessed an ability to describe symptoms, findings on inspection and clinical course as fully as is done today. This capacity may be gauged by consideration of the historical status of two conditions other than angina pectoris, as described in my earlier study.[42] The first selected was gout because it is an episodic complaint and now recognized as a risk factor for development of coronary heart disease.[43] Like the latter, it has been an affliction of the privileged, associated with eating to excess and the two conditions not infrequently occur in the same patient. The second disease chosen was migraine because, like angina pectoris, it too presents as a distinctive and episodic symptom complex with a state of well-being between the episodes, and usually without any obvious outward manifestations of disease during the attacks.[44]

The acute arthritis of gout was described in antiquity by a number of authorities including Hippocrates or a member of his school, and centuries later by Galen. It was certainly no rarity and distinguished sufferers included King Henry VII, Martin Luther, and Cardinal Wolsey.[45] Thomas Sydenham, himself a victim, not only described accurately the inflammatory features of the acute arthritis in the great toe, but also its general manifestations during subsequent years. These included the episodic recurrences, calcareous deposits in the region of affected joints, disturbances of urination, and an association with kidney stones. As with all early descriptions, his account made no mention of any patient with gout complaining of chest pain

[41] Jean Ward and Joan Yell (eds and transl.), *The medical casebook of William Brownrigg, M.D., F.R.S. (1712–1800) of the Town of Whitehaven in Cumberland*, Medical History, Supplement No. 13, London, Wellcome Institute for the History of Medicine, 1993, pp. 1–160.

[42] Leon Michaels, 'Aetiology of coronary heart disease: an historical approach', *Br Heart J*, 1966, **28**: 258–64, p. 258.

[43] Arthur P Hall, 'Correlations among hyperuricemia, hypercholesterolemia, coronary disease and hypertension', *Arthritis Rheum*, 1965, **8**: 846–64, p. 848.

[44] Michaels, op. cit, note 42 above, p. 259.

[45] Dudley Hart, 'Gout and non-gout through the ages', *Br J Clin Pract*, 1985, **39**: 91–2, pp. 91, 92.

on effort at any time during the course of the disease.[46] This silence contrasts with the subsequently recognized association with angina pectoris, beginning within five years of Heberden's 1772 publication, when Fothergill reported a history of a gouty foot in a patient with subsequent typical anginal pain on exertion.[47]

In past times migraine may have been confused on occasion with headaches due to other causes. Nevertheless, an association between paroxysmal one-sided headaches and coincident visual and abdominal disturbances was already recognized in antiquity by Galen. The descriptive term hemicrania and the name *migrana* were already being used in Roman times. In the sixth century, Alexander of Tralles described hemicrania, the concept of unilateral headaches being implicit in the term. Caelius Aurelianus too noted involvement of half of the head, including the temple and region of one eye. He recorded an association with nausea and bilious vomiting and described accompanying dizziness, disturbance of vision, a need to close the eyes in order to avoid the aggravating effect of light and the beneficial effects of rest in a dark room.[48] Heberden included an account of migraine in his *Commentaries* using the classical name hemicrania, and observed that liability to attacks may be life-long. He recorded that they were usually unilateral and recorded an association with "great disorder of the stomach" including vomiting and also transient visual disturbances, including flashes of light that would now be termed fortification spectra. Of greater relevance for the present discussion however, is the way in which he alluded to migraine as a well-known and familiar disease, "Very early distinguished by medical writers from other species of headaches".[49] In this respect, the contrast with his comments on the previous exceedingly great rarity of angina pectoris is striking. His medical predecessors were, as indicated, well able to recognize a condition that resembles angina pectoris in presenting with symptoms that are intermittent and unaccompanied by outward manifestations of disease, and with the patient well between the attacks.

Means of speedily alleviating the pain of angina are now readily to hand. In contrast, in Heberden's times availability of amyl nitrite was still a century away. Without it the relief with rest would inevitably have been somewhat delayed and recurrences of the pain with renewed exertion sooner. In an era in which no long-term medication for prevention or palliation was available, the course of angina pectoris was usually one of increasing severity, with the pain coming more frequently, earlier in the course of exertion, with ever greater intensity and longer in duration. Once fully established, the pain must have often been terrifying in its severity and understandably accompanied by fear of sudden death. The condition, as we know from some of Heberden's case records, could have continued episodically in individual patients for a decade or more. It would therefore seem hardly plausible that the pain of angina pectoris could have gone unnoticed by the medical community if indeed it had been anything but exceedingly rare before the mid-eighteenth century.

[46] Thomas Sydenham, *Compleat method of curing almost all diseases*, 4th ed., London, T Horne and R Parker, 1710, p. 104.

[47] Fothergill, op. cit., note 20 above, p. 237.

[48] F C Rose, *The history of migraine from Mesopotamia to medieval times*, Cephalalgia, Supplement No. 15, 1995, p. 1.

[49] Heberden, op. cit., note 15 above, pp. 75–7.

The virtual absence of earlier descriptions did not escape notice in the years that immediately followed the first widespread recognition of angina pectoris. Henry Bogart, for example, commented in 1813 that "It is somewhat singular that a disease characterized by such peculiar symptoms as belonged to that which is now generally known by physicians under the name of angina pectoris should have escaped the attention of the ancients and that we should be indebted to authors of comparatively late times for all that has been written on it. Yet such is the fact".[50]

Little less in significance is the absence during the Georgian era of any reference to chest pain on exertion by non-medical writers. Among the population of eighteenth-century England there was tremendous concern with matters of health, understandable in view of the great frequency of disease affecting people of all ages, and the high death rate in infancy, childhood and all stages of adult life. Members of the literate middle and upper classes often kept diaries and their personal experiences with disease were recorded. James Boswell's *London journal* for instance, is peppered with references to his own frailties, mental and physical, and their course and treatment.[51] Writers in general had no hesitation in describing their own symptoms and those of their families and friends in very great detail, and considerations of delicacy did not inhibit them when documenting complete accounts of any disturbances of bodily function. Among the educated members of English society at any rate there was much speculation about the causes of disease and acquaintance with medical writings and opinions was widespread. As a further example, an account of Heberden's description of angina was printed as early as March 1772 in *The Critical Review or Annals of Literature*, a magazine published by "A Society of Gentlemen" and with a predominantly nonmedical readership.[52] Nevertheless, prior to 1768, the Earl of Clarendon appears to have been the only layman to have described the pain in a way that could be understood readily as a variant of angina pectoris.[53]

Independent negative evidence for the extreme rarity of angina pectoris is provided by examination of the London Bills of Mortality. From Tudor times onward, every English parish had been compelled by law to record the numbers and the causes of all deaths as they occurred. Beginning in 1603, deaths in London were published weekly in the Bills. There were deficiencies of which contemporaries, including Heberden himself, were aware. The causes as they were listed are indicative of the way in which maladies were then categorized. Some designations such as smallpox, tuberculosis or asthma are readily recognizable from descriptions of that time. The diagnoses are therefore acceptable notwithstanding occasional uncertainties in individual patients. Frequently, however, symptoms or symptom complexes were listed as causes of death as if they were disease entities. In some such cases possible causes of disease may be inferred. For example, apoplexy as listed in the Bills could indicate an abnormality of limb movements including paralysis as now associated

---

[50] Bogart, op. cit., note 33 above, pp. 3–4.
[51] James Boswell, *The London journal 1762–1763*, ed. Frederick A Pottle, M K Danziger, and F Brady, London, McGraw-Hill, 1989.
[52] *The Critical Review or Annals of Literature*, A Society of Gentleman, 1772, **33**: 203–4.
[53] Leibowitz, op. cit., note 25 above, p. 65.

*Table II.1*
Causes of death, from London Bills of Mortality,
last three weeks of 1700
(Original spelling retained)

| | |
|---|---|
| Abortive | Liver grown |
| Accident | Lunatick |
| Aged | Mortification |
| Apoplexy | Murder |
| Bleeding | Overlaid |
| Cancer | Plurisie |
| Canker | Purples |
| Childbed | Rheumatism |
| Chrisoms[1] | Rickets |
| Collick | Rising of the Lights[5] |
| Consumption | Rupture |
| Dropsy | Spotted Fever |
| Fever | Stillborn |
| Fistula | Stone |
| Flux[2] and Smallpox | Stopping of the Stomach |
| Frenchpox[3] | Suddenly |
| Gangrene | Surfeit |
| Grief | Teeth |
| Griping in guts | Thrush |
| Impostume[4] | Tissick[6] |
| Infant | Wound |
| Jaundice | |

[1]Infants under 1 month. [2]Discharge. [3]Syphilis. [4]Abscess. [5]Asthma. [6]Phthisis.

with a stroke. Jaundice suggests either a haemolytic process, then undiagnosable as such, or a disease of the hepatobiliary system, the latter being the more likely in view of its greater prevalence. Examination of the Bills of Mortality of the London parishes from the early eighteenth century, a 1700 example of which is shown in Table II.1, reveals no conditions that could now be attributed to either accelerated angina pectoris or a myocardial infarct. The records of the next ninety-three years are equally silent in this respect. However, in 1794 a condition described as "palpitation of the heart" was recorded for the first time and once only. There was none reported during the next three years, but from 1798 onwards this condition was listed fairly regularly as a cause of death. It appeared in the Bills in sixteen of the next twenty years for a total of seventy entries. In 1816 there were eleven fatalities attributed to "palpitation of the heart", the largest number in a single year. In no other respect was there any noteworthy change in the pattern of deaths recorded in the Bills of Mortality during the years from 1794 to 1816. Although a relationship of "palpitation of the heart" to coronary heart disease cannot be proven, it is a frequent complication and the sudden appearance for the first time and the subsequent steady recurrence of an apparently cardiac cause of death is striking. It raises the possibility that a heart condition not present earlier had become manifest.

Sudden deaths, reported in the Bills without any elaboration, rose from 16.9 per 10,000 total deaths recorded in the period 1691–95 to 67.9 per 10,000 during the years 1771–79.[54] Whilst instantaneous death is almost invariably cardiac in origin, this is not true of "sudden" death, with the interval between the onset of symptoms and death either unstated or not known. In contemporary medical literature, it is usually defined as occurring within twenty-four hours of the onset of symptoms and it can be due to a variety of factors of which only one is cardiac. An eighteenth-century example of an infectious cause is fulminating smallpox, which could be fatal in hours and was not diagnosable clinically if death occurred before appearance of the characteristic skin lesions.[55] Heberden himself listed rupture of blood vessels, suffocation from "inundations" of phlegm and "breaking" lung abscesses among the causes of sudden death.[56] However, the fourfold *increase* that occurred at a time when angina pectoris, often with fatal outcome, was first becoming manifest raises the distinct possibility that a new cardiac cause of death was then emerging.

In contrast to a handful of possible cases noted in total by earlier physicians, Heberden in his 1768 presentation reported a history of angina pectoris in some twenty patients. These had been seen during about twenty of the years during which he had been engaged in practice.[57] In further contrast, between 1772, when his publication in the *Transactions* appeared, and 1782, when at age seventy-two he greatly reduced his practice and devoted his energies in large measure to writing his *Commentaries*, the total number had risen to nearly 100, an almost eightfold increase in average annual incidence.[58] The series incidentally included only three females. The greater frequency cannot be attributed to Heberden being less aware of the condition before 1768 but alerted to it afterwards. Perusal of his case records shows that his first patient with angina was seen in 1748 at the latest.[59] The second died suddenly in April of the same year, having by then suffered a fourteen-year history of chest pain on walking, after talking excessively or when experiencing emotional upsets. Even if Heberden had seen neither individual previously, he would have acquired twenty years of familiarity with angina pectoris by 1768. His earliest note of a patient with nocturnal chest pain dates from 1756, and his first recording of pain worsened by walking after a meal from some time between 1759 and 1765.[60] It follows that any failure to report more than twenty patients with angina pectoris before 1768 cannot be attributed to Heberden having been unaware of the symptom complex during the earlier years and therefore unable to recognize it when patients presented themselves. The contrast between a score of patients seen in the twenty years before 1768 and almost eighty more in less than half of that time afterwards strongly suggests that patients with angina pectoris had in fact been very few and far between in the earlier period, but increasingly common subsequently.

[54] Personal examination of the London Bills of Mortality, Guildhall Library, City of London.

[55] F W Price (ed.), *A textbook of the practice of medicine*, London, Oxford University Press, 1946, p. 161.

[56] Heberden, op. cit., note 16 above, manuscript 342.

[57] Heberden, op. cit., note 2 above, p. 61.

[58] Heberden, op. cit., note 15 above, p. 295.

[59] Heberden, op. cit., note 16 above, manuscript 342.

[60] Ibid.

*Historical Evidence*

## The Contemporaries of William Heberden

William Heberden's 1768 presentation was followed very closely by reports from the quills of many contemporary English physicians who, either retrospectively or prospectively, diagnosed from among their patients some who were suffering from angina pectoris. Dr John Wall of Worcester, for example, reported seeing no fewer than twelve or thirteen such patients.[61] By 1776 Fothergill was referring to angina pectoris as "a disease which I had too often met with".[62] Individual cases such as one reported by Edward Jenner of vaccination fame contributed to the total.[63] As remarked by Latham a century later, angina pectoris is "an assemblage of symptoms ... made to bear the name of a disease".[64] It is therefore necessary to examine critically all late-eighteenth-century clinical descriptions, as it was upon these alone that the diagnosis could be based and the extent estimated. Heberden himself pointed out the need to distinguish angina pectoris from other types of chest pain that were different in character and benign in their course.[65] This differentiation can be difficult even today when the purely descriptive term "chest wall pain" is *faute de mieux* used as a diagnosis. The diagnostic problem was well recognized before the end of the eighteenth century when Caleb Parry reviewed the recent literature and added some of his own experiences. He considered the condition common enough to be worthy of a book that he wrote and entitled *An inquiry into the symptoms and the causes of syncope anginosa, commonly called angina pectoris*. He accompanied one of his own patients on an uphill walk, the gentleman having volunteered to thus induce the pain so that he could be observed during the attack. Parry remarked on "considerable experience of my own with this disorder" and was able to distinguish what he considered to be true angina pectoris from the paroxysmal discomfort associated with asthma. He also excluded patients in whom either dyspnoea was the dominant symptom or the pain abdominal in location. Modern observers might also query some of Parry's examples in which "syncope" was the main feature, but with this exception his careful observations and critical judgement suggest to a contemporary physician that his patients and those of half a dozen other contemporary doctors whose diagnoses he accepted were in fact suffering from angina pectoris. Indeed modern physicians might regard as truly anginal instances of pain that were characteristic in nature, but tended to be dismissed by Parry because they occurred only in association with palpitations.[66] A rapid heart rate results in increased work for the heart and is now recognized as a frequent precursor of the typical pain.

Some of the diagnoses of angina pectoris made by late-eighteenth-century authors other than Parry do not stand up to modern critical appraisal. Indeed one of Heberden's original patients would appear from his description to have had some

[61] J Wall, 'Letter to Heberden', *Medical Observations and Inquiries by a Society of Physicians in London*, 1776, **5**: 233–51, quoted by W L Proudfit, 'Origin of concept of ischaemic heart disease', *Br Heart J*, 1983, **50**: 209–12, p. 209.

[62] Fothergill, op. cit., note 20 above, p. 235.

[63] Leibowitz, op. cit., note 25 above, p. 93.

[64] P M Latham, *Collected works*, vol. I, *Diseases of the heart*, London, New Sydenham Society, 1876, p. 445.

[65] Heberden, op. cit., note 15 above, p. 362.

[66] Parry, op. cit., note 24 above, p. 61.

form of purulent chest infection.[67] A man whose pain was attributed by J Hooper to angina pectoris would seem from both the clinical course and the autopsy findings to have suffered from acute pericarditis.[68] The stomach pains of which John Hunter complained in 1773 were quite unlike his later symptoms and may have had nothing to do with his heart.[69] However, after critical examination and exclusion of the reported complaints of some individual patients, there remain a considerable number of late-eighteenth-century descriptions of pain with the essential characteristics of angina pectoris, namely, location in the chest, jaw or arms, episodic attacks with a clear-cut relation to exertion, a sense of imminent death, relief with rest and, in contrast, a sense of well-being between the attacks. Frequently the authors identified the pain with that described by Heberden. Fothergill instanced two patients, one an obese man in his late fifties with a previous history of gout who developed "spasm in the breast" that occurred only with exercise, usually in the morning, particularly when walking quickly or into the wind, and initially with invariable relief with rest. Fothergill noted too that the pain on effort was particularly severe if walking uphill.[70] The symptoms of which John Hunter complained in the last eight years of his life were typical. His clinical course was recorded in detail by his brother-in-law who described how in 1785 Hunter developed unpleasant sensations in the left side of his face with radiation to the head, lower jaw, throat and left arm as far as the ball of his thumb. Occasionally the pain, as it was subsequently described, occurred in the right arm as well and it later extended to his sternum. It was often agonizing and on occasion accompanied by fainting. At the start, these episodes were brought on by exercise, such as walking up a slope or climbing up stairs, but never when going down. Eventually the pains occurred even at rest and on occasion they woke him from sleep. The attacks continued to occur with agitation and in particular when in difficult situations which he could not control. John Hunter foretold the possibility of his dying during an emotionally induced attack and in this he was prescient. In 1793 he did indeed pass away during one such episode.[71]

An anonymous individual wrote a letter to Heberden that was published with an addendum in 1785. In it the writer described the similarity of his own symptoms to the composite picture presented earlier by Heberden.[72] The patient was once thought to be Dr John Haygarth of Chester, but a careful study by Paul Kligfield and Konrad Filutowski suggests very strongly that he was John Mallet, a merchant of Exeter and London.[73] The writer, evidently therefore a layman, suffered attacks of pain in the left upper arm with radiation to the left chest and accompanied by slight faintness and shortness of breath. These attacks occurred when walking and in particular

[67] Heberden, op. cit., note 16 above, manuscript 342.
[68] J Hooper, 'A case of angina pectoris', *Memoirs of the Medical Society of London*, 1792, **1**: 238–43, p. 241.
[69] E Home, 'A short account of the author's life', in J Hunter, *A treatise on the blood, inflammation, and gunshot wounds*, London, John Richardson, 1794, p. lxi.
[70] Fothergill, op. cit., note 20 above, p. 234.
[71] Home, op. cit., note 69 above, p. 234.
[72] Anon., 'A letter to Dr. Heberden, concerning the angina pectoris; and an account of the dissection of one, who had been troubled with that disorder', *Med Trans Coll Physns Lond*, 1785, **3**: 1–11, p. 3.
[73] Paul Kligfield and Konrad Filutowski, '"Dr. Anonymous" unmasked: resolution of an eighteenth century mystery in the history of coronary artery disease', *Am J Cardiol*, 1995, **75**: 1166–9, p. 1168.

after dinner. Initially there was immediate relief with slowing, but the pains recurred after resumption of his usual pace. The attacks were worse in winter and accompanied by a sense of impending death, but remission was followed by a normal sense of wellbeing. In an addendum Heberden reported that three weeks after writing the letter, its author developed an episode of chest pain at rest that lasted half an hour and was followed by death.[74] The modern clinician would unhesitatingly diagnose the pain as anginal. It is all the more convincing as the description was apparently written by a layman after reading a single published description of the symptoms. Samuel Black, practising in Ulster, described one of his patients whose symptoms too were typical. He was a man of fifty-five, who in 1792 developed pain below the left breast while walking uphill. It cleared with rest, recurred repeatedly while walking, and remitted repeatedly on standing still. It was accompanied by anxiety and numbing in the left shoulder and arm.[75]

When describing the features of angina pectoris, many of these reports contained details of great diagnostic significance. They included the aggravating effects of walking in winter, a tendency for the pain to come on more readily with morning activity, with going upstairs rather than down and with taking exercise shortly after a meal. These are all features uniquely typical of angina pectoris. They could hardly be anything else. The diagnostic conclusions that can be drawn from William Heberden's initial description and from the subsequent review by Parry are therefore borne out by the majority of other reports by late-eighteenth-century English physicians. Some of these publications may not have added to an understanding of the symptom complex and individual authors may have been motivated on occasion by a desire to seek attention. Their recognition of their patients' pains as anginal may have been triggered in some measure by Heberden's verbal presentation and subsequent publication. However, with the exception of one patient of Fothergill, no contemporary of Heberden made retrospective mention of a single person with angina pectoris having been seen before 1768 and diagnosed in retrospect.[76] It is hard to conceive that symptoms as severe, characteristic and dramatic as those being described widely after 1768 could have gone completely unnoticed earlier. The accounts of the late-eighteenth-century collective clinical experiences combine to indicate that, in contrast to earlier years, patients who suffered from the pain of angina pectoris were no longer uncommon in late-eighteenth-century England.

"Ossification" or, to use the modern term, "calcification" was frequently reported in eighteenth-century autopsies of patients who had suffered from angina pectoris for varying periods of time, one a patient of Fothergill with typical symptoms in life.[77] In an autopsy description of a coronary artery, Jenner noted that a "firm fleshy tube ... did not appear to have any vascular connections with the coats of the artery, but seemed to lie merely in simple contact with it". This is clearly recognizable as a

---

[74] Anon., op. cit., note 72 above, p. 7.

[75] Samuel Black, 'Case of angina pectoris with remarks', *Memoirs of the Medical Society of London*, 1795, **4**: 261–79, p. 262.

[76] Fothergill, op. cit., note 20 above, p. 241.

[77] John Fothergill, 'Further account of the angina pectoris', *Medical Observations and Inquiries*, 1776, **5**: 252–8, p. 255.

description of a coronary thrombosis with occlusion of the vessel. Jenner also commented on "the importance of the coronary arteries and how much the heart must suffer from their not being able duly to perform their functions", thereby suggesting that the coronary artery blood flow was significantly impeded.[78] Post-mortem examination of a patient of Fothergill, performed in 1773, revealed the presence of "a small white spot as big as a sixpence resembling a cicatrix" located near the apex, the description being highly suggestive of an old myocardial infarction.[79] At other autopsies the heart muscle was described as "looser" and paler, as would now be associated with the fatty degeneration of chronic ischaemia. Cardiac rupture was also observed.[80] Together these findings indicate that not only angina pectoris as a symptom, but also its connection to virtually all major pathological manifestations of coronary arterial disease was being recognized before the end of the eighteenth century.

Little is known about the social status of William Heberden's patients, his case notes containing clinical details but little else. It is noteworthy, however, that he was a very prosperous physician, able in 1767 to spend over £5000 on the purchase of a house, merely to have it demolished in order to make way for a new home.[81] His practice included King George III, peers, knights, and members of parliament with their families. There is no record, however, of his seeing dispensary patients and, having failed to receive an appointment to the staff of St Bartholomew's Hospital, he did not attend hospital clinics.[82] It is likely, therefore, that apart from an occasional servant of a private patient, his practice was very largely confined to the ranks of the privileged. Black, writing in 1819, noted that angina pectoris was an affliction of the prosperous with the "poor and laborious" being unaffected.[83] This was reported by William Osler to have remained a feature of the condition a century later.[84] This characteristic of angina pectoris was observed for a further fifty years, Richard G Wilkinson remarking that "coronary heart disease in the first half of the twentieth century was regarded as a businessman's disease".[85] Although eighteenth-century physicians tended to favour "salubrious" locations and moneyed patients, there were dispensaries where doctors attended patients who were unable to pay and latterly the indigent received care in hospital outpatient clinics.[86] It is unlikely that if anything but very rare the complaint would have gone unobserved by physicians attending the needy. In having apparently been a rarity among the poor whilst not uncommon among the prosperous, angina pectoris has been exceptional among the afflictions

[78] Leibowitz, op. cit., note 25 above, p. 94.

[79] Fothergill, op. cit., note 20 above, p. 244.

[80] Morgagni, op. cit., note 8 above, epistle xxvii, pp. 837–8.

[81] Ernest Heberden, op. cit., note 17 above, p. 149.

[82] Ibid., p. 111.

[83] Samuel Black, *Clinical and pathological reports*, Newry, Alexander Wilkinson, 1819, p. 31.

[84] William Osler, 'The Lumleian lectures on angina pectoris, Lecture I', *Lancet*, 1910, **i**: 697–702, p. 698.

[85] Richard G Wilkinson, *Unhealthy societies: the afflictions of inequality*, London and New York, Routledge, 1996, p. 44.

[86] Joan Lane, 'The medical practitioners of provincial England in 1783', *Med Hist*, 1984, **28**: 353–71, p. 355.

of humankind. Possible reasons for this unusual feature are sought in subsequent chapters.

In contrast to the experience in England, there were almost no reports in the medical literature of any patients with angina pectoris having been seen elsewhere during almost half a century following Heberden's 1768 presentation. Eugène Desportes, writing in France in 1811, quoted five German publications which mentioned angina pectoris by name.[87] I have been able to trace only the earliest one of them, a dissertation by Schaeffer in 1787. This was devoted in large measure to descriptions of accounts by a total of fourteen British physicians.[88] There is extensive discussion of clinicopathological relationships, disagreements with the opinions of other writers being expressed forcibly and indeed undiplomatically.[89] However, there is but a single report of a German case, the patient of Friedrich Hoffmann, which antedated Heberden's presentation to the Royal College of Physicians of London and has been described earlier in this chapter.[90] It is evident from its title that one of the other German publications quoted by Desportes concerns but a single patient.[91] There is only one other reference to a possible Continental author, a physician with a Spanish name. In contrast, Desportes quoted no fewer than seventeen British authors, including William Heberden himself. The other sixteen included Dr Wall with his twelve or thirteen patients, the anonymous writer who had informed Heberden about his own experience of angina, Caleb Parry and Erasmus Darwin, the paternal grandfather of Charles. Two English case histories were quoted *in extenso* by Desportes, one a patient of Fothergill. In contrast, he reported no French cases from the eighteenth century.[92] The earliest possible one that he was able to find in the French medical literature was based on a description by M Baumes as late as 1808, forty years after Heberden's presentation to the Royal College of Physicians of London.[93] Jean Nicholas Corvisart, the leading physician in France at the beginning of the nineteenth century, and Napoleon's personal doctor, wrote an essay in 1811 specifically devoted to illnesses and organic lesions of the heart and great vessels without making any mention whatsoever of angina pectoris, even though he described the pathology of cardiac rupture in detail.[94] The failure of physicians in France to report patients with angina cannot be attributed to lack of clinical acumen. Auscultation was pioneered in France by René Théophile Hyacinthe Laënnec at this time.[95] The achievements of the galaxy of French physicians who throughout the nineteenth century provided eponyms for clinical features and disease

[87] Eugène H Desportes, *Traité de l'angine de poitrine, ou nouvelles recherches sur une maladie de la poitrine, que l'on a presque toujours confondue avec l'asthme, les maladies du coeur, etc.*, Paris, Méquignon, 1811, p. 4.

[88] G B Schaeffer, *De angina pectoris vulgo se dicta*, Dissertatio inauguralis medica, Gottingen, H M Grape, 1787, iii, p. 4.

[89] Ibid., xi, pp. 33–4.

[90] Hoffmann, op. cit., note 33 above, pp. 19–20.

[91] Desportes, op. cit., note 87 above, pp. 3ff.

[92] Ibid.

[93] Ibid., p. 5.

[94] Jean Nicholas Corvisart, *Essai sur les maladies et les lésions organiques du coeur et des gros vaisseaux*, Paris, Méquignon-Marvis, 1818, p. 266.

[95] Leibowitz, op. cit., note 25 above, p. 111.

entities in all branches of medicine attest to their ability. Neither can the failure be attributed to doctors in France being unaware of Rougnon's 1768 case description. This was reported initially in 1768 in a personal letter to Dr A-Ch Lorry, a well-known Paris physician, but published in abstract form later in the same year in the widely read publication *Journal de Sçavans* (*Savants* in modern French).[96] Most certainly lack of awareness of angina cannot be attributed to poor communication across the English Channel. Despite the periodic hostilities, a great deal of interchange of ideas and information took place. As noted earlier, Desportes was able to refer to the case reports of seventeen British physicians in a book published in Paris in 1811 at a time when the war between Britain and France had been raging for eight years.[97] Black, as early as 1819, suggested that Corvisart's failure to make mention of angina pectoris raised the possibility that it was a complaint not then being experienced in France.[98]

A similar silence characterized the American medical scene. Physicians practising in the main cities of the British American colonies and the subsequent United States had numerous contacts with England, notwithstanding interruption during the War of Independence, and communication with Europe was frequent. During his years in the American diplomatic service in Europe, Benjamin Franklin was instrumental in transmitting scientific ideas and information across the Atlantic Ocean. The results of Jenner's report on the effectiveness of vaccination was known in the United States within the year. Fothergill, of whom much mention has been made earlier, spent several years in America. Dr William Shippen Junior, who was one of his students, also studied in England under William Hunter before returning to Philadelphia in 1762, subsequently playing an important part in the establishment of the medical college of that city. Benjamin Rush, the outstanding Philadelphia physician of his day, had also travelled in Europe, and Dr John Morgan of Philadelphia had visited Italy, meeting Morgagni in Padua in 1764. However, the first reference to angina pectoris in the American medical literature appears to be that which was written by John Warren in 1812 and published on the first page of the very first issue of the *New England Journal of Medicine and Surgery*, the forerunner of the present *New England Journal of Medicine*. Warren reviewed the history of the condition and noted the relation to coronary ossification, quoting extensively from the work of English physicians, notably Heberden himself, Wall, Fothergill, John Hunter and Jenner. Warren reported four of his own cases, but made no mention of this symptom having occurred in the practices of any other American physicians.[99] Angina pectoris does not appear to have been observed in the United States in either the late eighteenth or the very early years of the nineteenth century.

During the last half of the eighteenth and the beginning of the nineteenth century the report of Hoffmann from Halle generated only five possible accounts of angina pectoris in any of the kingdoms or principalities of pre-unification Germany. Morgagni's description of two patients was followed by no other in the various

[96] Leibowitz, op. cit., note 25 above, p. 99.
[97] Desportes, op. cit., note 87 above, p. 344.
[98] Black, op. cit., note 75 above, p. 8.
[99] John Warren, 'Remarks on angina pectoris', *N Engl J Med Surg*, 1812, **1**: 1–11, pp. 1–4.

states of Italy even by 1804, when reference to fatty myocardial change was made by Antonio Scarpa, a pathological description unaccompanied by any recording of prior exertional chest pain.[100] None was reported from the Netherlands by the countrymen of Boerhaave. It is hardly credible that the silence of Western European and American medical writers could reflect a failure of recognition by physicians, fully acquainted as they were with the many descriptions of the symptom complex as documented in England. One can but conclude that for several decades after 1768 angina pectoris scarcely affected anyone living either on the Continent of Europe or in North America. W L Proudfit remarked that "a just appellation" for angina pectoris "would be a British disease".[101] Reasons for its exclusive geographical as well as its societal distribution must therefore be sought in conditions unique to eighteenth-century Britain.

[100] Antonio Scarpa, *Sull'aneurisma, riflessioni ed osservazioni anatomico-chirurgiche*, Pavia, 1804, quoted in Leibowitz, op. cit., note 25 above, p. 106.
[101] William L Proudfit, 'Origin of concept of ischaemic heart disease', *Br Heart J*, 1983, **50**: 209–12, p. 209.

# III

# Population Trends:
# The Eighteenth Century and Earlier

The proper study of mankind is man.[1]

In its early years angina pectoris was for the most part an affliction of middle-aged and elderly men, almost exclusively a complaint of the affluent and a "British disease".[2] It was first reported in 1768 and became prevalent by the 1770s, a time when the population of England was growing rapidly and its expectation of life lengthening. It is therefore pertinent to examine the contribution of these demographic changes together with their wellsprings, magnitude and precise timing in relation to the emergence of angina. Differences in the extent to which the sexes and various age and social groups were affected need to be ascertained and explained if possible. Finally, any demographic explanation for the early geographical localizing of angina must be sought in a comparison of eighteenth-century population changes in England with those occurring elsewhere.

Despite high death rates in infancy, childhood and early adult life, many people in earlier centuries did live to middle and even old age. This was the case as long ago as the Classical Era. As an example, some nineteen prominent ancient Greek writers and fifteen Roman historians whose years of birth and death are known with reasonable certainty lived to beyond the age of sixty (Table III.1).[3] Longevity was not then the good fortune of the famous alone. W R Macdonell surveyed inscriptions on memorial monuments in ancient Rome and its empire in Hispania and Lusitania, the modern Spain and Portugal respectively, and in Africa, the Morocco, Algeria and Tunisia of today. He showed, *inter alia,* that the age at death of males and females as recorded on each epitaph was over sixty years in about 5 per cent of the Roman inscriptions, 20 per cent of the Iberian and 22 per cent of the African. The numbers cannot be considered typical of life expectancy in the Roman empire generally. There are discrepancies between the findings in the three areas. The inscriptions appear to refer exclusively to Roman citizens and personal slaves, and therefore they probably memorialize persons of means. The scant number of early ages at death that were recorded on the inscriptions suggest that children who died were rarely remembered in this way (Table III.2).[4]

The expectation of life in Roman times that Macdonell calculated is very low by

---

[1] Alexander Pope, *An essay on man*, Epistle II.2.

[2] William L Proudfit, 'Origin of concept of ischaemic heart disease', *Br Heart J*, 1983, **50**: 209–12, p. 209.

[3] Michael Grant, 'Ancient writers bibliography', in *idem, The founders of the western world: a history of Greece and Rome*, New York, Charles Scribner and Sons, 1991, p. 303.

[4] W R Macdonell, 'On the expectation of life in ancient Rome and in the provinces of Hispania, Lusitania and Africa', *Biometrika*, 1913, **9**: 366–80, pp. 378–9.

*Table III.1*
Some classical era notables living to beyond age 60

| Greek Writers | | Roman Historians | |
|---|---|---|---|
| Name | Age at death | Name | Age at death |
| Aeschylus | 68 | Cassiodorus | 93 |
| Anaxagoras | 72 | St Jerome | 72 |
| Antisthenes | 85 | Livy | 76 |
| Aristotle | 62 | Nepos | 75 |
| Callimachus | 65/70 | Tacitus | about 61 |
| Demosthenes | 62 | Dio Cassius | 80 |
| Dionysius I | 63 | Eusebius | 86 |
| Empedocles | 60 | Plutarch | over 70 |
| Epicurus | 71 | Polybius | about 62 |
| Euclides | 70 | Theodoretus | 73 |
| Euripides | 74/79 | Cato the Elder | 85 |
| Isocrates | 98 | Pollio | 72 |
| Pindar | 80 | Varro | 89 |
| Plato | 82 | Emperor Claudius | 64 |
| Simonides | 88 | Posidonius | 85 |
| Sophocles | 90 | | |
| Theophrastus | 82/85 | | |
| Xenophon | 76 | | |
| Zeno | 72 | | |

Sources: M Grant, 'Ancient writers bibliography', in *idem, The founders of the western world: a history of Greece and Rome*, New York, Charles Scribner and Sons, 1991, p. 303; M Grant, *History of Rome*, New York, Charles Scribner and Sons, 1978, p. 508.

*Table III.2*
Some records of inscriptions of age at death on Roman empire monuments

| Ages | Rome | Iberia | Africa |
|---|---|---|---|
| 40–49 | 292 | 124 | 635 |
| 50–59 | 146 | 109 | 611 |
| 60–69 | 144 | 106 | 633 |
| 70–79 | 89 | 93 | 726 |
| All ages* | 4,469 | 1,005 | 6,061 |

* Includes deaths under 40 and over 80 years.

Source: W R Macdonell, 'On the expectation of life in ancient Rome and in the provinces of Hispania, Lusitania and Africa', *Biometrika*, 1913, **9**: 366–80, pp. 378–9.

current standards, but, whatever their shortcomings, his data show that it was by no means uncommon for ordinary Romans to live until late middle and even old age. A full life span as now understood was not unknown in the Middle Ages and three succeeding centuries. Of the twenty-four kings and queens of England who reigned between the Norman Conquest and 1768 and who escaped violent death, accidentally or at the hands of wartime enemies, rebellious subjects or usurpers, no fewer than fourteen lived to beyond the age of sixty years.[5] At the beginning of the eighteenth century, over a quarter of the population of England was aged forty-five years or more.[6]

From 1538 onwards, births and deaths were recorded in all English parish registers. This procedure was initiated shortly after the break with Rome and establishment of the Church of England. The imposition of uniformity in religious practice at that time ensured that the registers would be comprehensive, with the possible exception of some infants who died before baptism or whose births were concealed. The information contained in some 404 of the 530 possible parish registers in various parts of the country was used by E Anthony Wrigley and Roger Schofield of the Cambridge Group for the History of Population and Social Structure for calculation of English population data from 1541 to 1871. Techniques were developed for dealing with data that deviated markedly from the average, whether from parish to parish or within a single parish in any particular year. Wrigley and Schofield had some doubts about the reliability of the data compiled during periods of acute disturbance, such as the mid-seventeenth-century Civil War, but considered them fairly accurate otherwise.[7] Although religious diversity became widespread and increasingly tolerated during the eighteenth century, almost all births and deaths were still being recorded in Church of England parish registers, especially when this became compulsory in 1696.[8] A technique of back projection was used to calculate the yearly population size from 1541 onwards using totals of births and deaths, population numbers at a succession of points in time, and making allowance for individuals moving from one parish to another.[9] After 1801 data thus obtained could be checked against census results and, starting some thirty years later, against government registration of vital statistics. As evidence of the validity of their methods, the nineteenth-century numbers obtained by the Cambridge Group were found to be in fairly close agreement with the new official figures.[10]

The Group revised the initial 1981 analysis with a technique of family data reconstitution. As an example, any one individual's baptismal, marriage and burial records could be related and age at marriage and death deduced. With enough individuals, expectation of life at various ages and times could be calculated, together

---

[5] John Cannon and Ralph Griffiths, *The Oxford illustrated history of the British monarchy*, Oxford University Press, 1989.

[6] E Anthony Wrigley *et al.*, *English population history from family reconstitution 1580–1837*, Cambridge University Press, 1997, pp. 614–15.

[7] E Anthony Wrigley and R S Schofield, *The population history of England 1541–1871: a reconstruction*, Cambridge, MA, Harvard University Press, 1981, p. 31.

[8] Ibid., p. 28.

[9] Ibid., p. 8.

[10] Ibid., p. 199.

*Table III.3*
Total population of England in the eighteenth century

| Year | Thousands |
| --- | --- |
| 1701 | 5,211 |
| 1731 | 5,414 |
| 1751 | 5,922 |
| 1771 | 6,623 |
| 1791 | 7,846 |
| 1801 | 8,671 |

Source: E Anthony Wrigley *et al.*, *English population history from family reconstitution 1580–1837*, Cambridge University Press, 1997, p. 614 (with permission).

with other vital statistics. The great extent of the material that this yielded necessitated confining the later study to twenty-six parishes that were considered collectively to be representative of England as a whole. The newer technique facilitated effective use of the additional information and, pertinent to the present study, it resulted in some revision of the figures for the total population in any year and at various ages. For the eighteenth century the newer annual tabulations were for the most part the higher by about 3 per cent.[11]

The Cambridge Group estimated that during the eighteenth century the population of England rose by about two-thirds, from just under five and a quarter million in 1701 to over eight and a half million by 1801 (Table III.3). During the second quarter of the century there was a slight and transient fall in number coinciding with a series of epidemics, so that almost all of the increase took place after 1750.[12] Immigrants to England came mainly from other parts of the British Isles with small numbers from the Continent. These, however, were largely balanced by emigrants, to North America in particular. The latter numbered over half a million during the course of the eighteenth century.[13] The rise in population must therefore of necessity have resulted from natural increase, due in turn to a decline in the death rate, a rise in the birth rate, or a combination of the two.

Which of these causes predominated has a direct bearing on estimates of any demographic contribution to the initial emergence of angina pectoris in the 1760s and 1770s. Any increase in numbers of middle-aged and elderly people alive in these decades could have resulted only from a decline in adult death rates beginning in mid-century. A mid-eighteenth-century start in either a rise in the birth rate or a fall in infant and childhood mortality could not have had any appreciable effect on the numbers of the middle-aged and elderly until the 1790s at earliest, well past the critical period when angina pectoris first became manifest and then increasingly prevalent.

[11] Wrigley *et al.*, op. cit., note 6 above, p. 614.
[12] Ibid., p. 614.
[13] B R Mitchell, *British historical statistics*, Cambridge University Press, 1988, p. 76.

Based on their earlier data, the Cambridge Group concluded that an increase in the birth rate accounted for about two-thirds of the population increase during the last half of the eighteenth century.[14] This presupposes that fertility could have been controlled and therefore limited at an earlier period. T McKeown has postulated that prior to the recent introduction of efficient means of contraception, fertility rates, unless adversely affected by severe female malnutrition, were unavoidably maximal and consequently there was, apart from some improvement in diet of the very poor, little room for any increase.[15] However, there is evidence for limitations on fertility in earlier times, both voluntary and dictated by extraneous factors. Low illegitimacy rates in the eighteenth century indicate that abstinence was widely practised, as was coitus interruptus,[16] a form of birth control known since Biblical times.[17] Primitive barrier forms of contraception were not unknown and the wider birth spacing that follows prolonged breast feeding had been noted and possibly utilized as early as the seventeenth century.[18] Lactation is now known to inhibit ovulation for several months and thereby reduce the likelihood of early post-partum conception,[19] but reduced sexual activity while breast feeding and caring for an infant may also have contributed to deferment of a subsequent pregnancy.[20]

Dorothy George has suggested that a further, albeit one time contributory cause, was the decline in gin drinking after 1751, when duties on spirits were increased and their retailing controlled by Act of Parliament.[21] A consequent reduction in alcohol-induced ill health among women of reproductive age could well have led to an increase in fertility. There was also an eighteenth-century betterment in nutritional status that benefited part of the population at least. It is largely attributable to an improvement in the availability, constancy, variety and quality of the food supply that followed changes in agricultural practice during the Georgian era, as detailed in Chapter IV. A good indicator of improving nutritional status is provided by contemporary records of the heights of individuals during years of growth and at maturity. Roderick Floud and his co-authors reported on the heights of military recruits born during a succession of five-year periods extending throughout the second half of the eighteenth century (Table III.4). Comparison of mid- and end-century cohorts shows an average height increase at recruitment of 3.36 inches at age eighteen, 3.74 at nineteen, and 1.44 inches in men of twenty-four to twenty-nine years. The lower average heights of recruits in the earlier cohorts suggests suboptimal nutrition; the greater heights in the latest one is evidence of improvement. The increase in heights of men in the eighteen- and nineteen-year age groups over the course of half a century was greater than that of the older recruits. This suggests

[14] Wrigley and Schofield, op. cit., note 7 above, p. 245.

[15] T McKeown, *The modern rise of population*, London, Edward Arnold, 1976, p. 23.

[16] Gigi Santow, '*Coitus interruptus* and the control of natural fertility', *Popul Stud*, 1995, **49**: 19–43, p. 29.

[17] Genesis 38: 9.

[18] Santow, op. cit., note 16 above, p. 27.

[19] Iris Y Wang and Ian S Fraser, 'Reproductive function and contraception in the postpartum period', *Obstet Gynecol Surv.*, 1994, **49**: 56–63, 58–9.

[20] Santow, op. cit., note 16 above, p. 25.

[21] Dorothy M George, *London life in the eighteenth century*, New York, Harper and Row, 1965, pp. 516–17.

*Table III.4*

Average height (in inches) of military recruits: quinquennial averages

| 1st quinquennial year | Age at recruitment | | |
|---|---|---|---|
| | 18 | 19 | 24–29 |
| 1747 | 61.75 | 61.22 | 65.22 |
| 1752 | 63.29 | 63.53 | 65.12 |
| 1757 | 63.68 | 64.49 | 65.74 |
| 1762 | 63.91 | 64.59 | 66.84 |
| 1767 | 65.62 | 64.70 | 66.42 |
| 1772 | 64.42 | 66.59 | 66.37 |
| 1777 | 64.16 | 65.78 | 66.30 |
| 1782 | 65.16 | 65.53 | 65.97 |
| 1787 | 63.44 | 65.52 | 66.11 |
| 1792 | 64.11 | 64.67 | 65.84 |
| 1797 | 65.11 | 64.96 | 66.66 |

Source: Roderick Floud, A Gregory and K Wachter, *Height, health and history: nutritional status in the United Kingdom 1750–1980*, Cambridge University Press, 1990, pp. 506, 508 (with permission).

that in the earliest cohorts attainment of maximal height was delayed; in the latest ones it was sooner and thus further evidence of better nutrition.[22] Although there may have been a tendency for male family members to have priority at the table, it is unlikely that females failed to derive any benefit from the improving food supply. Deficiency states are associated with late menarche, early menopause and with diminished vigour and fertility, all of which can be corrected by better nutrition.[23]

The Cambridge Group associated an increase in female fertility with a fall in the age of marriage that they had documented. The change was quite modest during the period here under review, the Group's estimates of the mean age of females at first marriage being twenty-six years in the first decade of the eighteenth century and about a year and a half earlier during its third quarter.[24] However, because of the spread of the usually numerous births over many years, the youngest children would have been born during late years of female reproductive life and a time of fast declining fertility. A one year head start could have affected fertility favourably and appreciably by the end of, say, a twenty-year period of childbearing when the wife would have reached her forties, a time of rapidly diminishing likelihood of conception. This, for example, could have made the difference between having eleven rather than ten children. After a twenty-year interval, any initial increase in fertility would have raised both the numbers and the proportion of the population at ages

[22] Roderick Floud, A Gregory and K Wachter, *Height, health and history: nutritional status in the United Kingdom 1750–1980*, Cambridge University Press, 1990, pp. 506, 508.

[23] Susan Scott and C J Duncan, 'Nutrition, fertility and steady-state population dynamics in a pre-industrial community in Penrith, northern England', *J Biosoc Sci*, 1999, **31**: 505–23.

[24] Wrigley *et al.*, op. cit., note 6 above, p. 134.

*Table III.5*
Eighteenth-century infant and childhood mortality rate/1000/year

| Period | Age (in years) | | | |
|---|---|---|---|---|
| | 0–1 | 1–4 | 5–10 | 0–15 |
| 1700–1724 | 195.1 | 107.9 | 27.0 | 333.8 |
| 1725–1749 | 196.3 | 121.0 | 28.4 | 348.1 |
| 1750–1774 | 170.4 | 107.3 | 25.7 | 308.1 |
| 1775–1779 | 166.0 | 107.7 | 22.7 | 297.9 |

Source: E Anthony Wrigley *et al.*, *English population history from family reconstitution 1580–1837*, Cambridge University Press, 1997, p. 262 (with permission).

of maximal reproductive activity, thereby initiating a cyclical course of rising birth rates.

The conclusions of the Cambridge Group have been disputed by proponents of decrease in mortality rates, especially in infancy and childhood, as the main cause of the rise in population numbers. Peter E Razzell has queried the completeness and reliability of the baptismal registration data on which the Cambridge Group's conclusions were based. He has also highlighted some difficulty in correcting for absence of birth entries of nonconformist families in the parish registers and also the problems arising as a result of people moving, and births, marriages and deaths being registered in different parishes as a result.[25] Razzell has also drawn attention to the common eighteenth-century practice of memorializing a deceased child by giving his or her name to the next sibling of the same sex. The recorded marriage and death of the surviving brother or sister could therefore be linked erroneously with the birth of the *deceased* child. As a result, calculation of the surviving namesake's age at marriage and death would be over-estimated by the length of the interval between the births of the deceased and the next living siblings.[26] Wrigley and his colleagues have included a detailed refutation of this critique in their 1997 publication. They point out, *inter alia*, that the same first name was not infrequently given to a younger *sibling* of a living child. Resulting errors in these circumstances would therefore have been random, and with adequate numbers they would have tended to cancel out.[27]

Data published by the Cambridge Group itself do indicate a modest fall in infant and child mortality between the first and last quarters of the eighteenth century (Table III.5).[28] Razzell has produced evidence to suggest that the mortality rates of adults also declined during the same period. A spinster marrying by licence when below the age of twenty-one was required to have the consent of her father, the mother if her father were dead, or a guardian if both parents were deceased. Registers

[25] P E Razzell, 'The growth of population in eighteenth century England. A critical reappraisal', *J Econ Hist*, 1993, **53**: 743–71, p. 744.
[26] Ibid., p. 750.
[27] Wrigley *et al.*, op. cit., note 6 above, p. 100.
[28] Ibid., p. 262.

recording this form of marriage consequently noted whether one or both parents of the bride were alive or not on her wedding day. If alive, the parental age must have been thirty-five years at least. Between the periods 1677–1700 and 1751–1779 the percentage of brides with living fathers rose from 59 to 74; in the case of widowed mothers, there was almost no change, 20 and 21 per cent respectively, but the percentage of brides with both parents dead fell dramatically, from 21 to 4 per cent. The findings are convincing, but whether they are applicable to the whole country is problematic as the investigation was confined to the Canterbury area and the sources of similar studies that Razzell quoted were also localized.[29]

Several reasons for a decline in mortality rates have been suggested. Apart from a beneficial effect on fertility, Dorothy George has pointed out that there was a potential for improvements in maternal health following the decline in gin drinking. Alcohol related deaths among women could have become fewer, and with increasing sobriety there was scope for improvement in infant care and their survival to follow.[30] Other possible reasons for falling mortality rates include the overall improved nutrition mentioned earlier and a rise in standards of cleanliness. For example, the newly introduced cotton replaced in part the use of wool and made the washing of clothes much easier.[31] Razzell has also suggested that improved housing construction played a part, in particular with brick or stone replacing floors of bare earth.[32] In addition, slates and tiles were being substituted for thatch in roofs. Both the roof and floor changes would have reduced contact with vermin.[33] The late eighteenth century also saw some improvement in the physical environment of towns, especially in the better districts. Streets were being paved, piped water introduced, sewers constructed and exposure to waterborne infections consequently reduced. The differences between the protagonists of each of the two possible reasons for the eighteenth-century population increase are mainly questions of emphasis. They have between them produced causes of and evidence for both increased fecundity *and* a decrease in mortality, whether in infancy, childhood or adult life.

The demographics of the capital are of special significance because it was in the metropolis that a disproportionately large number of the country's physicians then lived and where William Heberden practised for most of his professional life. During the Georgian era, death rates in London were greater than in the country as a whole.[34] This reflected the appalling conditions under which most of the population of the burgeoning cities lived,[35] the endemic fevers[36] and periodic epidemics[37] that ravaged the metropolis, and the probable lack of resistance to infection among the new arrivals from the relatively disease free countryside.[38] Until 1775, London

[29] Razzell, op. cit., note 25 above, p. 759.
[30] George, op. cit., note 21 above, p. 28.
[31] Ibid., p. 60.
[32] Razzell, op. cit., note 25 above, p. 766.
[33] Bill Breckon and Jeffrey Parker, *Tracing the history of houses*, Newbury, Countryside Books, 1991, p. 72.
[34] J Landers, *Death and the metropolis*, Cambridge University Press, 1993, p. 175.
[35] Ibid., pp. 68–70.
[36] Ibid, p. 122.
[37] Ibid., p. 282.
[38] Ibid., p. 123.

consistently suffered an excess of deaths over births, and it was only because of immigration from rural areas and the smaller towns that its population rose in number.[39] In the early years of the eighteenth century, many Londoners did live to be elderly, but during the forty years leading to the time when angina pectoris was first reported, their numbers actually declined slightly. From December 1728 onwards, the London Bills of Mortality tabulated the number of deaths at various ages in ten-year groupings. My own perusal of the Bills for the first of these groupings, i.e. the decade ending in December 1738, showed that during this period 33,935 persons were aged sixty years or over at death. During the ten-year period that ended in December 1770 and encompassed the time when angina pectoris was first being described, the number of Londoners who were sixty or more at death had fallen marginally to 33,573.

The eighteenth-century population trends in England as a whole diverged from those of the metropolis. In contrast to London, the overall number of individuals in the entire country who were aged sixty and over increased between the same two decades (1728–38 and 1760–70) by about one-fifth, from about 518,000 to 620,000. In 1771 their percentage of the total population was 7.38 in contrast to 9.95 in 1701, the former being a smaller percentage of a far larger total number.[40] The impact of rising fertility and fewer deaths in infancy and childhood apparently outweighed the more modest effects of declining mortality in adult life. The greater increase in the numbers of younger people had "diluted" the proportion of the older ones. Between the start of the century and 1771 the numbers of all English middle aged and elderly (defined somewhat arbitrarily as persons over forty-five), rose from 1,319,000 to 1,493,000, a modest 13.2 per cent. This group encompassed almost all of the people vulnerable to coronary disease by reason of age.[41]

In light of the characterization of angina as a "British disease", the demographic differences between England and elsewhere are modest. For example, mortality rates were greater in late-eighteenth-century France than in England (Table III.6), but the differences were not enough to have precluded many French men and women from living to middle life and beyond.[42]

There is evidence to indicate that the average life span of the British nobility increased considerably between the late seventeenth and late eighteenth centuries and in doing so overtook the expectation of life of the general population, the comparative changes being shown in Table III.7. T H Hollingsworth's data indicate that the percentage of the peerage who lived to *fifty* years during the last half of the eighteenth century was half as great again as the percentage of the general population who then only reached the age of *forty-five*.[43] Although there are some deficiencies, data concerning the nobility are close to comprehensive as there are records giving

[39] Wrigley *et al.*, op. cit., note 6 above, p. 615.

[40] Ibid., pp. 614–15.

[41] Ibid., pp. 614–15.

[42] Wrigley *et al.*, op. cit., note 6 above, p. 291.

[43] T H Hollingsworth, *The demography of the British peerage, Population Studies*, **18**: Supplement No. 2, London, Population Investigation Committee, London School of Economics, 1964, pp. 56–7; Wrigley *et al.*, op. cit., note 6 above, pp. 614–15.

*Table III.6*
Adult mortality/1000/year.
Sexes combined, England and France, ages 30–70

| Age | England 1750–1809 | France 1740–1789 |
|---|---|---|
| 30–34 | 54.1 | 62.7 |
| 35–39 | 62.3 | 71.9 |
| 40–44 | 68.1 | 86.2 |
| 45–49 | 89.0 | 101.1 |
| 50–54 | 101.1 | 119.1 |
| 55–59 | 124.1 | 148.6 |
| 60–64 | 172.1 | 203.4 |
| 65–69 | 237.7 | 285.5 |

Source: E Anthony Wrigley *et al.*, *English population history from family reconstitution 1580–1837*, Cambridge University Press, 1997, p. 291 (with permission).

*Table III.7*
Expectation of life at birth: 1650–1774
Total population of England and British peerage

| Cohort year of birth | Life expectancy (years) | | | |
|---|---|---|---|---|
| | Total population* | | British peerage† | |
| | Male | Female | Male | Female |
| 1650–74 | 38.1 | 36.3 | 29.6 | 30.7 |
| 1675–99 | 35.4 | 35.4 | 32.9 | 34.2 |
| 1700–24 | 36.6 | 36.8 | 36.6 | 36.3 |
| 1725–49 | 35.8 | 37.4 | 38.6 | 36.7 |
| 1750–74 | 40.8 | 40.0 | 44.5 | 45.7 |

* Source: E Anthony Wrigley *et al.*, *English population history from family reconstitution 1580–1837*, Cambridge University Press, 1997, p. 308 (with permission).
† Source: T H Hollingsworth, *The demography of the British peerage*, *Populations Studies*, **18**, Supplement No. 2, London, Population Investigation Committee, London School of Economics, 1964, pp. 56–7 (with permission).

the dates of birth and death of individual members of the peerage and their immediate families.

There are several possible reasons why members of the peerage ultimately had a greater expectation of life than the general population. A small part of the credit may be due to improvements in medical practice. The peerage had greater access to the very limited number of physicians practising in the mid-eighteenth century. In 1752 there were in England but 52 Fellows of the Royal College of Physicians of London, 3 candidates, 23 licentiates and a limited number of Edinburgh and foreign trained doctors, perhaps 100 in all. They became more numerous subsequently, but by 1783, when the first comprehensive register was established, the total number of physicians for the whole of England was still only 363.[44] Their availability for serving the general population was limited, although some doctors did attend indigent patients in newly established dispensaries.[45] To a very large extent the population as a whole used the services of the more numerous apothecaries or lay practitioners who were regarded by licensed physicians as quacks. Their diagnoses and treatments were in all probability even less substantiated than those of the Fellows of the Royal College.

The most notable eighteenth-century medical development was the introduction of measures to prevent smallpox, which had previously been the scourge of rich and poor alike. Its impact on the highest in the land during the seventeenth century can be gauged by its incidence in the Stuart royal family. Mary II, joint sovereign with William III, died of smallpox, as did two of the six children of Charles I, two of the five children of James II and the eldest son of Queen Anne.[46] Lady Mary Wortley Montagu learnt of inoculation against smallpox while living in Constantinople, where her husband was the English ambassador to the Ottoman empire. She introduced the practice into England in 1721 and variolation (introduction of material from smallpox patients' pustules beneath the skin of the persons being immunized) became widespread among the well-to-do, especially after King George II and his family, including the royal princesses, consented to being inoculated.[47] The side effects were far more severe than the vaccination using cowpox vaccine introduced by Jenner towards the end of the century. Risk of local abscesses was not inconsiderable and the live virus in the inoculum could on occasion induce a severe attack of smallpox. Nevertheless, variolation became increasingly popular, initially with the upper classes, among whom its effect on the incidence and mortality of smallpox became evident. A modified and safer technique of variolation came into widespread use by about the 1760s, still well before its replacement by vaccination after 1798.[48]

Since at least early Stuart times ague or marsh fever had been prevalent in England, possibly as a "new disease" that resulted from opening up of contacts with tropical Africa and America.[49] Unlike so many fevers, it is clearly recognizable as malaria in the contemporary descriptions which detailed the periodicity of the febrile episodes.[50] It was especially concentrated in marshy parts of south-east England,[51] including low-lying areas of London.[52] Recovery was usual, but the debilitating effects contributed

---

[44] Joan Lane, 'The medical practitioners of provincial England in 1783', *Med Hist*, 1984, **28**: 353–71, p. 353.

[45] Ibid., p. 362.

[46] D R Hopkins, *Princes and peasants: smallpox in history*, University of Chicago Press, 1983, p. 40.

[47] P E Razzell, 'Population change in eighteenth-century England: a reinterpretation', *Econ Hist Rev*, 2nd series, 1965, **18**: 312–32, p. 318.

[48] Ibid., p. 318.

[49] M J Dobson, *Contours of death and disease in early modern England*, Cambridge University Press, 1997, pp. 328–9.

[50] Ibid., p. 295.

[51] Ibid., p. 321.

[52] Ibid., p. 315.

indirectly to deaths from other causes. The introduction of cinchona or Peruvian bark in the late seventeenth century proved to be an effective remedy, this responsiveness further identifying the disease with malaria.[53] It is probable that here too the aristocracy gained the most benefit, not only because proportionally fewer of them lived in the most swampy parts of the country, but also because they could the more readily afford the new treatment. Ultimately, drainage of the marshes was of general benefit in the affected areas.

The third change in medical practice that was of selective class advantage was the changing attitude of physicians to bleeding. Phlebotomy continued to be practised throughout the eighteenth century, but licensed physicians of the time adopted an increasingly conservative approach. The number of conditions for which their patients were bled tended to lessen and, if there were no immediate benefits, patients were the more frequently spared repeated venesections.[54] There was a growing tendency to refrain from excessive bleeding if there were any untoward effects such as faintness, and to interrupt the procedure if the contralateral radial pulse became weak. The amount of blood removed was adapted increasingly to the body size and "strength" of the patient.[55] The privileged, who had the more ready access to physicians, gained the most from these advances. The general population had limited access to professional care, continued to be bled uncritically, often by friends or neighbours, and consequently suffered more frequent exposure to the attendant hazards.

Probably more important than medical advances, eighteenth-century improvement in hygiene was a cause of declining mortality among the privileged. Cleanliness became valued to an extent unknown previously. The lack of running water was not a problem for those fortunate enough to have an unlimited number of servants to fetch and carry. Soap was coming into wider use and among the upper classes it became customary to wash, bathe and have clothes laundered regularly. The newly available cotton garments could be cleaned more easily than the woollen ones that they replaced.[56] With lessening civil strife in England, homes became less fortresslike with larger windows and better ventilation. The aristocracy were also among the first to benefit from the improvements in water supply and waste disposal of which mention has already been made. The improved hygiene was reflected primarily in a decline in mortality in infancy and early childhood. Among male children born to the English peerage, the probability of dying in the first five years of life fell from 338 per thousand in the 1650–74 cohort to 191 in that of the 1750–74 quinquennium. The female equivalents were 323 and 187 respectively.[57] The changes in living styles over the intervening hundred years were apparently proving beneficial.

In 1696 Gregory King placed the number of families whose head was either a nobleman or engaged in "middle class" occupations at a little over 80,000 (Table

---

[53] L S King, *The medical world of the eighteenth century*, University of Chicago Press, 1958, p. 129.
[54] Ibid., p. 319.
[55] George, op. cit., note 21 above, p. 60.
[56] Razzell, op. cit., note 25 above, p. 744.
[57] Hollingsworth, op. cit., note 43 above, pp. 54–5.

*Table III.8*

English upper- and middle-class families 1688 (to nearest thousand)

|  | Number of families |
|---|---|
| Nobility and gentry | 18,000 |
| Persons in office | 10,000 |
| Merchants and traders | 7,000 |
| Persons in law | 10,000 |
| Clergymen | 10,000 |
| Persons in sciences and liberal arts | 16,000 |
| Naval and military officers | 9,000 |
| TOTAL | 80,000 |

Source: Gregory King, *Natural and political observations and conclusions upon the state and condition of England 1696*, ed. G E Barnett, Baltimore, Johns Hopkins Press, 1936, p. 31.

*Table III.9*

English upper- and middle-class families mid-eighteenth century (to nearest thousand). Estimate by Joseph Massie 1759

|  | Number of families |
|---|---|
| Nobility and gentry | 18,000 |
| Civil offices | 16,000 |
| Military and naval officers | 8,000 |
| Merchants | 13,000 |
| Manufacturers | 80,000 |
| Law | 12,000 |
| Eminent clergy | 2,000 |
| Lesser clergy | 9,000 |
| Arts and sciences | 18,000 |
| TOTAL | 176,000 |

Adapted from: P Mathias, *The transformation of England: essays in the economic and social history of England in the eighteenth century*, New York, Columbia University Press, 1979, pp. 186–7 (with permission).

III.8).[58] During the eighteenth century there was a considerable increase in the size of the middle classes, comprised principally of the families of the more prosperous farmers, professional men, notably lawyers and clergymen, and persons engaged in manufacturing and commerce and finally their dependents. An estimate of the social structure of England in 1759–60, shown in Table III.9, indicates that during the intervening years there was more than a doubling to a total of 176,000 households, perhaps an increase from 500,000 to one million persons, or from about one-tenth

[58] Gregory King, *Natural and political observations and conclusions upon the state and condition of England 1696*, ed. George E Barnett, Baltimore, Johns Hopkins Press, 1936, p. 31.

to about one-sixth of the total population of England.[59] During the Georgian era these families, sometimes then designated as "the middling sort" considered the gap between themselves and the nobility to be much narrower than the gulf which separated them from the labouring classes. They therefore sought, to the extent that their means allowed, to emulate upper-class lifestyles. The families of the people in middle-class occupations would rarely have been as wealthy as members of the nobility, and incomes within any one occupation could vary widely.[60] However, the "middling sort" as a class enjoyed freedom from overcrowding. Increasingly they were living away from their places of work and in more and well-ventilated, spacious, better constructed homes in ever more salubrious neighbourhoods. They were acquiring reasonable standards of cleanliness of person and clothes, and access to professional medical attention. In most instances they had diets that were adequate if not more than adequate. Whilst the large proportion of the middling sort living in London remained in some measure exposed to the adverse health consequences, their lifestyles and location would have conferred some degree of protection from the epidemic and endemic diseases that ravaged the metropolis.[61] It is likely therefore that the growing life expectancy of the nobility was accompanied by a more or less corresponding increase among the middle classes. A rise in middle class expectation of life during the course of the Georgian era is attested by the findings of Southwood Smith who compared the course of insured lives of persons born between 1690 and 1790, and calculated an extension of some 25 per cent during this time. His data were based on records of families whose heads could afford to lend money to the government through purchase of a tontine, that is an annuity shared by a number of subscribers and successively transferred after each death to the survivors in the group.[62] Razzell, using the same method, found that during the Georgian era a considerable reduction in mortality was demonstrable among members of parliament and Scottish advocates.[63] As noted earlier, he also documented an eighteenth-century rise in the proportion of parents who lived to see their under 21-year-old daughters marrying, an age of thirty-five at least. As his conclusions were based on information in records of marriage by licence, which was more costly than marriage by banns, the information he obtained probably related to families with means.[64] The overall evidence presented suggests that the proportion of middle-class people who lived well into adult life and beyond probably exceeded that of the population as a whole, even though the extent cannot be quantified in the way that is possible for the entire population.

Twentieth-century epidemiological surveys have consistently established that, notwithstanding female vulnerability to the traditional risk factors, the frequency of

[59] P Mathias, *The transformation of England: essays in the economic and social history of England in the eighteenth century*, New York, Columbia University Press, 1979, pp. 186–7.

[60] P Langford, *A polite and commercial people: England 1727–1783*, Oxford University Press, 1992, pp. 61–3.

[61] Landers, op. cit., note 34 above, pp. 282, 347.

[62] Southwood Smith, 'On the evidence of the prolongation of life during the eighteenth century', *Trans Nat Assoc Promotion Social Sci*, 1857, p. 498.

[63] Razzell, op. cit., note 25 above, p. 765.

[64] Ibid., p. 759.

coronary heart disease is much lower in women than in men until the age of about fifty-five. After fifty-five years, the female incidence approaches that of males.[65] Currently, many more women than men now live beyond that age. As a consequence, the overall incidence among women is today less than among men but not greatly so. Conversely, in any society, the lower the proportion of women living beyond fifty-five and the smaller the ratio of women to men in older age groups, the lower would be the overall ratio of women to men vulnerable to coronary heart disease. Such was the situation in the eighteenth century because numerous pregnancies were the rule and maternal mortality rates high. Female expectation of life at birth was consequently no greater than that of males and the proportion of women living to fifty-five and beyond was about the same as that of men.[66] These factors would have resulted in the proportion of Georgian era women among sufferers from coronary heart disease being lower than today. This was indeed the situation exemplified by Heberden's own series. Amongst nearly 100 of his patients with angina, there were only three females.[67]

In conclusion, there were 1,319,000 people in England aged forty-five or more at the start of the eighteenth century. By 1771 their numbers had increased to 1,493,000, a modest 13 per cent,[68] reflecting the impact on population growth of declining adult death rates from the early mid-eighteenth century onwards. The contribution made by a rising birth rate and a fall in infant and childhood mortality beginning in the mid-1700s would not have impacted on the number of over forty-fives until near the end of the century. The evidence presented earlier suggests that although the large numbers of the middle class who lived in London could not wholly escape its health hazards, the percentage of their over forty-fives probably rose by more than the national average. In addition, the actual numbers of middle class in that age bracket must have more than doubled because of their growing population base. The middle-class heads of family increased in number more than twofold between 1696 and 1759.[69] However, the large-scale population growth that began in mid-century was due mainly to an increase in fertility and a decline in mortality in infancy and early childhood.[70] These changes could not have impacted on growth in numbers of the middle aged until well after the 1770s when angina pectoris had already first been recognized and was apparently increasing in prevalence. The really substantial increase of the middle-class and middle-aged population came two or more decades later. Unfortunately these changes cannot be quantified with the degree of accuracy possible for the total population.

By the beginning of the eighteenth century only two possible instances of angina pectoris had been described in England during the whole of its recorded history.

---

[65] William B Kannel and Thomas J Thom, 'Statistical data of clinical importance, incidence, prevalence and mortality of cardiovascular disease', in J Willis Hurst and Robert C Schlant (eds), *The heart, arteries and veins*, 7th ed., New York, McGraw-Hill, 1990, pp. 627–8.

[66] Wrigley *et al.*, op. cit., note 6 above, p. 308.

[67] William Heberden, *Commentaries on the history and cure of diseases*, London, T Payne, 1802, p. 295.

[68] Wrigley *et al.*, op. cit., note 6 above, p. 614–15.

[69] King, op. cit., note 58 above, p. 31; Mathias, op. cit., note 59 above, pp. 186–7.

[70] Wrigley and Schofield, op. cit., note 7 above, p. 245.

## Population Trends

The twenty or so people with the characteristic pain seen by Heberden alone between 1748 and 1768 were followed by a near fourfold rise in his numbers in half that time, and by case reports by close to a score of contemporary physicians. All the while it remained uniquely "a British disease" and confined almost exclusively to affluent middle-aged and elderly men. The eighteenth-century increase in their numbers cannot alone explain the initial emergence of angina pectoris virtually *ex nihilo* and is insufficient to account in more than part for the extent of its subsequently rapid growing incidence. The demographic differences between Britain and elsewhere are also insufficient to explain by themselves the unique geographical distribution. The select group of patients with angina pectoris could have become susceptible to it only if other factors had emerged concurrently during the Georgian era and these must be sought. The demographics can contribute only some of the soil. It remains to find the seeds.

# IV

# The Agricultural Revolution

## Cows and Plows

The most significant development in eighteenth-century England that relates to the present enquiry was the Agricultural Revolution. The resulting changes in farming practices impacted on crop production, the biological characteristics of domesticated animals and eventually on human eating habits. These warrant consideration in some detail, with emphasis on the changes in animal husbandry. In medieval times, as in many developing countries today, sheep and cattle grazed on communal grasslands left in their natural state. As the lands were held jointly there was very little attempt either to avoid overgrazing or to effect improvements, for example by appropriate drainage.[1] Cows were also allowed to roam untended in the forests, then much more extensive than now. Pigs were left to forage in the woods, feeding for the most part on acorns and beech masts. Deer roamed in the woodlands and subsisted on branches of trees and shrubs. Poultry scratched the ground in the farmyards, such as they were, subsisting on whatever seeds or scraps they could find.

There was no attempt at selective breeding, which would have been impossible anyway in the absence of any fencing and with the stock of the entire community mingling together. Unsupervised and free to roam, cattle, sheep and pigs were not fastidious in choice of sexual partners with the resulting "promiscuous unions of nobody's son with everybody's daughter".[2] The animals were almost invariably stunted and underweight (Illustrations 1 and 2). Rams were described as having skin that rattled on the ribs. The milk yield of cows was both low and erratic. The arable lands were cultivated in accordance with the strip system. This ensured that allocations between better and poorer land was fair, but compelled each individual to waste much time walking between his isolated allotments, which were usually dispersed widely. Much land was wasted in order to keep the strips clearly separated. The good farmer could not maintain his lands free of weeds if his neighbour was neglectful in this respect. Attempts at improving the land such as by better drainage was frustrated by need for general agreement and the sequence of crop rotation did not allow for individual variation. With its innate inefficiencies, the strip system could barely supply enough for human consumption and little or none was available for winter feeding of the animals.[3] Stock with breeding potential could be maintained, although with difficulty, over the winter, but because of limited availability of feed,

---

[1] R E Prothero, *The pioneers and progress of English farming*, London, Longmans Green, 1888, p. 6.
[2] Ibid., p. 50.
[3] Lord Ernle, *The land and its people: chapters in rural life and history*, London, Hutchinson, 1925, pp. 5, 9, 10.

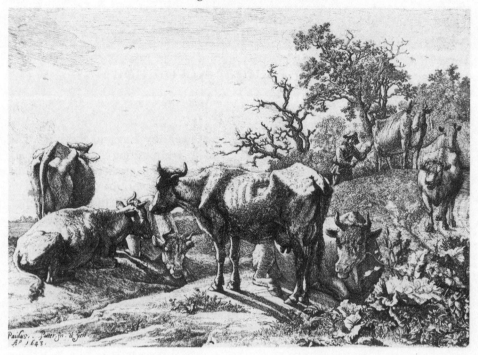

*Illustration 1:* Cattle roaming on common land. Etching by P Potter, 1643. (Wellcome Library, London.)

most other animals had to be killed in the autumn.[4] The meat was then salted as no other methods of preservation were available. The supply of meat, even if considered edible when tainted, would rarely last until the spring, and the availability of milk in winter was very limited.

Improvements in agricultural practices in association with the enclosure movement had their beginnings late in the medieval period and continued at a very slow pace in Tudor times.[5] The changes involved replacing widely separated strips of land by consolidated fields of equivalent area with each individual receiving an additional allotment equal to his share of the common and waste lands.[6] The newly allocated fields were enclosed with walls or hedges and the owners had the right to farm their consolidated lands in accordance with their own personal wishes, resources and abilities.[7] The enclosure movement continued piecemeal in the Stuart era[8] but became dramatically more rapid during Georgian times when the need for unanimous agreement to the changes was circumvented by introduction of private bills submitted

[4] Ibid., p. 6.

[5] Prothero, op. cit., note 1 above, p. 65.

[6] Ibid., p. 18.

[7] Ibid., p. 19.

[8] Joan Thirsk, 'Agricultural policy: public debate and legislation', in Joan Thirsk (ed.), *The agrarian history of England and Wales, Volume V: 1640–1750. II. Agrarian change,* Cambridge University Press, 1985, p. 379.

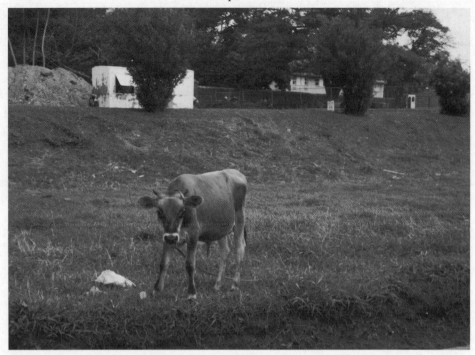

*Illustration 2:* A calf grazing on public lands. Barbados (photograph: L Michaels).

to parliament. There were eight Enclosure Acts passed during the years 1724 to 1729 and thirty-nine during both the 1740s and 1750s,[9] but a subsequent surge followed so that by the end of the century the total exceeded 2,000.[10] The status of over five million acres was changed in this way, but the total acreage affected was considerably greater as much land was enclosed by mutual agreement and without recourse to sanction by Acts of Parliament.[11] Although often causing considerable and perhaps avoidable suffering to the small farmer, the overall effect on agricultural output was dramatic. The efficiency of the landholder or the farm labourer was increased because the new consolidated fields were far more compact than the old strips. Time was no longer spent walking between dispersed landholdings and the unused land that had formerly separated the many individual holdings was brought into cultivation. Protection of crops from uncontrolled grazing became possible. By separating the animals of individual farmers, enclosures had the potential for limiting the spread of epizootic diseases and providing an assured supply of manure. Long and secure leases or outright ownership provided motivation for improvement of the land, both for the raising of crops and for animal husbandry.

During the early eighteenth century the pace of change was rapid. The nobility

[9] Ibid., pp. 380–2.
[10] Frank O'Gorman, *The long eighteenth century: British political and social history 1688–1832*, London, Arnold, 1997, p. 122.
[11] Thirsk, op. cit., note 8 above, p. 379.

and gentry, although despising income earned through trade, were not averse to increasing the income from their estates and they were in the forefront when it came to developing new agricultural techniques. Viscount Townshend propagated a system of crop rotation that included clover, silage and root crops, notably turnips, thereby earning himself the sobriquet "Turnip Townshend".[12] As a result of his innovations, it was no longer necessary to leave fields fallow. Henceforth they could be cultivated every year. Rye and other "artificial" grasses were introduced, fields were manured intensively, marled regularly and overgrazing reduced. Iron ploughs and harrows were brought into use and Jethro Tull advanced the use of drills for sowing. As a result it was possible to cut deep furrows and implant seeds directly into the soil at predetermined intervals, thereby eliminating the wastage associated with the previous practice of broadcasting the seed.[13] Horses, notably Clydesdales, replaced oxen, and with their greater strength and speed they were more effective when pulling the newly developed implements.[14] Drainage systems were introduced and increasingly well maintained.[15] While all of these changes resulted in greater productivity per acre, marginal and waste lands were brought into use and some of the forests cleared so that the area under cultivation in England increased by some two million acres between 1696 and 1797.

As a result of these changes, crushed rapeseed residues, cattle cake, oil cake, crushed oats, clover and cabbage became available as cattle feed, and sheep were given turnips, oil cake made from clover, vetches and mustard to supplement their grazing.[16] Deer were domesticated by being kept in parks, often under licence, and given supplemental feeds of grain. Hogs were fattened with brewers' grain, beans and pulses, and also from the increasingly available buttermilk and curds.[17] Poultry were kept in enclosed farmyards or coops and fed grain in regular and adequate amounts. The supply of animal feed became not only more assured but also more varied and plentiful. Its abundance, and the housing of cows in stalls and sheep in folds, meant that they could be kept in better health in summer and alive and well nourished over the winter. In consequence meat became available throughout the year. Manure produced in winter in stalls or folds could be used as a supplementary fertilizer for application to summer grazing lands.

The exemplars of improved farming practice were frequently prominent in society. The first three Hanoverian kings were greatly interested in agriculture, George III taking great delight in being known to his subjects as "Farmer George".[18] An example of improved management of estates was set by Sir Robert Walpole, First Lord of the Treasury and *de facto* Prime Minister for twenty-one years. He was reported to

[12] Prothero, op. cit., note 1 above, pp. 44–7.

[13] Ibid., p. 47.

[14] Jonathan Brown and H A Beecham, 'Farming techniques', in G E Mingay (ed.), *The agrarian history of England and Wales, Volume VI: 1750–1850*, Cambridge University Press, 1989, p. 289.

[15] Prothero, op. cit., note 1 above, p. 43.

[16] Ibid., p. 33.

[17] Peter J Bowden, 'Agricultural prices, wages, farm profits and rents', in Joan Thirsk (ed.), *The agrarian history of England and Wales, Volume V: 1640–1750. II. Agrarian change,* Cambridge University Press, 1985, p. 32.

[18] Prothero, op. cit., note 1 above, p. 79.

have given attention to his stewards' reports on the state of his farmlands priority over the contents of government dispatch boxes.[19] Turnip Townshend, whose innovations have already been described, had been Lord Privy Seal and played an important part in the negotiations that led to the 1707 Union of England and Scotland. He had also served as Secretary of State for Foreign Affairs during the War of the Spanish Succession. Thomas Coke of Norfolk, who set an example in consolidating his 43,000 acre estate and applying the new farming techniques, was a descendant of one of England's most famous Lords Chief Justice and eventually became Earl of Leicester. When it came to making improvements in farming methods, the gentry as well as members of the nobility were in the forefront. Eighteenth-century English society was very class-conscious. The small-scale farmer respected and looked up to his "betters" and at the same time sought to emulate them. Large-scale landowners, such as Coke of Norfolk, often made renewal of the leases of their tenants dependent on good farming practice and increases in rents made raising agricultural productivity a necessity for survival on the land.[20] Establishment of farming societies and regular agricultural shows facilitated wide dissemination of the new knowledge. This all helped to overcome inertia and any resistance to change so that the new methods became widely adopted by small as well as large-scale farmers.

Animals were bred selectively to some extent by the early 1700s and this practice continued on an increasing scale as the century advanced, largely under the influence of Robert Bakewell. The enclosures had made it possible to hedge or fence pastures to which farm animals could be confined and this made selective breeding feasible for the first time. Bakewell's methods included crossing breeds with different characteristics and then selectively mating animals with qualities considered desirable, to the total exclusion of strains judged to be inferior.[21]

Selective breeding was motivated almost exclusively by the desire to increase the mature weight of cows, sheep and pigs and the speed with which this could be attained. These considerations took precedence over all others. "Size was the only criterion of merit".[22] As horses replaced oxen at the plough, the need to strengthen cattle as draught animals diminished. Regard for appearance lessened and features such as colouring and horn structure ceased to be matters of concern. Hardihood when driven became less important as improved road surfaces made for easier movement (see pages 140–1). Often driven in early life from the Midlands and beyond to the vicinity of London, they were then fattened close to their place of ultimate slaughter by farmers who specialized in managing feed lots for this purpose. The untoward weight loss with lengthy road transfer before killing was thereby avoided.[23] Docility became less important once animals were kept in enclosed fields in summer and in stalls in winter. When selectively breeding sheep, quality of fleece

[19] Ibid., p. 18.

[20] R A C Parker, 'Coke of Norfolk and the agrarian revolution', *Econ Hist Rev.*, 2nd series, 1955–6, **8**: 156–66, pp. 157, 159.

[21] Prothero, op. cit., note 1 above, p. 51.

[22] G E Fussell, 'The size of English cattle in the eighteenth century', *Agric Hist*, 1929, **3**: 160–81, p. 163.

[23] Brown and Beecham, op. cit., note 14 above, p. 247.

Table IV.1
Average weight of animals sold at Smithfield (lbs)

| Year | Beeves | Calves | Year | Sheep | Lambs |
|------|--------|--------|------|-------|-------|
| 1710 | 370    | 50     | 1710 | 28    | 18    |
| 1785 | 800    | 148    | 1790 | 80    | 50    |

Sources: G E Fussell, 'The size of English cattle in the eighteenth century', *Agric Hist*, 1929, **3**: 160–81, pp. 160–1; G E Fussell and Constance Goodman, 'Eighteenth century estimates of British sheep and wool production', *Agric Hist*, 1930, **4**: 131–51, p. 134.

and quantity of wool were subordinated to amount and speed of weight gain. Wool became relatively less important commercially after 1614 when its export was banned in order to reduce Continental competition with the English clothing industry. Meanwhile, improved techniques of processing wool made length and fineness of fibre less important.

The new breeding, feeding and management techniques produced generations of farm animals that could mature at earlier ages, gaining weight extremely rapidly and, by modern standards, to excess. There was close to a threefold increase in weight in cows and calves, sheep and lambs sold in Smithfield (London's central meat market) during the eighteenth century (Table IV.1).[24] As there was no recorded tendency for the age at which lambs and calves were sold to change during this time, their greater weights at slaughter as the century progressed can be explained by a faster rate at which they could be fattened before reaching maturity.

The increasing weight of adult cattle sold at Smithfield was part of a general tendency for them to become heavier throughout England during the course of the eighteenth century. Records for its earlier years are rather scanty, but become more plentiful later, the changes being documented to a greater extent and county by county by interested individuals, notably Arthur Young, and later by a newly constituted, government-sponsored Board of Agriculture, of which he was one of the originators.[25] James Thorold Rogers reported that at the beginning of the century the average weight of oxen was about 400 lbs after evisceration and removal of the head, the figure agreeing reasonably well with Gregory King's 1696 estimate of 370 lbs.[26] By 1770, Arthur Young was reporting cows of 700 lbs and oxen of 1,120 to 1,400 lbs. Later he listed shorthorn and Devon cattle with weights ranging from 840 to 1,120 lbs and 1,400 lbs respectively.[27] George Fussell documented English cattle weights during the years 1786–96. Hereford, Devon, long- and shorthorns ranged

[24] Fussell, op. cit., note 22 above, pp. 160–1; G E Fussell and Constance Goodman, 'Eighteenth century estimates of British sheep and wool production', *Agric Hist*, 1930, **4**: 131–51, p. 134.

[25] Arthur Young, *The farmers' tour through the north of England or the northern tour*, vols 1–4, London, W Strachan, 1770, p. 151.

[26] James E Thorold Rogers, *Six centuries of work and wages: the history of English labour*, London, Swan Sonneschein, 1909, p. 77 fn; Gregory King, *Natural and political observations and conclusions upon the state and condition of England 1696*, ed. George E Barnett, Baltimore, Johns Hopkins Press, 1936, p. 38.

[27] Young, op. cit., note 25 above, vol. 4, p. 190.

widely, from 420 to 1,568 lbs. The range of weights varied with the breed, longhorns for example being lighter than the others. All, however, were substantially heavier than recorded at the start of the century.[28]

Limitations of eighteenth-century records of cattle weights apply equally to sheep, but, as was the case with cattle, the increases in weight of sheep sold at Smithfield appear indicative of a growth trend throughout the country. George Fussell and Constance Goodman quoted a 1710 report by Davenant of sheep of 28 lbs.[29] By 1774, John Campbell was reporting average weights of 40 to 50 and 64 to 88 lbs for small and large ewes respectively, but 144 to 160 lbs for the largest wethers.[30] Fussell and Goodman documented weights of sheep that varied from 40 lbs to as much as 190 lbs during the years between 1790 and 1800. There were variations from breed to breed, with ewes a little lighter than wethers. All were heavier than indicated in records from the beginning of the century.[31]

With all their limitations, the records appear to indicate a very substantial increase in the weight of cattle and sheep during this period. As drawings show (Illustrations 3–4), some of the increase in weight of cattle and sheep could be not only obvious, but even result in appearances that were grotesque. Even allowing for the possibility that exceptionally heavy animals were selected for their portraits, the result on paper reflects a degree of obesity previously unknown. On occasion the animals had difficulty walking because they were so heavy.

Some increase in bone and muscle mass does accompany greater obesity but a rise in the weight of cattle and sheep over only one or two generations meant relatively little increase in lean body mass. Anything more would have been dependent in large measure on genetic factors and would only have become manifest over a longer period of selective breeding. The increase that resulted from feeding in excess of energy requirements would have been predominantly fat, whether interspersed between muscle fibres or stored in depots. These effects of the changes in animal husbandry were demonstrated a century and a half ago in a remarkable investigation conducted by J B Lawes and J H Gilbert, with the help of some highly co-operative farmers. Numbers of mature heifers, bullocks, oxen, sheep, and pigs were separated into two groups. One of each group was slaughtered immediately; the other was fattened by then conventional practices and slaughtered at a later date when the weight eventually stabilized. Carcass weight, and as far as possible the dry weight of the members of each pair were obtained and the fat content estimated after a combination of mechanical expression, melting and extraction with ether. Among the animals kept for later slaughter, there was an average weight gain of between one-quarter and one-half of the weight at pairing (Table IV.2). Fat accounted for about two-thirds of the weight increase. The control animals had been fed in accordance with changes already introduced during the Agricultural Revolution and they were therefore likely to have been heavier than their early eighteenth-century

---

[28] Fussell, op. cit., note 22 above, pp. 170–4.
[29] Fussell and Goodman, op. cit., note 24 above, p. 138.
[30] John Campbell, *Political survey of Britain*, London, printed by the author, 1774, vol. 2, p. 157.
[31] Fussell and Goodman, op. cit, note 24 above, p. 138.

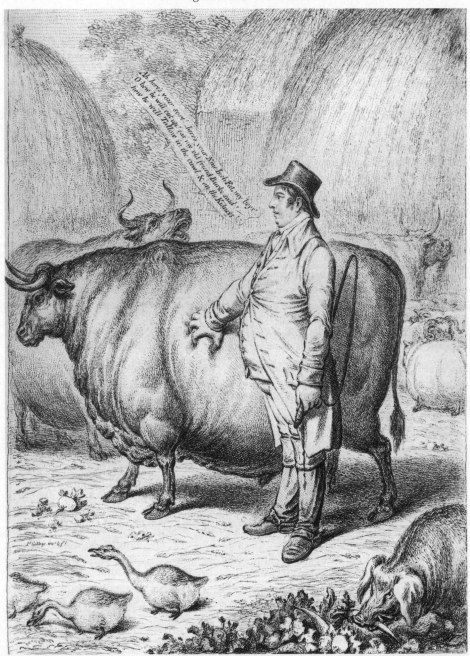

*Illustration 3:* A fat judge admiring a fat bullock. Etching by James Gillray, *c.* 1802. (Wellcome Library, London.)

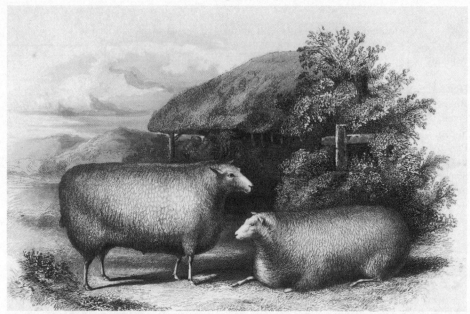

*Illustration 4:* Two prize winning Leicester rams. Etching by H Beckwith, *c.* 1849, after H Strafford. (Wellcome Library, London.)

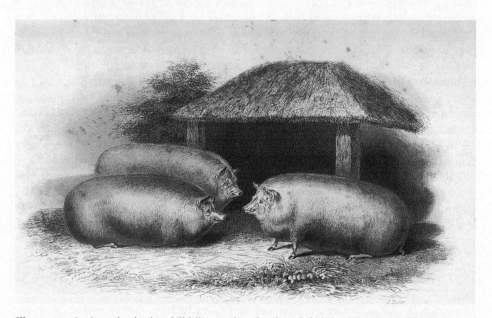

*Illustration 5:* Award winning Middlesex pigs, bred and fed by Mr Wm Mills Barber of Uxbridge. December 1848. Etching by E Hacker, *c.* 1848, after H Strafford. (Wellcome Library, London.)

*Table IV.2*
Comparison of controls with animals managed in special feed lots

| Animal | Number | % Fat Increase |
|---|---|---|
| Heifers | 12 | 72.5 |
| Bullocks | 86 | 65.4 |
| Oxen | 98 | 66.2 |
| Sheep | 348 | 70.4 |
| Pigs | 80 | 71.5 |

Source: J B Lawes and J H Gilbert, 'Experimental inquiry into the composition of some of the animals fed and slaughtered as human food', *Philos Trans Roy Soc*, London, 1859, **149**: 493–680, pp. 529, 537.

counterparts. Consequently, the differences between the weights of early eighteenth-century farm animals and the ones selected for special fattening in Lawes and Gilbert's trials probably reflect a much greater difference in fat content than was observed when the authors' control animals were compared with the ones selected for continued fattening.[32]

Although in general shortening the time taken to reach maturity, the effect of the new feeding techniques on the weight of pigs varied from breed to breed. While some strains remained fairly constant in weight, others tended to become heavier during the course of the eighteenth century. On the whole pigs respond to increased feeding with rapid weight gain.[33] The overall changes in the average weight of the swine population of England cannot be ascertained readily because to a large extent the animals were raised by individual home owners who kept one or two animals for family consumption. Fat pigs were certainly esteemed at agricultural shows and weights of several hundredweight were recorded not infrequently during the late eighteenth century.[34] Mark Overton devised a ratio between the sale prices of pigs and the cost per pound of their meat in order to obtain an indication of the average weight at slaughter of animals raised on a commercial scale. On this basis he calculated an approximately 50 per cent average increase in weight between the 1670s and the 1740s.[35] This is much less than the change based on comparison of King's estimate of 46 lbs in 1696[36] with Young's records of ranges from 140 to 350 lbs by the 1770s.[37] Notwithstanding the wide range of weights, they do suggest a considerable gain in pig weight during the intervening years. Eighteenth-century paintings depicted pigs that were grossly overweight and grotesque in appearance and even if the nineteenth-century examples shown in illustration 5 are exceptional, they certainly reflect a trend.

[32] J B Lawes and J H Gilbert, 'Experimental inquiry into the composition of some of the animals fed and slaughtered as human food', *Philos Trans Roy Soc*, London, 1859, **149**: 493–680, pp. 529, 537.
[33] Julian Wiseman, *A history of the British pig*, London, Duckworth, 1986, pp. 39–40.
[34] Young, op. cit., note 25 above, pp. 178, 189.
[35] M Overton, *Agricultural revolution in England: the transformation of the agrarian economy 1500–1850*, Cambridge University Press, 1996, pp. 115–16.
[36] King, op. cit., note 26 above, p. 38.
[37] Young, op. cit., note 25 above, vol. 2, p. 223.

*Chapter IV*

*Table IV.3*

Five-year average cattle and sheep sales at Smithfield (thousands)

| Period | Cattle | Sheep |
|--------|--------|-------|
| 1732–36 | 81.4 | 536.0 |
| 1737–41 | 85.4 | 560.4 |
| 1742–46 | 75.8 | 529.4 |
| 1747–51 | 70.6 | 628.8 |
| 1752–56 | 74.0 | 638.6 |
| 1757–61 | 85.0 | 599.2 |
| 1762–66 | 83.4 | 596.6 |
| 1767–71 | 84.0 | 624.8 |
| 1772–76 | 92.4 | 620.2 |
| 1777–81 | 98.6 | 700.2 |
| 1782–86 | 98.4 | 670.8 |
| 1787–91 | 99.2 | 706.4 |
| 1792–96 | 116.2 | 742.6 |

Abstracted from B R Mitchell, *British historical statistics*, Cambridge University Press, 1988, p. 708.

In 1696 Gregory King reckoned that the cattle population of England was 4,500,000.[38] There was a decline during the next eighty years to an estimated 3,500,000 in 1779, the reduction being largely a consequence of outbreaks of cattle plague during the second and fourth decades of the eighteenth century.[39] Although the absolute number of cattle was less in 1779 than in 1696, the individual animals were much heavier and the proportion of the total that became available for human consumption in any one year became higher as they reached mature weight more quickly and horses were replacing oxen at the plough. As a result, the availability of meat was greater in the late eighteenth century than at the end of the seventeenth. In any case, the fall in numbers was only temporary. Towards the end of the eighteenth century the cattle population increased, the trend being reflected in consistently rising cattle sales at Smithfield after 1766 (Table IV.3).[40] Needless to say, the moneyed classes would not have been unduly affected by any passing shortfall in numbers even if this was reflected in higher prices of meat. The number of sheep in England rose fairly consistently during the eighteenth century. Gregory King reckoned their number to be 11 million in 1696.[41] By 1770, Arthur Young's estimate was almost 29 million.[42]

Gauging changes in the pig population has been difficult as production was highly localized, but their commercial importance grew with the price of pigs relative to cattle increasing considerably between the sixteenth and mid-eighteenth centuries.

[38] King, op. cit., note 26 above, p. 37.
[39] Fussell, op. cit., note 22 above, p. 178.
[40] B R Mitchell, *British historical statistics*, Cambridge University Press, 1988, p. 708.
[41] King, op. cit., note 26 above, p. 37.
[42] Fussell and Goodman, op. cit., note 24 above, p. 132.

Poultry production rose by about 25 per cent in the first half of the eighteenth century.[43] Egg production per bird became greater with better feeding and management. When compared to the present day, the overall increase in the amount of fat in poultry at the time of slaughter was all the greater because ducks and geese then formed a higher proportion of the poultry consumed than is now the case. Ducks tend to become fatter than chickens, as do geese as they instinctively eat to an unlimited extent whenever the opportunity arises, because of their need to build up reserves of energy for migration.

With controlled serving of cows, which come on heat about once a month, calving could be spread over the entire year and with assured and improved cattle nutrition milk yields increased and lactation after each calving could be prolonged by twenty to thirty days. As a result, milk became more plentiful and available throughout the year. In the late eighteenth century it was not uncommon for the middle and upper classes to keep a cow or two in a stall or field adjacent to their homes in order to ensure a continuous and abundant fresh milk supply for their households. Breeding of dairy cattle had as its main objective increase in the richness as well as the quantities of the milk produced. Specifically, Jersey and Guernsey cows were imported from the Channel Islands and bred in the south of England on an increasing scale. Guernsey cows were often crossed with Devon bulls, the offspring being particularly good milkers. Animals with poor milk yields were culled unhesitatingly. As a result of these changes early eighteenth-century annual milk yields of about 150 to 300 gallons per cow rose by the end of the century to 350 to 500, and even on occasion 600 gallons a year.[44] Milk was used increasingly for large-scale commercial production of cheese, butter and cream, as these were easier to transport than liquid milk.

Variations of up to 3 per cent in the fat concentration of milk can be produced by diet modification,[45] and analyses conducted in the twentieth century showed that by selective breeding and appropriate feeding the fat content can be raised in some instances to over 5.1 per cent, Jerseys and Guernseys in particular being noted for high fat content.[46] It is therefore probable that the eighteenth-century developments that have been described resulted in milk becoming creamier as well as more plentiful.

All the changes that have been described were driven in large measure by consumer demand for fatty foods. Notwithstanding current warnings about associated cardio-vascular health risks, even contemporary consumers have been found to show a liking for fatty foods and to choose them preferentially. Lean meat tends to be dry and somewhat tough, whilst marbled meat is more tender. Fatty meat has a pleasant moist taste and a smooth feel to the tongue. The texture of meat as sensed in the mouth is enhanced by frying and the aroma makes it all the more appetizing.[47] It is

[43] J A Chartres, 'The marketing of agricultural produce', in Joan Thirsk (ed.), *The agrarian history of England and Wales, Volume V: 1640–1750. II. Agrarian change*, Cambridge University Press, 1985, p. 446.

[44] C H Eckles, *Dairy cattle and milk production*, 5th ed., revised by E L Anthony, New York, Macmillan, 1956, p. 206.

[45] J D Sutton, 'Altering milk composition by feeding', *J Dairy Sci*, 1989, **72**: 2801–14, p. 2802.

[46] J P Gibson, 'Altering milk composition through genetic selection', *J Dairy Sci*, 1989, **72**: 2815–25, p. 2816.

[47] Adam Drewnowski, 'Sensory properties of fats and fat replacements', *Nutr Rev*, 1992, **50** (4, Part 2), pp. 17–20.

unlikely that these preferences were any different 250 years ago. In the late eighteenth century, butchered carcasses were sold by weight with relatively little influence of other meat qualities on price. Dairy products and baked foods with a high animal fat content were similarly appreciated and in demand. Valuing foods for freedom from fat is a modern trend driven mainly by concern for health.

The production of ever greater amounts of animal produce was accompanied by an increasingly efficient distribution system. Coastal traffic, an ever more extensive canal network and better roads made transport of all commodities easier.[48] Growth in importance of market towns further facilitated movement of produce from farmer to consumer. The financial instruments needed to back these movements were being developed at the same time. They included growing use of paper transactions and increasing availability of credit with the beginnings of a banking system.[49] With all of these changes periods of food shortage became less frequent, less severe and more localized in their effects when they did occur.

It can be concluded that the eighteenth-century Agricultural Revolution in England resulted in better care and nutrition and an increase in the numbers and weights of farm animals, with a resulting greater and year-round availability of fatty meat, pure animal fat, eggs and increasingly creamy dairy products. The quantitative increase in production exceeded the rate of human population growth. As a consequence, the amount of meat and fat of animal origin available per person became very much greater and for both the upper and the growing middle classes they were usually readily affordable. The impact of these changes upon English everyday eighteenth-century eating habits and their potential cardiac consequences are discussed in the next chapter.

It has been noted earlier that angina pectoris appeared to have been uniquely a "British disease" for about half a century following its first recognition.[50] As pointed out in the previous chapter, country to country demographic differences are insufficient to account alone for this singularity. Parenthetically, a genetic basis is also unlikely. The peoples of eighteenth-century England were akin to those of northern and western Europe, whence they had migrated in waves from prehistoric times onwards and the European population of the eastern American seaboard consisted very largely of migrants from Britain. The cases reported in the UK in the late eighteenth century were dispersed as far apart as London, Bath, the west country and Ulster.[51] Any predisposing mutational changes are therefore highly improbable. In the next chapter reasons are given for concluding that of all the changes in Georgian England that contributed to the early emergence there of angina pectoris, the impact of the Agricultural Revolution on diet played the leading role. However,

[48] J A Sharpe, *Early modern England: a social history 1550–1760*, London, Edward Arnold, 1988, p. 141.

[49] Christopher Clay, 'Landlords and estate management in England', in Joan Thirsk (ed.), *The agrarian history of England and Wales, Volume V: 1640–1750. II. Agrarian change*, Cambridge University Press, 1985, p. 178.

[50] William L Proudfit, 'Origin of concept of ischaemic heart disease', *Br Heart J*, 1983, **50**: 209–12, p. 209.

[51] J O Leibowitz, *The history of coronary heart disease*, London, Wellcome Institute of the History of Medicine, 1970, pp. 83, 94, 96, 97.

Table IV.4
Absolute and relative risk of death according to use of wine, beer or liquor (abstainers 1.0;
confidence limits bracketed)

| Number | Deaths | Cause | Wine | Beer | Liquor |
|--------|--------|-------|------|------|--------|
| 28,488 | 426 | All | 0.8 (0.7–0.9) | 0.9 (0.8–1.1) | 1.0 (0.8–1.1) |
| 21,152 | 318 | CHD | 0.5 (0.4–0.7) | 0.7 (0.5–0.9) | 0.6 (0.5–0.8) |
| 20,492 | 597 | Liver Disease | 5.6 (1.1–27.7) | 5.1 (0.9–28.5) | 4.8 (0.9–24.6) |

Reprinted from A L Klatsky, M A Armstrong and G D Friedman, 'Risk of cardiovascular mortality in alcohol drinkers, ex-drinkers and non-drinkers', *Am J Cardiol*, 1990, **66**: 1237–42, p. 1240, with permission from Excerpta Medica Inc.

before examining in detail the differences between England and other countries with respect to agricultural practice at that time, it is necessary to review briefly one other reason that has been proposed. It was advanced by Samuel Black as early as 1819. Having observed that angina pectoris was a complaint that had not been observed in France, he suggested that this was attributable to a protective effect of the red wine of which its inhabitants partook liberally.[52] This belief has survived to the present day, but closer examination suggests that it is a very unlikely explanation. Firstly, the privileged English classes themselves drank large quantities of French wines during the late eighteenth century whilst claret, sherry and port, which are all basically variations of red wine, also enjoyed very great popularity among them. Secondly, there is recent evidence to suggest that any protective effect of alcohol is attributable to the alcohol itself irrespective of the type of drink and then only when consumed in moderation, hardly a characteristic of the eighteenth-century drinker (Table IV.4).[53] Finally, it would not explain the then virtual absence of angina pectoris as a complaint in other countries where red wine was not the usual alcoholic drink.

With rare exceptions, the changes accompanying the Agricultural Revolution in England and their consequences were delayed elsewhere for at least half a century. The social and political climate in the British North American colonies and in the subsequent United States were conducive to the development of farming societies that resembled English rather than Continental European patterns. However, agricultural commerce was hampered by trade barriers between the colonies of British North America and between the thirteen states during the years between the securing of independence and establishment of federal government in 1789. Inevitably too, disruptions to farming accompanied Indian raids, French incursions and the War of American Independence. Eighteenth-century settlement was confined to areas east of the Appalachians. The prairies, with their wide expanses suitable for raising cattle, were as yet unexplored. Machinery was not then available and land for agriculture had to be carved out of the forests by hand labour. Much of the farmland that

[52] Samuel Black, *Clinical and pathological reports*, Newry, Alexander Wilkinson, 1819, p. 8.
[53] A L Klatsky, M A Armstrong and G D Friedman, 'Risk of cardiovascular mortality in alcohol drinkers, ex-drinkers and non-drinkers', *Am J Cardiol*, 1990, **66**: 1237–42, p. 1240.

became available was set aside for cash crops such as cotton and tobacco.[54] Time was necessary for improvement of pastures by measures that included the planting of appropriate grasses and liberal manuring. Optimal feeding of large numbers of farm animals with a resulting increase in weight and fat content had to await the future opening up of the West.

In most of western and central Europe feudal patterns of land tenure survived until the early nineteenth century. Landowners rarely took any personal interest in either their properties or in the welfare of their tenants, both being viewed exclusively as sources of income. Concerns with day-to-day farming problems were considered beneath the dignity of the absentee seigneur. In pre-revolutionary France, in particular, the nobles "had little desire to manage their farms themselves as was done in England" and "considered seigneurial rights a more attractive source of income than agricultural improvement".[55] In most of mainland Europe the peasants who cultivated the land had the status of serfs in practice, if not formally and legally. Their obligations to the seigneur were onerous and numerous, their security of tenure minimal.[56] Feudal bonds usually ended with the death of the peasant when the seigneur had the right to repossess the land and to choose a successor, who would in turn be bound to assume all the obligations and restrictions of serfdom.[57] The inherent inefficiencies of strip farming were frequently compounded by the requirement that the individual peasant conform to communal farming patterns. As a consequence of all these factors, there was little incentive or possibility for any one peasant to improve either his land or his farming practices. An authoritarian system of government and a rigidly stratified and legally enforced structure of society contributed further to the stifling of any initiative that might have remained. Strip farming was the rule on the Continent until the end of the eighteenth century and even beyond.[58] Rulers occasionally attempted to end serfdom, either under the influence of the Enlightenment or, less altruistically, in order to weaken the power of overmighty nobles. These endeavours were usually brought to naught by resistance on the part of the nobility, even when the French Revolution was followed by abolition of serfdom in France and in its European conquests. The lands formerly owned by the nobility were then confiscated but frequently bought back by "men of straw" who were acting as intermediaries for the former owners; there was little change in farming methods. In any case, the liberalizing tendencies were reversed to a large extent after Napoleon's final defeat at Waterloo and the restoration of the ancien régime.[59]

In comparison to England, the various support systems needed to facilitate changes in agricultural practice were much less developed on the Continent. During the period from 1754 to 1784, 81 per cent of yeoman farmers and 54 per cent of

[54] Samuel Eliot Morison, *The Oxford history of the American people*, New York, Oxford University Press, 1965, p. 304.
[55] B H Slicher van Bath, *The agrarian history of western Europe* A.D. 500–1800, transl. Olive Ordish, London, Edward Arnold, 1965, p. 322.
[56] Ibid., p. 189.
[57] Ibid., p. 52.
[58] Ibid., pp. 55ff.
[59] Ibid., p. 322.

husbandmen were literate in England. The literacy rate of rural Europe was much lower. In 1800 the percentage of husbandmen who could sign their names was 62 in England, 47 in France and 40 in East Prussia.[60] In the eighteenth century reading was frequently taught well before writing, and the latter often confined to a signature. Ability to sign one's name was consequently a frequent marker of ability to read adequately.[61] It was only those who could read who could benefit from the books and pamphlets describing the new agricultural practices. The banking system and other means of obtaining credit were relatively advanced in England, but on the Continent borrowing at other than usurious rates of interest was much more difficult. The backward state of Continental industrialization meant that many of the new agricultural implements which became available in England were simply not obtainable elsewhere, even in the unlikely event that knowledge of their existence and means for their purchase were available. Movement of farm produce was impeded by the condition of the roads, which were in much poorer state than in England. In contrast to England where there were no internal restrictions upon the freedom of movement of commerce, there were in France a variety of internal tariffs and protectionist barriers to trade that hampered movement of farm produce for sale in any but local markets. A similar situation existed in eighteenth-century Germany and Italy, but in aggravated form as both countries were fragmented into many small states.[62] Lastly, the very frequent wars of the period were accompanied by considerable setbacks to farming as a result of both physical destruction and the depredations of armies. Seed grain was frequently seized, breed stock slaughtered and horses commandeered. There were a few exceptions to the prevailing backward patterns, notably in the Netherlands where agriculture was relatively more advanced. However, that country was fought over repeatedly and its small size and high population density dictated an emphasis on growing cereals and vegetables for human consumption. Animal husbandry requires large areas of land for pasturing and these were simply not available.

In southern Europe, the Mediterranean climate had long determined the pattern of farming. In particular, the long dry summers and frequent droughts often affected crop yields adversely, hampered production of fodder and impoverished pasture lands, limiting the number of farm animals that could be grazed and the extent to which they could be fattened. As early as the Renaissance, travellers from northern Europe who visited Mediterranean countries commented on how lean the cattle and sheep were. Cattle at slaughter yielded a mere average of 148 kilograms of meat and sheep as little as 12 kilograms.[63] Agricultural practices in Mediterranean lands consequently placed relatively little emphasis on raising farm animals. Most of the available acreage was devoted to cereal production, orchards, olive groves and vineyards.

[60] D Grigg, *The transformation of agriculture in the west*, Oxford, Blackwell, 1992, p. 118–19.

[61] R S Schofield, 'Dimensions of illiteracy 1750–1850', *Explorations in Economic History*, 1972–3, **10**: 437–54, pp. 440–1.

[62] Carlton J Hayes, Marshall W Baldwin and Charles W Cole, *History of Europe*, 2 vols, New York, Macmillan, 1956, vol. 2, p. 98.

[63] Fernand Braudel, *The Mediterranean and the Mediterranean world in the age of Philip II*, transl. S Reynold, 2 vols, Berkeley, University of California Press, 1995, vol. 1, pp. 238–44.

## Chapter IV

As the historian H A L Fisher has written, "Earlier by more than half a century than any other country in Europe, England assumed the character of a modern high-farming industrial state".[64] Half a century is roughly the interval that separates the emergence of angina pectoris in England from its first manifestation in any other country on the European mainland. A connection between these two is postulated in this and succeeding chapters.

[64] H A L Fisher, *A history of Europe*, London, Edward Arnold, 1946, p. 777.

# V

# The Impact of the Agricultural Revolution on Food: The Cardiac Consequences

Felix qui potuit rerum cognoscere causas.[1]

## Fats: Saturated and Unsaturated

It is obviously impossible to measure directly the impact of the eighteenth-century changes in English farming practices on the fat content and fatty acid characteristics of the animals that were then raised for human consumption. The necessary analytic techniques had yet to be developed. However, some cautious deductions can be made from studies during the last century. As detailed in Chapter IV, the food available to animals and birds farmed in England before the Agricultural Revolution, or more currently in developing societies, was not very different from that of free living herbivorous birds and animals. It is probable therefore that some 300 and more years ago the fat composition of English domestic animals and birds corresponded roughly to that of their twentieth-century descendants, either foraging in the wild or herded in developing societies where animal husbandry has been unaffected by the Agricultural Revolution. The fat characteristics of these last two categories have been studied,[2] as have the lipid profiles of domestic animals and birds farmed in developed societies in the mid-twentieth century.[3] This was before consumption of animal fat was considered to be a potential health hazard and western world farming practices began to be modified in order deliberately to produce leaner cattle, sheep, pigs and poultry. It follows that comparisons drawn from all of these sources should give some measure of the differences between the pre- and post-Agricultural Revolution on the status of English farm animals with respect to total carcass fat as a percentage of total weight, the amount of fat in muscle and its fatty acid composition.

In general, it can be said that until the middle of the last century domesticated

---

[1] Virgil, *Georgics*, 2.490.

[2] M A Crawford, 'Fatty-acid ratios in free-living and domestic animals. Possible implications for atheroma', *Lancet*, 1968, i: 1329–33, pp. 1331–2; H P Ledger, 'Body composition as a basis for comparative study of some East African mammals', in M A Crawford (ed.), *Comparative nutrition of wild animals: the proceedings of a symposium held at the Zoological Society of London held on 10 and 11 November 1966*, London, published for the Zoological Society of London by Academic Press, 1968, pp. 289–310, pp. 306–7.

[3] Andrew J Sinclair, W J Slattery and K J O'Dea, 'The analysis of polyunsaturated fatty acids in meat by capillary gas-liquid chromatography', *J Sci Food Agric*, 1982, **33**: 771–6, p. 772.

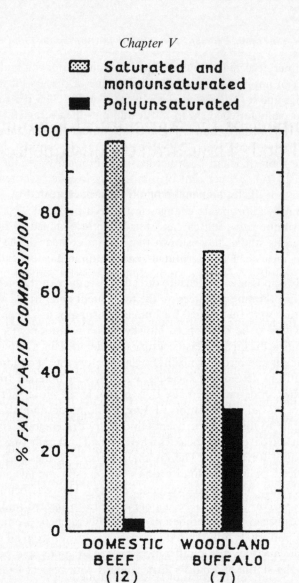

*Figure V.1:* Fatty acid composition of free living woodland buffalo and domestic beef compared. Number of animals in brackets. Reproduced from M A Crawford, 'Fatty-acid ratios in free living and domestic animals. Possible implications for atheroma', *Lancet*, 1968, **i**: 1329–33, p. 1331. (Permission granted by The *Lancet* Ltd.)

animals and birds in the developed world were far more adipose than their twentieth-century counterparts that either grazed in the wild (Figure V.1) or were reared in developing countries. Evidence cited earlier (pages 50, 53) indicated that the increase in weight of domestic animals subsequent to the introduction of late-eighteenth-century feeding techniques consisted largely of fat. In the mid-nineteenth century Lawes and Gilbert estimated the percentage of fat in the carcasses of a number of animals that either received the usual feed for that period or had been specially fattened as part of an investigation. The percentage of carcass fat in a "store", i.e. standard fed pig, and a "store" fed sheep were 28.1 and 23.8 per cent respectively. Among eight specially fattened sheep, cattle and pigs the average fat percentage was 36.5 per cent.[4] H P Ledger found that the fat content of four ranch-fed zebu, an East African variety of cow, was 32.9 ± 3.3 per cent. In contrast, he found that in a group of nine zebu that had been herded in traditional ways, the fat constituted a mean of only 13.4 ± 5.9 per cent of total carcass weight.[5] Contemporary studies have shown too that the fat content of poultry can be increased by over 50 per cent in any one strain by appropriate changes in the feed provided.[6]

The fat contribution to total carcass weight is not confined to obviously visible deposits. Numerous studies have shown that the fat content of the muscle, i.e. the apparently lean meat, can contain fat in varying quantities depending on feeding practices. As examples, Australian studies showed the fat content of pork leg to be almost 50 per cent greater than in corresponding tissues obtained from wild pigs. The muscle content of pastured beef was four times that of buffalo and that of lamb over five times the fat content of free ranging deer.[7] M A Crawford found even more extreme differences; the fat content of wild bovid never exceeded 3 per cent; domestic meat fat ranged from 3 to 18 per cent.[8]

The fat of pastured animals and birds is not only greater in amount than that of their free ranging cousins. There are significant qualitative differences as well. The proportion of polyunsaturated fatty acids (PUFA) is higher and that of saturated and monounsaturated fatty acids (SFA and MUFA) lower in free living animals and birds when compared with those raised on farms. A study of wild buffalo and warthogs showed that the percentage of polyunsaturated fatty acids were 30 and 44 per cent respectively. In contrast, the PUFA percentages of fat-tailed sheep and samples of pork and beef obtained from slaughterhouses were very much lower, 4, 8 and 2 per cent respectively (Table V.1). These differences in fat composition have even been found when closely related species were compared.[9] The PUFA also form a significantly greater proportion of total fat among birds reared in the wild. Forty per cent of wild grouse fat was found to be polyunsaturated whilst among domestic chickens this percentage was 17. Similar chemical differences have been found in a comparison of the fat composition of wild and farmed pigs.

Although polyunsaturated fat as a proportion of the total lipid content was higher among wild animals, the absolute amounts were, weight for weight, less than in those that were pastured. The polyunsaturated fatty acids constituted a higher

[4] J B Lawes and J H Gilbert, 'Experimental inquiry into the composition of some of the animals fed and slaughtered as human food', *Philos Trans Roy Soc*, London, 1859, **149**: 493–680, p. 520.

[5] Ledger, op. cit., note 2 above, pp. 306–7.

[6] G Havenstein, personal communication, quoted by Peter Hunton, 'The broiler industry. Thirty-four years of progress', *Poultry International*, 1995, **34**: 28–30, p. 28.

[7] Sinclair, Slattery, O'Dea, op. cit., note 3 above, p. 772; A J Sinclair and K J O'Dea, 'The lipid levels and fatty composition of the lean portions of pork, chicken and rabbit meats', *Food Technol*, Australia, 1987, **39**: 232–3, 240.

[8] M A Crawford *et al.*, 'Comparative studies on fatty acid composition of wild and domesticated meats', *Int J Biochem*, 1970, **1**: 295–305, p. 302.

[9] Crawford, 'Fatty-acid ratios', op. cit., note 2 above, p. 1331.

## Chapter V

### Table V.1
Fatty acid composition of muscle as percentages: wild and farmed animals and birds

|  | SFA and MUFA combined | PUFA |
|---|---|---|
| Wild Buffalo | 71 | 30 |
| Pastured Beef | 99 | 2 |
| Wild Pig Leg | 71 | 28 |
| Pork (farmed pig) | 92 | 8 |
| Fat-tailed Sheep | 96 | 4 |
| Wild Giraffe | 61 | 39 |
| Captive Giraffe | 96 | 4 |
| Wild Grouse | 60 | 40 |
| Domestic Chickens | 83 | 17 |

Source: M A Crawford, 'Fatty-acid ratios in free living and domestic animals. Possible implications for atheroma', *Lancet*, 1968, i: 1329–33. (Permission granted by The *Lancet* Ltd.)

proportion of a much lower total carcass fat content. The differences in the chemical composition of fat that have been described appear to be general. They have even been found when wild and captive giraffes were compared, the former having a higher PUFA percentage than the latter. Of possible significance, the polyunsaturated fat of wild animals is predominantly phospholipid. In twentieth-century farm animals it is mainly triglyceride.[10]

Crawford and his colleagues found too that the fat of free living animals contained significant amounts of long chain (C20-5 N3 and C20-6 N3) polyunsaturated fatty acids. These were scarcely detectable in the fat of domesticated animals.[11] This is of possible significance in view of the mildly inhibitory action on human blood co-agulation and clotting detected in similar long chain fatty acids derived from fatty fish and marine mammal oils.[12]

The results obtained in the wild animals and the example cited from a developing society give an approximate indication of what would have been the fat content and characteristics of animals reared before the English eighteenth-century changes in animal husbandry, i.e. low in the amount of total fat and with the PUFA proportion high. In contrast, the lipid content of domesticated animals reared in mid-twentieth-century developed societies provides some indication of what would have been the fat content and characteristics of animals farmed in England after the eighteenth-century agricultural changes, high in total fat content and with the PUFA proportion low and probably different qualitatively.

As observed in the previous chapter, there is evidence to suggest that with the better feeding techniques some breeds of pig did increase in weight. Twentieth-century studies show that saturated fatty acids predominate over unsaturated in the

[10] Crawford *et al.*, op. cit., note 8 above, p. 299.
[11] Ibid., p. 300.
[12] Clemens von Schacky and Peter C Weber, 'Metabolism and effects on platelet function of the purified eicosapentaenoic and docosahexaenoic acids in humans', *J Clin Invest*, 1985, **76**: 2446–50, pp. 2447–8.

adipose tissue of pigs reared in the developed world. As they are not ruminants, their body lipid composition tends to reflect closely that of the fats in their diet. As dairy products (now known to be high in saturated fat content) were increasingly used for feed during the course of the eighteenth century, it is likely that porcine fats were consequently high in SFA at that time too.[13]

As noted earlier, poultry production rose during the early eighteenth century and the increase continued thereafter. Twentieth-century studies have shown that egg yolk characteristics are subject to variations in response to the type of feed provided. Thus a study of 18 differing genetic lines of experimental chickens showed that mean yolk weights in each line could vary from a low of 14.55 g to a high of 18.71 g and the cholesterol content, expressed as mg/g yolk, from a low of 13.30 to a high of 15.58.[14] Changes in feeding techniques, including addition of cholesterol to the feed, could increase yolk weight by up to 3.29 g in any one strain and yolk cholesterol content by up to 2.01 mg/g. Although there was a tendency for heavier yolks to be associated with somewhat lower cholesterol concentrations, the overall effect was for the larger yolks to contain greater absolute amounts of cholesterol. The latter also responds positively to cholesterol in the hens' diet and to their total energy intake.[15] The changes that can result from improved feeding methods can be gauged by comparing the yolk cholesterol content of currently domesticated birds with that of their cousins in the wild. In one typical study, the egg yolks of domestically raised turkeys and ducks were found to have a mean cholesterol content almost 2 mg greater than that of free ranging birds.[16] These twentieth-century differences give some indication of the possible impact of eighteenth-century changes in poultry management on the cholesterol content of eggs. Probably much more important than the chemical characteristics of individual yolks was the impact of eighteenth-century farming improvements on the number and continuous availability of eggs. The rate of increase in the number of laying fowl during the early eighteenth century probably exceeded the rate of human population increase in England and Wales at that time.[17] Productivity of the individual birds became greater, notwithstanding an unavoidable fall in the number of eggs laid during winter with its reduced hours of sunlight and the absence then of effective forms of artificial lighting. In so far as conclusions can be drawn from twentieth-century studies, the data reported raise the possibility that eighteenth-century changes in poultry management resulted in greater availability of eggs with higher average SFA and cholesterol contents and a consequent increase in atherogenic potential.

In conclusion, the data presented suggest that English farmed animals were a

[13] Peter W Bowden, 'Agricultural prices, wages, farm profits, and rents', in Joan Thirsk (ed.), *The agrarian history of England and Wales, Volume V: 1640–1750. II. Agrarian change*, Cambridge University Press, 1985, p. 32.

[14] Craig W Bair and William M Marion, 'Yolk cholesterol in eggs from various species', *Poult Sci*, 1978, **57**: 1260–5, p. 1264.

[15] P Stewart Hargis, 'Modifying egg yolk cholesterol in the domestic fowl', *World Poult Sci J*, 1988, **44**: 17–29, p. 19.

[16] Bair and Marion, op. cit., note 14 above, p. 1261.

[17] E Anthony Wrigley *et al.*, *English population history from family reconstitution 1580–1837*, Cambridge University Press, 1997, p. 614.

## Table V.2

Effect of varying PUFA as percentage of constant total fat intake. Lipid profile at beginning and end of trial

| PUFA % | LDL Cholesterol (mmol/L) | | VLDL Cholesterol (mmol/L) | | Apo B (mg/L) | | HDL/Total | |
|---|---|---|---|---|---|---|---|---|
| | Initial | Final | Initial | Final | Initial | Final | Initial | Final |
| 3 | 2.07±0.08 | 2.33±0.59* | 0.22±0.05 | 0.27±0.12 | 664±202 | 718±175 | 0.36±0.06 | 0.35±0.05 |
| 19 | 1.91±0.40 | 1.98±0.60 | 0.27±0.13 | 0.23±0.12 | 580±103 | 574±120* | 0.35±0.06 | 0.38±0.06 |

* P<0.05: change from initial values.

Source: Jantine A Brussaard *et al.*, 'Effects of amount and type of dietary fat on serum lipids, lipoproteins and apolipoproteins in man. A controlled 8-week trial', *Atherosclerosis*, 1980, **36**: 515–27, 515. (With permission from Elsevier Science.)

scant source of fats prior to the Agricultural Revolution, but the changes that it brought about resulted in a very great increase in the availability of the animal fats associated with meat, poultry, eggs and dairy produce. There is indirect evidence to suggest that there was an accompanying increase in predominance of saturated as opposed to unsaturated fatty acids. It remains to consider the consequences.

### Dietary Fats and Coronary Heart Disease

In the present study it is thought adequate for the most part to provide evidence for a considerable eighteenth-century increase in the availability of animal fats in general and saturated fats in particular. It is not considered necessary to marshall in any more than summary form the now well-established reasons for associating high animal fat intake with a lipid profile conducive to development of coronary heart disease. Reference to a limited number of late-twentieth-century landmark studies should suffice.

A direct relationship between high saturated animal fat consumption and raised serum cholesterol levels has long been established, dietary changes altering the lipid profile significantly in little over a month. For example, as part of a wider study, Jantine H Brussaard and his colleagues studied forty healthy young subjects of both sexes. Following a run-in period on identical diets, two groups took 40 per cent of their energy requirements as fat. For one-half of the subjects, 3 per cent of the fats were polyunsaturated. Saturated and monounsaturated animal fats constituted the remainder. For the second group, the polyunsaturated fats, mainly of vegetable origin, were raised to 19 per cent and the saturated animal fats correspondingly reduced. Initially the lipid profiles of the two groups were almost identical. After five weeks the mean serum total cholesterol, triglycerides, apolipoprotein-B and low density lipoprotein (LDL) cholesterol levels were all significantly higher in the group with the higher saturated fat intake. The HDL/cholesterol ratios were minimally lower (Table V.2).[18] *Mann ist was mann isst.* The Seven Countries Investigation

[18] Jantine H Brussaard *et al.*, 'Effects of amount and type of dietary fat on serum lipids, lipoproteins and apolipoproteins in man. A controlled 8-week trial', *Atherosclerosis*, 1980, **36**: 515–27, pp. 520–3.

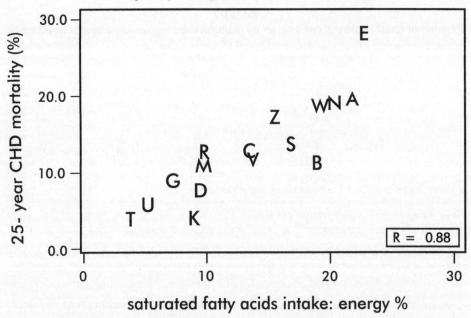

*Figure V.2:* Correlation between average intake of saturated fats and 25-year mortality from coronary heart disease (%) in the Seven Countries study. The letters relate to location (not listed). Source: Daan Kromhout *et al.*, 'Dietary saturated and trans-fatty acids and cholesterol and 25-year mortality from coronary heart disease. The Seven Countries Study', *Prev Med*, 1995, **24**, 308–15, p. 311. (With permission by Academic Press.)

involved 12,763 middle-aged men living in Greece, the Netherlands, Yugoslavia, Italy, Japan, USA and Finland. The follow-up, which lasted some twenty-five years, showed that the higher the animal fat consumption was in any one location, the higher were the overall serum cholesterol levels and the incidence of coronary heart disease (CHD) (Figure V.2).[19] In the multiple risk factor intervention trial (MRFIT) study over one-third of a million men aged from thirty-five to thirty-seven years at entry were followed for twelve years. At entry, risk factors were present in some instances, but none had a history of heart disease. During the follow-up there was an aged-adjusted CHD mortality that was positively and continuously related to the total serum cholesterol concentrations.[20]

In contrast, there is evidence to indicate that reductions in total fat intake in general, and saturated fats in particular, are followed by lessening risk of myocardial infarction, both fatal and non-fatal. As an example, Thomas Lyon and his colleagues compared survivors of a myocardial infarction whose fat intake was restricted to 50 g daily with a control group of survivors among whom no such limits were

[19] Daan Kromhout *et al.*, 'Dietary saturated and trans-fatty acids and cholesterol and 25-year mortality from coronary heart disease. The Seven Countries Study', *Prev Med*, 1995, **24**: 308–15, pp. 310ff.

[20] J M Martin *et al.*, 'Serum cholesterol, blood pressure, and mortality: implications from a cohort of 361,662 men', *Lancet*, 1986, **ii**: 933–6, p. 934.

*Table V.3*
Relation of CHD deaths to diet and serum cholesterol levels (mg/dl), Helsinki heart study

| Hospital Designation | | 1st Period | Number of deaths | 2nd Period | Number of deaths |
|---|---|---|---|---|---|
| N | Males | L 217 | 20 | H 266 | 52 |
| K | | H 268 | 24 | L 234 | 14 |
| N | Females | L 245 | 52 | H 278 | 107 |
| K | | H 270 | 22 | L 236 | 21 |

L: Low Cholesterol Diet H: High Cholesterol Diet.

Source: Matti Miettinen *et al.*, 'Effect of cholesterol-lowering diet on mortality from coronary heart-disease and other causes', *Lancet*, 1972, **ii**: 835–8, p. 836. (Permission granted by The *Lancet* Ltd.)

imposed. During a 3.8 year follow-up of the 155 subjects on the low fat diet, there were a total of 15 recurrent myocardial infarctions, of which 4 were fatal. In contrast, the 125 unrestricted subjects, albeit during a slightly longer 4.2 year follow-up, suffered 51 recurrences, of which 13 were fatal.[21] In the Helsinki heart study polyunsaturated fats were substituted for saturated in the diet of the participants in a cross-over study involving two institutionalized populations, some of whom had already had CHD. In both diets the percentage of energy requirements supplied by one or the other form of fat was higher than is currently considered optimal. Despite this, the polyunsaturated fat regime was associated with a reduction in male and female coronary heart disease mortality of about one-half among the men and one-third in the women (Table V.3).[22] In a prevention study of a free living population without any evidence of CHD at entry, J N Morris, Jean W Marr and D G Clayton examined the relationship of diet to the incidence of coronary heart disease among 337 middle-aged men who lived in either London or other parts of south-east England and who participated in a dietary survey. The subjects were stratified into lowest, middle and highest ranges of polyunsaturated/saturated fat (P/S) ratios. The differences in the ratios were not great and even among the highest third the proportion of polyunsaturated fat was suboptimal by standards generally adopted later. The study began in 1956 and by 1976 forty-five men had developed clinical coronary heart disease. Although the dietary differences between the groups was modest, the incidence of coronary heart disease during the first five years was significantly lower among the men with the highest P/S ratios. Although no longer

[21] Thomas P Lyon *et al.*, 'Lipoproteins and diet in coronary heart disease: a five-year study', *Calif Med*, 1956, **84**: 325–8, p. 328.
[22] Matti Miettinen *et al.*, 'Effect of cholesterol-lowering diet on mortality from coronary heart-disease and other causes', *Lancet*, 1972, **ii**: 835–8, p. 836.

statistically significant, benefits were still present at ten and twenty years. By the end of the twenty-year follow-up, deaths from coronary heart disease totalled 11, 10 and 5 in the lowest, middle and highest tertiles of P/S ratio respectively, i.e. an inverse relationship between polyunsaturated fatty acid intake and coronary heart disease incidence was demonstrated.[23] Whether these benefits were due to the increase in polyunsaturated or the decrease in saturated fat intake is not readily determinable, but the benefits of substituting the former for the latter are evident. Conversely these studies demonstrate that diets low in polyunsaturates but unrestricted in saturated fatty acids are associated with an *increased* incidence of coronary heart disease.

Thus far, emphasis has been placed on the relationship between diets high in animal fats and the incidence of major coronary events, notably myocardial infarction and cardiac deaths. Stress has been placed on the connection between liberal consumption of saturated fats and the adverse cardiac consequences of *structural* coronary arterial disease, notably plaque formation and coronary arterial narrowing and blockage. However, of late a clear-cut and significant relationship has been established between elevation of serum cholesterol levels and deleterious changes, notably loss of coronary arterial and arteriolar capacity to dilate (see Table V.4). The endothelial lining of the coronary arteries has active metabolic properties and *inter alia* produces an endothelial derived relaxing factor that makes possible a response to the increased demands of exercise by blood flow increases of up to four times the basal requirements of the heart. Demonstration of the ability of normal arterial walls to produce nitric oxide and its role as a simple inorganic vasodilator earned Robert Furchgott, Louis Ignarro and Ferid Murad the 1998 Nobel Prize in physiology or medicine.

In the presence of a raised serum total cholesterol, the coronary arterial capacity for vasodilatation is impaired and the possibility of increasing coronary blood flow in response to demand is impeded. This functional impairment has been demonstrated even in coronary arteries with no macroscopic abnormalities or nothing other than fatty streaks in the vessel wall. The consequences of failure of normal parts of the arterial wall to relax are necessarily more profound if structural narrowing is present as well.[24] Andreas M Zeiher and his colleagues used quantitative coronary angiography (a means of outlining a blood vessel radiologically after injection with radiopaque dye) to compare the responses of subjects with either a normal or a raised serum cholesterol to intra-arterial acetylcholine infusion.[25] The latter is a naturally occurring chemical secreted at certain nerve endings and linked with activation of the parasympathetic nervous system. Zeiher and his colleagues found that the coronary arteries of subjects with a normal total serum cholesterol had a larger pre-infusion cross-sectional area on average and they responded to acetylcholine by dilatation. On the other hand, the coronary arteries of the subjects with a raised serum cholesterol had a smaller initial cross-sectional area on average and they

[23] J N Morris, Jean W Marr and D G Clayton, 'Diet and heart: a postscript', *Br Med J*, 1977, **ii**: 1307–14, pp. 1311–12.

[24] Andreas M Zeiher *et al.*, 'Endothelium mediated coronary flow modulation in humans: effects of age, atherosclerosis, hypercholesterolemia and hypertension', *J Clin Invest*, 1993, **92**: 652–62, p. 657.

[25] Ibid., p. 652.

*Table V.4*
Serum cholesterol status and coronary artery responsiveness

Comparison of angiographic responses of left anterior descending coronary artery (on which the left ventricle is largely dependent for its blood supply) to **1** 72 g/mm acetylcholine (AC) infusion, and **2** papaverine induced maximal coronary flow. Subjects with normal or elevated serum cholesterol.

|   |   |   | Cholesterol | |
|---|---|---|---|---|
|   |   |   | Normal | Elevated |
|   | No. of subjects | | 18 | 20 |
|   | Age (years) | | $50.2 \pm 6.7$ | $52.7 \pm 11.7$ |
| **1** | LAD Status at angiography | | Normal | 13 normal<br>7 lumen irregular |
|   | Cross-sectional area mm$^2$ | Pre AC infusion | $10.6 \pm 7.3$ | $7.0 \pm 4.0$ |
|   |   | During AC infusion | $12.8 \pm 7.9$ | $4.9 \pm 3.9$ |
| **2** | Maximal coronary blood flow increase (%) | | $476.1 \pm 127.7$ | $356.9 \pm 150.6$ |

Source: Andreas M Zeiher *et al.*, 'Endothelium mediated coronary flow modulation in humans: effect of age, atherosclerosis, hypercholesterolemia and hypertension', *J Clin Invest*, 1993, **92**: 652–62, pp. 654, 656 (by permission of the American Society for Clinical Investigation).

responded to the infusion by constriction of the artery (Figure V.3).[26] There was a direct relationship between elevation of serum cholesterol levels and the degree of impairment of the vasodilator response. In addition, the maximal inducible increase in coronary artery flow, as established by intra-arterial infusion of the pharmacological agent papaverine, was the less in the group with a raised serum cholesterol.[27]

These effects have also been demonstrated experimentally in pigs in which diet-induced elevation of serum cholesterol resulted in increases in concentration of plasma endothelin. This substance too is generated by the endothelium (the innermost lining of the artery) and has a vasoconstrictor action. In these pigs direct infusion of acetylcholine into coronary arteries resulted in vasoconstriction, in contrast to the absence of coronary artery diameter change in animals with normal serum cholesterol levels.[28]

In the Regress investigation, the effects of administering the cholesterol-lowering medication pravastatin on serum cholesterol levels and the clinical course were

[26] Ibid., p. 652.
[27] Ibid., pp. 654–8.
[28] A Lerman *et al.*, 'Circulating and tissue endothelin immunoreactivity in hypercholesterolaemic pigs', *Circulation*, 1993, **88**: 2923–8, p. 2925.

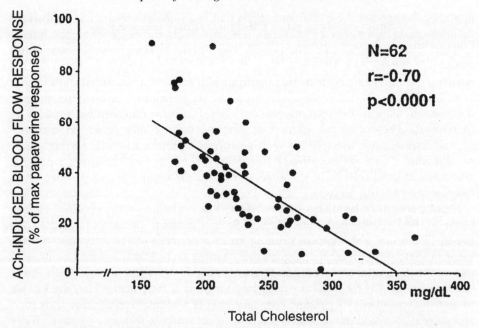

*Figure V.3:* Correlation between total serum cholesterol level and acetylcholine induced dilator capacity of the coronary system. Source: Andreas M Zeiher *et al.*, 'Endothelium mediated coronary flow modulation in humans: effects of age, atherosclerosis, hypercholesterolaemia and hypertension', *J Clin Invest*, 1993, **92**: 652–62, p. 657. (By permission of the American Society for Clinical Investigation.)

studied. It was found that when compared with the controls who were given a placebo, the patients in the active treatment arm and whose serum total cholesterol was lowered significantly had a correspondingly significant reduction in the total ischaemic burden. This was defined electrocardiographically as the product of the duration of S-T segment depression (an indicator of deficient heart muscle blood flow) in minutes and its extent in millimetres. These changes could be either asymptomatic or accompanied by angina pectoris. The total ischaemic burden decreased from an average of 34.6 millimetre-minutes at baseline to 26.4 in the placebo arm, but from 41.5 to 22.5 millimetre-minutes in the pravastatin treated group, a 23 per cent lowering in the former as opposed to 46 per cent in the latter. The Regress investigators found that after some five months a functional and cholesterol-related vasoconstrictor basis for periodic spontaneous reductions in myocardial blood flow was countered by cholesterol lowering, a concept now widely accepted.[29] Lessening of serum total cholesterol levels has also been shown by coronary angiography to be followed by a beneficial effect on coronary arterial responsiveness to the effects of acetylcholine, constriction being replaced by moderate

[29] Ad J van Boven *et al.*, 'Reduction of transient myocardial ischemia with pravastatin in addition to the conventional treatment in patients with angina pectoris. REGRESS Study Group', *Circulation*, 1996, **94**: 1503–5.

dilatation.[30] Together these findings suggest that in a population with a low saturated fat intake and resulting low serum total cholesterol levels, the incidence of functionally induced transient ischaemic events with their possible symptomatic associations would be relatively low. By implication, these conclusions suggest the converse: the eighteenth-century English increase in saturated fat consumption, with its now known association with serum cholesterol elevation, had the potential to result in functionally induced imbalances between myocardial blood supply and cardiac muscle requirements. These changes, occurring independently of any structural coronary arterial disease, could precipitate angina pectoris in a patient otherwise asymptomatic or aggravate it in a person already susceptible. They thereby constitute a possible additional link between dietary changes during the Georgian era and the concurrent emergence of angina pectoris.

Finally, note must be made of the nearly complete absence of the very long carbon chain PUFAs (C20:5 N-3 and C20:6 N-3) in the lipids of cattle farmed in the twentieth century, although constituting up to 8 per cent of the fatty acids of free living bovids.[31] This difference suggests that changes in cattle management as initiated during the Agricultural Revolution could account for very considerable falls in the concentrations of these naturally occurring long chain fatty acids. They are known to improve endothelial dependent coronary arterial and microvasculature relaxation and thereby facilitate increase in blood flow to the heart in response to need.[32] They also have mildly anticoagulant properties[33] and are, incidentally, plentiful in fatty fish and the blubber of marine mammals. They may therefore contribute to a lowered incidence of coronary heart disease among peoples who eat large amounts of these foods (see pages 64, 182). Conversely, the disappearance of these beneficial long chain PUFAs from the fats of land animals with changing eighteenth-century feeding practices could have been one more factor contributing to development of coronary heart disease in that period.

During the 1960s saturated fat consumption in the United States started to fall and coronary heart disease rates to decline. The Framingham study compared CHD incidence and mortality in a ten-year follow-up of 1950 and 1970 cohorts of men who were aged fifty to fifty-nine and free of heart disease at entry into the study. The end points included myocardial infarction, whether fatal or otherwise, stable or unstable angina pectoris, sudden death, congestive heart failure and any other clinical presentations. The authors were able to separate the fall in CHD incidence from the effects of recently introduced treatment on survival after the disease had become established. They were thereby able to show that the *incidence* of coronary heart disease with its first manifestations was lower in the 1970 than in the 1950 cohort (Table I.1).[34] Lee Goldman and E Francis Cook came to similar conclusions. They

[30] Charles B Treasure *et al.*, 'Beneficial effects of cholesterol-lowering therapy on the coronary endothelium in patients with coronary artery disease', *N Engl J Med*, 1995, **332**: 481–7, p. 484.

[31] Crawford *et al.*, op. cit., note 8 above, p. 297.

[32] Vladimir I Vekshtein *et al.*, 'Fish oil improves endothelial dependent relaxation in patients with coronary arterial disease (abstract 1727)', *Circulation*, 1989, Suppl II, p. 434.

[33] Schacky and Weber, op. cit., note 12 above, pp. 2447–8.

[34] Pamela A Sytkowski, William B Kannel and Ralph B D'Agostino, 'Changes in risk factors and the decline in mortality from cardiovascular disease. The Framingham Heart Study', *N Engl J Med*, 1990, **322**: 1635–41, pp. 1637–8.

studied the decline in CHD death rates between 1968 and 1976. They first calculated the contribution to falling mortality made by intervening changes in the clinical management of established disease. These included the introduction of intensive care units and resuscitation procedures, prevention of serious heart rhythm disturbances, widespread use of beta adrenergic receptor blocking drugs to counter excessive sympathetic nervous system activity, treatment of high blood pressure and introduction of surgical coronary artery bypass grafting.[35] The authors then reviewed epidemiological studies reporting the effect of various primary preventive measures, such as those aimed at lowering serum cholesterol and reduction in smoking.[36] In conclusion, Goldman and Cook calculated that newer lifestyles, including low fat diets, accounted for about 54 per cent of the reduction in mortality observed during the eight-year study.[37] It would be equally reasonable to conclude that the reverse is true and that the substantially higher previous CHD incidence was associated in large measure with the earlier lifestyles that included higher consumption of animal fats.

During the late twentieth century the death rate from coronary heart disease began to fall not only in the United States[38] but in countries as disparate as Finland,[39] New Zealand,[40] Iceland,[41] Australia and, albeit to a lesser extent, the United Kingdom.[42] Although improved management of established disease played an important part, there was, as noted in the case of the USA, a reduction in incidence as well as in mortality. Concurrently, there were changes in lifestyle risk factors in all of these five countries, among them a fall in saturated fat consumption that was taking place in the developed world generally. Thus in Finland, selected as the country whose eastern regions once had the world's highest CHD death rate, there was a reduction in mortality of over 50 per cent. During the 25-year period in which this decline occurred, the average total fat content of the Finnish diet fell from 38 per cent of energy intake to 34, and saturated fat from 21 to 16 per cent.[43] The Finnish investigators applied previously established epidemiological data relating dietary fat to total serum cholesterol levels and the effect of their reduction on coronary heart death rates. On this basis they calculated that almost half of the observed fall in mortality could be attributed to the reduction in total and saturated fat consumption and the concomitant increase in intake of polyunsaturated fats, as

[35] Lee Goldman and E Francis Cook, 'The decline in ischemic heart disease mortality rates. An analysis of the comparative effects of medical interventions and changes in lifestyle', *Ann Intern Med*, 1984, **101**: 825–36, pp. 825–31.

[36] Ibid., pp. 831–2.

[37] Ibid., pp. 832–4.

[38] Sytkowski, Kannel, D'Agostino, op. cit. note 34 above, p. 1638.

[39] Pirjo Pietinen *et al.*, 'Changes in diet in Finland from 1972 to 1992: impact on coronary heart disease risk', *Prev Med*, 1996, **25**: 243–50, p. 243.

[40] Rodney Jackson and Robert Beaglehole, 'Trends in dietary fat and cigarette smoking and the decline in coronary heart disease in New Zealand', *Int J Epidemiol*, 1987, **16**: 377–82, p. 378.

[41] Nikulas Sigfusson *et al.*, 'Decline in ischaemic heart disease in Iceland and changes in risk factor levels', *Br Med J*, 1991, **302**: 1371–5, p. 1373.

[42] Terry Dwyer and Basil S Hetzel, 'A comparison of trends in coronary heart disease mortality in Australia, USA and England and Wales with reference to three major risk factors—hypertension, cigarette smoking and diet', *Int J Epidemiol*, 1980, **9**: 65–71, p. 66.

[43] Pietinen *et al.*, op. cit., note 39, pp. 244–6.

in soft margarines. Their findings thus conformed closely to those of Goldman and Cook.[44] The conclusions from the comparable studies conducted in the United Kingdom, Australia, New Zealand and Iceland have been similar.[45]

In eighteenth-century England the dietary changes were in the reverse direction to the twentieth as animal fats then became available in greatly increased quantities. In so far as twentieth-century findings can be applied to that time, it is probable, as pointed out earlier, that these fats were for the most part saturated. It therefore seems probable that the eighteenth-century dietary changes, which were in the opposite direction to recent trends, had correspondingly opposite and therefore adverse effects on the lipid profile in general and on the serum total cholesterol levels in particular. The richer diet could have thereby contributed significantly to the eighteenth-century development of clinically recognizable coronary heart disease. As part of the present postulate, the changes in fat consumption are considered the most conclusive and the most important of all the eighteenth-century developments examined either in this or later sections where the role of changes in ancillary risk factors is analysed. The evidence cited indicates that excessive fat consumption, as characterized the eating habits of the affluent during the late eighteenth century, results in serum cholesterol abnormalities that are conducive to development of coronary heart disease, even in the absence of other risk factors. The Seven Countries study results showed that over 40 per cent of the variance in the ten-year CHD death rate could be accounted for by differences in serum total cholesterol levels.[46] The authors of the MRFIT study concluded that by themselves serum total cholesterol levels in excess of 4.68 mmol/L could alone account for about half of the observed coronary heart disease mortality.[47] As discussed later under their respective headings, the effects of other dietary factors, protective in the case of fish and fibre, deleterious in the case of sugar and coffee, are associated with corresponding changes, harmful or beneficial, in the lipid profile. This is one important way in which their effects are produced. Conversely, the effects of non-dietary risk factors, notably smoking, high blood pressure and stress, are greatly reduced or even nullified when fat intake and serum cholesterol are low. A striking example of this is provided by early post-Second World War Japan. It was and is a developed society where in the 1950s the fat intake was very low and what there was came from fish and was therefore very high in unsaturated fatty acid content. During this time the annual male death rate from heart disease was 363/100,000 in England and Wales, but only 131 in Japan. The corresponding numbers for females were 158 and 81 respectively. Heart disease was then more likely to be reported in Japan than in England and Wales and about a quarter of the Japanese cardiac deaths were due to conditions other than CHD. The incidence of the latter was low despite heavy smoking, severe stresses, aggravated by the course and outcome of the Second World War and its aftermath, and a severe

---

[44] Ibid., p. 246; Goldman and Cook, op. cit., note 35 above, p. 832.

[45] Dwyer and Hetzel, op. cit., note 42 above, p. 65; Jackson and Beaglehole, op. cit., note 40 above, p. 378; Sigfusson *et al.*, op. cit., note 41 above, p. 1374.

[46] Kromhout *et al.*, op. cit., note 19 above, p. 319.

[47] Martin *et al.*, op. cit, note 20 above, p. 935.

*Table V.5*

Average systolic blood pressures: Japanese* and American** applicants for life insurance.
Age groups 45–65 (mmHg)

| Age Group | United States | | Japan | |
|---|---|---|---|---|
| | Systolic BP | % ≥ 150 | Systolic BP | % ≥ 150 |
| 45 + | 130.0 | 13.4 | 130.6 | 17.3 |
| 50 + | 134.5 | 20.2 | 137.2 | 26.3 |
| 55 + | 137.8 | 26.3 | 138.2 | 29.7 |
| 60 + | 141.8 | 34.9 | 144.0 | 39.8 |

* 75,000 (including females; not separately tabulated).
** 269,583 males (86% of applicants).

Reprinted from Henry A Schroeder, 'Degenerative cardiovascular disease in the Orient. II hypertension', *J Chron Dis*, 1958, **8**: 312–33, p. 315. (With permission from Elsevier Science.)

housing shortage.[48] Salt intake was high in Japan, estimated at 10 to 15 g daily per person, and may have been a factor contributing to the proportion of middle-aged men with elevated systolic blood pressures being higher in Japan than in the United States (Table V.5), possibly a cause for the then very high Japanese incidence of cerebral haemorrhage.[49] In the balance, the role of animal fat intake, harmful when excessive but beneficial when restricted, overrides other lifestyle risk factors in importance.

**Faith and Fish**

Some further developments in eighteenth-century English dietary practices may have had their origins in changes in religious observance. The Reformation in England resulted initially in establishment of a national church that retained many features of Catholicism, and even after the Elizabethan modifications, it resulted in a form of Protestantism less extreme than was usual on the continent.[50] There was consequently a tendency to retain some Roman Catholic dietary laws, particularly periodic abstinence from meat. These restrictions were reinforced by sixteenth-century civil laws designed to protect the fishing fleet, a potential source of men for the navy. Eating meat was prohibited during Lent, on all Fridays and on occasion on Wednesday. These were designated fish days. The laws were civil, but the choice of days and times Roman Catholic in origin.[51] All of this resulted in over a quarter

[48] Michael G Marmot and George Davey Smith, 'Why are the Japanese living longer', *Br Med J*, 1989, **299**: 1547–51, p. 1547.

[49] Henry A Schroeder, 'Degenerative cardiovascular disease in the Orient. II Hypertension', *J Chron Dis*, 1958, **8**: 312–33, pp. 315, 320.

[50] G R Elton, *England under the Tudors*, London, Methuen, 1974, pp. 156, 271–6.

[51] George Macaulay Trevelyan, *English social history*, London, Longman, 1978, p. 189.

of the year, a total of about 100 days, on which meat could not be eaten and fish was to be substituted.

During the late seventeenth and the eighteenth centuries the civil dietary restrictions lapsed and there was a considerable decline in Anglican religious observances, especially those of a ritual nature. This occurred to some extent when the Hanoverian succession became imminent and High Church practices aroused suspicion of Jacobite sympathies. However, following the failure of the 1745 uprising led by Bonny Prince Charlie, the need for militant Protestantism lessened as the High Church became fully reconciled to the House of Hanover.[52] As the possibility of a Stuart restoration faded so did the intensity of Protestant held attitudes. At this time the Church of England also lost followers to the growing nonconformist movements, possibly in part because of complacency in the face of challenges by dissenting communities and more certainly because of failure of the Church to move its physical presence into the new and growing centres of population.[53] The influence of rationalist movements grew during the late Stuart and the Georgian eras and amongst religious intellectuals there was increasing emphasis on personal integrity rather than strict belief and ritual orthodoxy. As a measure of its extent, no less a person than John Tillotson, Archbishop of Canterbury in the years following the Glorious Revolution of 1689, considered that doctrine stood or fell by its consonance with reason.[54] Meanwhile, the Toleration Act of 1689 had resulted in lessened coercion in connection with the observance of Anglican rites, and led ultimately to their 1779 removal by a further Act of Parliament.[55] All of these factors contributed to a decline in adherence to religious dietary practices. As a result there were about 100 days in the year when eating meat (with its attendant high fat content) became allowable.

This increase might well of itself have contributed appreciably to the development of coronary heart disease. Whether the concurrent fall in consumption of fish is to be judged contributory as well depends on an assessment of any possible protective role of fish, the evidence for which warrants consideration. Comparisons have been made between CHD incidence in populations with varying fish intake but the results of studies based on responses of individuals to questionnaires about food intake, with all their accompanying uncertainties, have not been consistent. Studies based on nationwide estimates of consumption have also yielded varying results. A recent review by M B Katan attempted to reconcile the inconsistencies by suggesting an all or none threshold effect. It was noted that groups having a fairly low fish intake, perhaps one or two servings a week, appeared to enjoy a lessening in coronary disease incidence, but no further reduction with greater fish consumption was evident.[56] It would be hard therefore to demonstrate any benefits of increasing fish intake in a population in which the lowest level of consumption was already above

[52] Ibid., pp. 356, 55.

[53] Frank O'Gorman, *The long eighteenth century: British political and social history 1688–1832*, London, Arnold, 1997, p. 295.

[54] Mark Goldie and John Locke, 'Jonas Proast and religious toleration 1688–92', in John Walsh, Colin Haydon and Stephen Taylor (eds), *The Church of England c.1689–c. 1833: from toleration to tractarianism*, Cambridge University Press, 1993, p. 161.

[55] O'Gorman, op. cit., note 53 above, p. 308.

[56] M B Katan, 'Fish and heart disease', *N Engl J Med*, 1995, **332**: 1024–5, pp. 1024, 1025.

Table V.6
Age adjusted death rates per 10,000 person-years according to baseline fish consumption

| Fish consumption (g/day) | Death rates/10,000 person-years |
| --- | --- |
| 0 | 78.6 |
| 1–17 | 69.2 |
| 18–34 | 57.9 |
| ≥35 | 45.3 |

Adapted from data published by M L Daviglus et al., 'Fish consumption and the 30-year risk of fatal myocardial infarction', in N Engl J Med, 1997, **336**: 1046–53, p. 1049.

any theoretical threshold. Support for the threshold concept was also provided by an analysis of findings reported by Alberto Ascherio and co-workers. This showed that during the period under review the death rate from coronary heart disease was about 25 per cent lower among men who regularly ate at least some fish when compared to those who ate none at all, but the mortality rate was not lower still in a third group of men who consumed larger amounts.[57]

The findings of Daan Kromhout and his colleagues contrasted with those of Katan and Ascherio. They compared, *inter alia*, the outcomes when elderly Dutch subjects who ate varying amounts of fish regularly were compared with "no-fish" eaters. In the course of a twenty-year follow-up, the risk ratio for CHD of the latter was 1.0 by definition, but the former only 0.60. The difference remained significant after correction for the usual confounders. More importantly, among the entire group of fish eaters, the risk ratio for coronary heart disease decreased progressively with increasing amounts of fish consumed, a finding which casts doubt on the threshold concept.[58] Several other investigations involving large numbers of subjects and with long term follow-up have also been able to demonstrate progressive benefits with increasing consumption. A further noteworthy example in this respect is provided by the results of the Chicago Western Electric Company study which involved 1,822 men, 47,153 person-years of follow-up and 430 deaths from coronary heart disease that became available for analysis. A significant reduction in CHD death rates that could be related to fish consumption was demonstrated, with benefits directly proportional to the amount consumed (Table V.6).[59] In general more findings negate rather than favour the concept of a threshold, but irrespective of this, the investigations are, by and large, in agreement in indicating that, as far as coronary heart disease is concerned, fish has a protective role.

There is also evidence to suggest that fatty fish, such as mackerel or herring,

[57] Alberto Ascherio et al., 'Dietary intake of marine n-3 fatty acids, fish intake, and the risk of coronary heart disease among men', N Engl J Med, 1995, **332**: 977–82, p. 979.

[58] Daan Kromhout, Edward B Bosschieter and C de Lezenne Coulander, 'The inverse relation between fish consumption and 20-year mortality from coronary heart disease', N Engl J Med, 1985, **312**: 1205–9, p. 1206.

[59] M L Daviglus et al., 'Fish consumption and the 30-year risk of fatal myocardial infarction', N Engl J Med, 1997, **336**: 1046–53, p. 1049.

*Chapter V*

have a specific beneficial effect.[60] Fish consumption does not directly affect serum cholesterol levels significantly.[61] However, the long carbon chain fatty acids present in fish have been found to reduce platelet aggregation in response to contact with the physiological stimulants collagen and adenosine diphosphate. They have therefore a mild anticoagulant effect of potential value in protecting against clot formation in coronary arteries.[62] Such fatty acids are important constituents of fish oil and this may be a basis for beneficial effects of fish consumption on CHD incidence. Lastly, fish oil has been found to improve endothelium dependent coronary arterial relaxation in patients with established coronary heart disease (page 72), thus facilitating an increase in blood flow to the heart in response to need.[63]

In conclusion, eighteenth-century changes in eating habits with a decline in religious observance of dietary constraints and a fall into abeyance of legal restrictions on meat consumption may have resulted in an appreciable fall in fish consumption, possibly to below a suggested critical threshold level. Reduced intake of fish with loss of its various beneficial effects could have contributed to the rising eighteenth-century coronary heart disease incidence, with its concurrent replacement by fatty animal foods constituting an inter-related additional risk factor.

**Fibre**

Some of the greatest changes in farming in Georgian England related to the growing of cereals and, in particular, to a shift in emphasis from coarse grains to wheat; the relative importance of oats and rye declining while that of wheat rose. With abandonment of the strip system and other improvements in methods of cultivation during the eighteenth century, yields of wheat and oats, as measured in bushels per acre, increased in roughly similar proportions, by about one-eighth in the case of the former and one-sixth in the latter. However, the acreage under wheat rose between 1695 and 1750 from about one and a third million to over 2 million acres, but the increase under oats was much less, from 1.22 to 1.44 million acres. As a result, wheat production increased by 73.5 per cent, almost exactly double the 37.5 per cent rise in the yield of oats. During the last half of the eighteenth century the rate of increase in the amount of wheat harvested rose sharply while the rate of rise in oat production lessened somewhat (Table V.7).[64] As a result oat production fell considerably as a proportion of total cereal output while that of wheat rose. The absolute amount of oats available for human consumption actually declined during this time. In 1696 the horse population of England was estimated by Gregory King

[60] M L Burr *et al.*, 'Effect of changes in fat, fish and fibre intakes on death and myocardial reinfarction: diet and reinfarction trial', *Lancet*, 1989, ii: 757–61, p. 759.

[61] Kromhout, Bosschieter, Coulander, op. cit., note 58 above, p. 1206.

[62] Schacky and Weber, op. cit., note 33 above, pp. 2447–8.

[63] Vekshtein *et al.*, op. cit., note 32 above, p. 434.

[64] B A Holderness, 'Prices, production and output', in G E Mingay (ed.), *The agrarian history of England and Wales, Volume VI: 1750–1850*, Cambridge University Press, 1989, p. 145.

Table V.7
English arable cereal yields, 1750–1800

| Crop | Area cultivated (acres × 10⁶) | | Yield/acre (quarters) | | Total yield (quarters × 10⁶) | | % Change 1750–1800 |
|---|---|---|---|---|---|---|---|
| | 1750 | 1800 | 1750 | 1800 | 1750 | 1800 | |
| Wheat | 1.8 | 2.5 | 3.6 | 6.1 | 6.5 | 15.3 | +135 |
| Rye | 0.5 | 0.3 | 1.0 | 0.9 | 0.5 | 0.27 | −48 |
| Barley | 1.4 | 1.3 | 3.8 | 4.5 | 5.3 | 5.9 | +10 |
| Oats | 2.0 | 2.0 | 6.0 | 7.8 | 12.0 | 15.6 | +30 |

Source: B A Holderness, 'Prices, production and output', in G E Mingay (ed.), *The agrarian history of England and Wales, Volume VI: 1750–1850*, Cambridge University Press, 1989, p. 145 (with permission).

at 1.2 million.[65] A corresponding estimate for 1750 was close to 1.5 million.[66] More importantly, as they replaced oxen at the plough, the number of draught horses with their high energy needs doubled, with consequent diversion of oats from human consumption to animal feed.[67] During this time the production of rye, a coarse grain, declined by some 48 per cent.[68] As described below, these changes were reflected, notably among the affluent, in increasing consumption of the more expensive white bread and diminishing intake of high fibre staples.

As with other risk factors, any contribution of these changes to eighteenth-century emergence of overt clinical manifestations of coronary heart disease cannot be measured directly. They must be inferred from relevant twentieth-century studies, which have taken two forms. One is based on observation of the effect of a deliberately varied fibre intake on the lipid profile. The other involves epidemiological studies that relate differing levels of fibre consumption to the incidence of CHD morbidity and mortality. Studies of the effects of experimentally varying fibre intake on lipid profiles involve fewer problems than do the epidemiological studies. Randomizing is possible, and fairly precise regulation of intake can be maintained during the short time needed to detect any biochemical changes. Compliance for a limited time is the more easily assured and regulation of the type of fibre to be consumed is not difficult. Other risk factors, notably those that involve diet, can be held constant throughout the study. Epidemiological studies do not have these advantages, but can use the incidence of clinical coronary heart disease events or deaths as the gold standard by which to gauge the possible effectiveness of high fibre consumption as a preventive measure. Furthermore, epidemiological studies have the potential for determining whether the effect of fibre on the lipid profile is or is not the only mechanism of any

[65] Gregory King, *Natural and political observations and conclusions upon the state and condition of England 1696*, ed. George E Barnett, Baltimore, Johns Hopkins Press, 1936, p. 37.

[66] J A Chartres, 'The marketing of agricultural produce', Joan Thirsk (ed.) *The agrarian history of England and Wales, Volume V: 1640–1750. II. Agrarian change*, Cambridge University Press, 1985, p. 446.

[67] Jonathan Brown and H A Beecham, 'Farming practices', in G E Mingay (ed.), *The agrarian history of England and Wales, Volume VI: 1750–1850*, Cambridge University Press, 1989, p. 289.

[68] Holderness, op. cit., note 64 above, p. 145.

benefit. These investigations too have taken two forms. One is prospective observation of the incidence of coronary heart disease in populations whose fibre consumption has been varied deliberately. The other is a retrospective dietary survey of fibre intake by patients who had suffered manifestations of CHD and who are compared with apparently healthy control subjects.

Observations of the effect of varying fibre intake on the lipid profile are now numerous and on the whole consistent. K Storch and colleagues studied twelve healthy college students in a cross-over investigation. Their diet was supplemented by either oat or wheat bran during a six-week period. The reduction in total serum cholesterol with oat bran was about double the modest lowering achieved with the wheat equivalent.[69] Kurt Gold and Dennis Davidson reviewed six investigations apart from their own (Table V.8). All showed falls in serum total cholesterol with experimental diets in which oats were the source of the designated high fibre. The reductions ranged from 3 to 26 per cent.[70]

The mechanisms by which fibre produces a favourable effect on the serum lipid profile have been reviewed by R C Spiller who has pointed out that the changes are more than can be explained by coincident reduction in total energy and saturated fat intake. They can also be dissociated from the laxative action and the increase in stool bulk associated with high bran diets. It was concluded that in the case of oat bran, the effects are probably related to its breakdown products trapping water in a gel and thereby reducing mixing movements. This has a slight negative effect on cholesterol absorption by lessening its contact with the walls of the small intestine. In addition, fibre derived from oats results indirectly in bile acid sequestration by bacteria normally present in the colon. This reduces the enterohepatic cycle, a process by which bile acids pass from the liver to the small intestine where they facilitate fat absorption and are themselves subsequently re-absorbed into the bloodstream.[71]

There are many studies of the relationship between fibre intake and coronary heart disease incidence. These include the Ireland–Boston diet-heart study in which, as part of their investigation, L H Kushi and colleagues recorded the diet history of 390 men resident in Ireland, 386 Irish immigrants to the Boston area and 225 first generation immigrants born in the United States to Irish immigrant parents. At entry into the study they were aged from thirty to sixty-nine years. A dietician recorded each man's initial diet history. When the study population was classified by tertiles, an inverse relationship between fibre intake and CHD mortality was demonstrated, the differences actually becoming greater after adjustment for other coronary risk factors (Table V.9) and just reaching statistical significance. Even the highest mean fibre intake of the three groups was low by current recommendations and during the follow-up period the overall risk factor profile was changing, so that in these circumstances the significance of the differences is especially noteworthy. In this study it was not possible to adjust for an observed inverse relationship between

[69] K Storch, J W Anderson and V R Young, 'Oat bran muffins lower serum cholesterol of healthy young people', *Clin Res*, 1984, **32**: 740A (abstract).

[70] Kurt V Gold and Dennis M Davidson, 'Oat bran as a cholesterol-reducing dietary adjunct in a young, healthy population', *West J Med*, 1988, **148**: 299–302, p. 301.

[71] R C Spiller, 'Cholesterol, fibre and bile acids', *Lancet*, 1996, **347**: 415–16, p. 415.

Table V.8
Human studies evaluating oat products and lipid effects

| Studies and grain(s) | Subjects No. | Amount g/day | No. of Days on Diet | Prestudy S. Cholesterol (mg/dl) | Cholesterol Reduction (%) |
|---|---|---|---|---|---|
| De Groot et al. 1963[a] | | | | | |
| Rolled Oats | 21 | 140 | 21 | 251 | 11 |
| Judd & Truswell, 1981[b] | | | | | |
| Rolled Oats | 10 | 125 | 21 | 203 | 8 |
| Kirby et al. 1981[c] | | | | | |
| Oat Bran | 8 | 94 | 10 | 269 | 13 |
| Anderson et al. 1984[d] | | | | | |
| Oat Bran | 10 | 100 | 21 | 257 | 19 |
| Chen & Anderson, 1986[e] | | | | | |
| Oat Bran/Beans | 10 | 41/145 | 182 | 257 | 26 |
| Oat Bran/Beans | 4 | 41/145 | 693 | 257 | 22 |
| Van Horn et al. 1986[f] | | | | | |
| Oat Bran | 69 | 39 | 28 | 196 | 3 |
| Rolled Oats | 69 | 35 | 28 | 195 | 3 |

[a] A P De Groot, R Luyken and N A Pikaar, 'Cholesterol lowering effect of rolled oats', *Lancet*, 1963, **ii**: 303–4.
[b] P A Judd and A S Truswell, 'The effect of rolled oats on blood lipids and fecal steroid excretion in man', *Am J Clin Nutr*, 1981, **34**: 2061–7.
[c] R W Kirby et al., 'Oat-bran intake selectively lowers low-density lipoprotein cholesterol concentrations of hypercholesterolemic men', *Am J Clin Nutr*, 1981, **34**: 824–9.
[d] J W Anderson et al., 'Hypocholesterolemic effects of oat bran or bean intake for hypercholesterolemic men', *Am J Clin Nutr*, 1984, **40**: 1146–55.
[e] W J L Chen and J W Anderson, 'Hypocholesterolemic effects of soluble fibres', in G V Vahouny and D Kritchevsky (eds), *Washington symposium on dietary fibre*, New York, Plenum Press, 1986, pp. 275–86.
[f] L V Van Horn et al., 'Serum lipid response to oat product intake with a fat modified diet', *J Am Diet Assoc*, 1986, **86**: 759–64.

Reproduced from Kurt V Gold and Dennis M Davidson, 'Oat bran as a cholesterol-reducing dietary adjunct in a young, healthy population', *West J Med*, 1988, **148**: 299–302, p. 301. (With permission from the BMJ Publishing Group.)

fibre and fat consumption, but any such tendency constitutes an additional if indirect cardioprotective benefit of high fibre intake.[72]

M G Marmot and colleagues showed that between 1951 and 1971 there was a slight increase in heart disease mortality in the two highest British social classes, but a more rapid rate of rise in the lowest two. In 1931 heart disease mortality was greater among men in social classes I and II when compared with classes IV and V.

[72] L H Kushi et al., 'Diet and 20-year mortality from coronary heart disease. The Ireland–Boston diet-heart study', *N Engl J Med*, 1985, **312**: 811–18, pp. 813–14.

*Table V.9*

Relationship between fibre intake tertiles and male CHD mortality expressed as relative risk (RR) males. 17–23 year follow-up.

| Fibre intake tertile | | CHD mortality | | |
|---|---|---|---|---|
| | | Lowest 3rd | Middle 3rd | Highest 3rd |
| RR | Crude * | 1.0 | 0.73 | 0.46 |
| | Adjusted ** | 1.0 | 0.88 | 0.57[1] |

* Adjusted for cohort and age
** Adjusted additionally for systolic BP, total serum cholesterol, EKG abnormalities, cigarette smoking and alcohol intake
[1] Difference from reference RR significant (P<0.05).

Adapted from data published by L H Kushi *et al.*, 'Diet and 20-year mortality from coronary heart disease. The Ireland–Boston diet-heart study', in *New Engl J Med*, 1985, **312**: 811–18, p. 816.

By 1961 the situation had become reversed. The fibre consumption of the highest income groups relative to that of the lowest increased steadily during this period. When compared to the lowest two social classes the highest two with the *higher* overall fibre intake emerged with a *lower* incidence of CHD over the twenty years.[73] Finally, in a prospective secondary prevention study, Daan Kromhout and his colleagues obtained a dietary history with respect to fibre intake in a group of 871 men who were followed for six to twelve months. The twenty-seven men who died from CHD during the period under review had an average daily fibre intake of 27.2 $\pm$ 8.1 g per day, appreciably less than the 30.8 $\pm$ 9.7 g per day of the survivors. When corrected for other factors by multivariate analysis, the difference approached conventional levels of significance, the P value being 0.06.[74]

In conclusion, the fibre intake of the English middle and upper classes declined during the Georgian era. Recent studies have shown that a low fibre intake affects the lipid profile and incidence of coronary heart disease adversely. The decline in oat fibre intake, in particular, during the eighteenth century could therefore be considered a contributory cause for angina pectoris then becoming manifest in England as a disease of the affluent and increasingly common thereafter.

## Sugar

Wild cane sugar plants probably grew originally on the island of New Guinea, which was possibly the site of its first cultivation.[75] By the end of the fifteenth century

[73] M G Marmot *et al.*, 'Changing social-class distribution of heart disease', *Br Med J*, 1978, **ii**: 1109–12, p. 1110.
[74] D Kromhout, E B Bosschieter and C de Lezenne Coulander, 'Dietary fibre and 10-year mortality from coronary heart disease, cancer, and all causes. The Zutphen study', *Lancet*, 1982, **ii**: 518–22, p. 519.
[75] N Deerr, *History of sugar*, 2 vols, London, Chapman and Hall, 1949–50, vol. 1, p. 44.

they had become disseminated, although to a very limited extent, throughout the Middle East and the Mediterranean littoral. The sweetness of beets was known from classical times and recognized in medieval Europe, but the sugar they contained made only a small contribution to diet, the mixture of glucose with fructose in honey then being the principal source of sweetening. The large-scale production of sucrose from the sugar cane began only after the European colonization of the Caribbean Islands. From the English standpoint it assumed significance only with the annexation of Jamaica, Barbados and other West Indian islands by England in the mid-seventeenth century.[76] The climate and soil in the Caribbean were ideal for growing sugar cane and large plantations developed, manned mostly by slave labour that was imported from West Africa. In addition to large-scale cultivation, factory style techniques were developed for harvesting and crushing the cane and for extracting and refining the sugar, which was then despatched to Europe in the form of loaves.[77] Mercantilist economic policies ensured that production in the colonies resulted in preferential trade with the mother country and bulk importation was facilitated by improvement in ship design. The West India Docks in London became known as the sugar docks because sugar grown in the Caribbean English colonies was the principal commodity that they handled. Production in Jamaica alone, slightly less than 1,000 tons a year during the 1670s, rose to 3,586 tons by 1684 and 19,641 by 1739, and virtually all of the output was exported to England.[78]

The developments described resulted in a dramatic increase in cane sugar (specifically sucrose) consumption in England during the eighteenth century. The period from 1713 to 1739 has been selected to illustrate trends, as this was the longest period in the century during which England was not involved in any major wars, with their attendant disruptions of trade. The earlier date is that in which the Treaty of Utrecht was signed, ending the War of the Spanish Succession, and the later year is that which preceded the outbreak of the War of the Austrian Succession. Net imports of sugar rose from 15,771 tons in 1713 to 43,103 tons by 1739. The figures for this have been obtained by subtraction of re-export tonnage from that of imports, both of which were well documented when subjected to customs inspection for taxation purposes. No cane sugar was produced at home. Only about 20 per cent of the sugar brought into the country was re-exported so that minor inaccuracies in the import and re-export figures would not have affected unduly the differences between them, i.e. the net imports.[79] Independent corroboration of the legitimate trade estimates is available for the year 1731 when N Deerr's figure for net imports was 35,063 tons[80] whilst W Reed arrived at the figure of 36,123 tons,[81] a difference of under 3 per cent. There is, however, some probable underestimation because of smuggling which took place on a very large scale, often using remote coastal inlets but also through ports and with either intimidation or the connivance of the revenue

---

[76] Ibid., p. 150.
[77] Ibid., p. 162.
[78] Ibid., vol. 2, p. 423.
[79] Ibid., p. 423.
[80] Ibid., p. 423.
[81] W Reed, *The history of sugar and sugar yielding plants*, London, Longmans, Green, 1866, p. 188.

officers. With the rise in volume of commerce with foreign lands "the eighteenth century marked the classic epoch of illicit trade".[82] As the population increased by barely one-tenth during 1713 and 1739,[83] the figures indicate a marked increase in English per capita sugar consumption. Despite two intervening wars, imports continued to rise, Reed reporting that they reached 69,146 tons by 1768,[84] the year of Heberden's presentation to the Royal College of Physicians of London. Deerr estimated that the amount consumed per capita rose from about 4 pounds a year during the first decade of the eighteenth century to 13 pounds annually during the last ten years, a greater than threefold increase.[85] Sugar was used in baking, in desserts and above all to sweeten the coffee and tea which were being drunk in ever greater amounts.

When the present project was first considered in the early 1960s, sugar was under suspicion as a CHD risk factor and its rising eighteenth-century usage considered a contributor to the emergence of angina as a recognizable complaint. John Yudkin had published a series of papers showing a relationship between sugar consumption at varying times and in different countries and the incidence of coronary heart disease.[86] However, J N Morris and others reported absence of any such association in a ten-year prospective study[87] and Yudkin's findings were challenged by Ancel Keys. The latter demonstated that the relationship appeared initially to be very similar to that previously established for fat consumption and CHD. When standardized for sugar consumption, the relationship between fat intake and coronary heart disease continued to hold. However, the reverse was not true, because when standardized for fat consumption, the relationship between sugar intake and incidence of ischaemic heart disease ceased to be significant.[88] Keys also pointed out that there was a dramatic rise in the incidence of CHD deaths in Great Britain during the first half of the twentieth century when fat consumption increased dramatically but sugar consumption rose a mere 25 per cent.[89] The importance of sugar as a possible risk factor was subsequently discounted to such an extent that a recent exhaustive epidemiological survey of coronary heart disease risk factors did not even see fit to mention sugar, even if only to question its significance.[90]

However, before dismissing the dramatic rise in eighteenth-century English sugar consumption and the appearance and subsequent increase in frequency of angina pectoris as merely coincidental, several factors need consideration. Carbohydrate

[82] G D Ramsay, 'The smugglers trade, a neglected aspect of English commercial development', *Royal Hist Soc Trans*, 5th series, 1952, **2**: 131–157, p. 132.

[83] Wrigley *et al.*, op. cit., note 17 above p. 614.

[84] Reed, op. cit, note 81 above, p. 190.

[85] Deerr, op. cit. note 75 above, vol. 2, p. 532.

[86] John Yudkin, 'Diet and coronary thrombosis: hypothesis and fact', *Lancet*, 1957, **ii**: 155–62, p. 157; John Yudkin, 'Dietary fat and dietary sugar in relation to ischaemic heart disease and diabetes', *Lancet*, 1964, **ii**: 4–5; John Yudkin and Janet Roddy, 'Levels of dietary sucrose in patients with occlusive atherosclerotic disease', *Lancet*, 1964, **ii**: 6–8.

[87] Morris, Marr and Clayton, op. cit., note 23 above, p. 1311.

[88] Ancel Keys, 'Sucrose in the diet and coronary heart disease', *Atherosclerosis*, 1971, **14**: 193–202, pp. 194–5.

[89] Ibid., p. 196.

[90] M Lawrence *et al.* (eds), *Prevention of cardiovascular disease: an evidence-based approach*, Oxford General Practice series No. 33, Oxford University Press, 1996.

*Table V.10*
Comparative effects of starch and sugar intake on lipid profile. Mean and SD (mg/dl)

| Serum lipid (mg/dl) | Week | Males | | Females | |
|---|---|---|---|---|---|
| | | Starch | Sugar | Starch | Sugar |
| Total | 0 | 798 ± 85 | 782 ± 81 | 711 ± 42 | 716 ± 52 |
| | 6 | 766 ± 67 | 883 ± 113 | 744 ± 46 | 802 ± 34 |
| Triglycerides | 0 | 113 ± 11 | 136 ± 30 | 94 ± 7 | 94 ± 8 |
| | 6 | 126 ± 23 | 165 ± 31 | 87 ± 6 | 109 ± 9 |
| Total cholesterol Pooled male and female results | 0 | 178 ± 12 | 176 ± 8 | | |
| | 6 | 191 ± 12 | 217 ± 19 | | |

Source: S Reiser *et al.*, 'Isocaloric exchange of dietary starch and sucrose in humans. Effects on levels of fasting blood lipids', *Am J Clin Nutr*, 1979, **32**: 1659–68, pp. 1663–4. (With permission © American Society for Clinical Nutrition.)

taken in excess of energy requirements is converted in the body into saturated fats in which form it is stored in adipose tissues. Sucrose, possibly because of its speed of absorption from the gut, has a propensity to elevate serum cholesterol. Thus, Sheldon Reiser and his colleagues compared the effects of sucrose with those of wheat starch when one or the other constituted the principal source of carbohydrate during a six-week dietary trial. It was conducted in volunteers with a normal lipid profile and for whom 43 per cent of the energy requirements was supplied as carbohydrate, of which 30 per cent was either sucrose or wheat starch. No significant weight gains were recorded during the period of observation. When compared with starch administration, sucrose intake was associated with significantly higher serum total cholesterol levels (Table V.10).[91] M A Antar and colleagues had comparable results when fourteen patients with various lipoprotein abnormalities consumed experimental diets during two four-week periods and a cross-over sequence was used. Either sucrose or starch constituted 40 per cent of the energy intake. In other respects the diets "simulated a typical North American diet". During both the starch and sugar phases 35 per cent of the energy intake was in the form of fat, predominantly saturated. The serum cholesterol levels, initially about the same, fell during the period of starch intake but rose with sucrose with final means of 285 and 328 mg/dl respectively. The differences were highly significant.[92]

High sugar consumption results in elevation of serum triglycerides as well as

[91] S Reiser *et al.*, 'Isocaloric exchange of dietary starch and sucrose in humans. Effects on levels of fasting blood lipids', *Am J Clin Nutr*, 1979, **32**: 1659–69, pp. 1663–4.

[92] M A Antar *et al.*, 'Interrelationship between the kinds of dietary carbohydrate and fat in hyperlipoproteinemic patients, Part 3: Synergistic effect of sucrose and animal fat on serum lipids', *Atherosclerosis*, 1970, **11**: 191–201, p. 199.

cholesterol, as has been shown by Reiser and his colleagues.[93] In a prospective study, Meir Stampfer and his colleagues have recently shown that serum triglyceride levels *are* related directly to risk of coronary heart disease. In a seven-year follow-up of 14,916 men aged forty to eighty-four years who were enrolled in a physicians' health study they found a positive linear association between non-fasting serum triglyceride levels and myocardial infarction rates. Men in the highest quintile had a relative risk about two and a half times greater than males in the lowest one.[94] Michael Miller and his colleagues showed that particularly when above 100 mg/dl, fasting serum triglyceride levels are significantly predictive of CHD events.[95] Finally, Melissa Austin, in an extensive meta-analysis, has shown that among men serum triglyceride elevation is a significant risk factor for coronary heart disease, even when adjusted for the serum HDL levels with which triglyceride concentrations have an inverse relationship.[96] The one time benign perception of elevated serum triglycerides would therefore seem to need revision. The interaction between cane sugar consumption and elevation of serum triglyceride levels provides a further possible basis for linking sucrose intake with predisposition to development of coronary heart disease.

Ingestion of sugar is also followed by surges in pancreatic production of insulin which is associated with sympathetic nervous system activation and a rise in blood pressure.[97] Although high serum insulin levels were not found to be significant a risk factor for atherosclerotic cardiovascular disease in Edinburgh and Swedish men,[98] prospective long-term studies in Finland, France, and among Australian men tended to show a positive association, as have investigations involving immigrant South Asians in England.[99] The divergent results of these studies arise in large measure from difficulties in isolating the effects of raised serum insulin levels when it is associated, as is frequently the case, with other factors, notably excessive consumption of animal fats, obesity, elevation of serum triglycerides, Type II diabetes mellitus (the form which usually arises in middle life and is associated with insulin resistance rather than insulin deficiency) and hypertension.

[93] Reiser *et al.*, op. cit., note 91 above, pp. 1663–4.
[94] Meir J Stampfer *et al.*, 'A prospective study of triglyceride level, low-density lipoprotein particle diameter, and risk of myocardial infarction', *JAMA*, 1996, **276**: 882–8, p. 882.
[95] Michael Miller *et al.*, 'Normal triglyceride levels and coronary heart disease events: the Baltimore coronary observational long-term study', *J Am Coll Cardiol*, 1998, **31**: 1252–7, p. 1253.
[96] Melissa A Austin, 'Plasma triglyceride and coronary heart disease', *Arterioscler Thromb*, 1991, **11**: 2–14, p. 9.
[97] Gerald M Reaven, Hans Lithell and Lewis Landsberg, 'Hypertension and associated metabolic abnormalities—the role of insulin resistance and the sympathoadrenal system', *N Engl J Med*, 1996, **334**: 374–81, p. 376.
[98] A D Hargreaves *et al.*, 'Glucose tolerance, plasma insulin, HDL cholesterol and obesity: 12-year follow-up and development of coronary heart disease in Edinburgh men', *Atherosclerosis*, 1992, **94**: 61–9, p. 66; L Welin *et al.*, 'Hyperinsulinemia is not a major coronary risk factor in elderly men. The study of men born in 1913', *Diabetologia*, 1992, **35**: 766–70, p. 768.
[99] Kalevi Pyörälä, 'Relationship of glucose tolerance and plasma insulin to the incidence of coronary heart disease: results from two population studies in Finland', *Diabetes Care*, 1979, **2**: 131–41, p. 136; P Ducimetiere *et al.*, 'Relationship of plasma insulin levels to the incidence of myocardial infarction and coronary heart disease mortality in a middle-aged population', *Diabetologia*, 1980, **19**: 205–10, p. 206; T A Welborn and K Wearne, 'Coronary heart disease incidence and cardiovascular mortality in Busselton with reference to glucose and insulin concentrations', *Diabetes Care*, 1979, **2**: 154–60, p. 156; Jatinder Dhawan *et al.*, 'Insulin resistance, high prevalence of diabetes, and cardiovascular risk in immigrant Asians. Genetic or environmental effect?', *Br Heart J*, 1994, **72**: 413–21, p. 418.

To a large extent these difficulties were overcome by J P Després, who measured the fasting plasma insulin of 2,103 men aged thirty-five to sixty-four years who were free of ischaemic heart disease at entry into a five-year follow-up study. At the start of the follow-up the plasma insulin was 92.1 $\pm$ 27.5 µU/mL in the group of 114 men who subsequently developed at least one manifestation of CHD, significantly higher than the 78.2 $\pm$ 20.8 µU/mL in the group who remained free of coronary heart disease. The association of insulin with CHD was independent of differences in lipid profile, systolic blood pressure, body mass index and smoking.[100] Kalevi Pyörälä and colleagues obtained similar results in a nine and a half year follow-up of 982 men aged thirty-five to sixty-four years and free of coronary heart disease at entry. The initial fasting plasma insulin levels, and the ones at one and two hours after a standard glucose drink all correlated positively with the subsequent incidence of both coronary heart disease death and non-fatal myocardial infarction.[101] Finally, high insulin levels in the blood are frequently associated with insulin resistance. Evidence reviewed by Peter Savage and Mohammed Saad suggests that the latter may be an important link between abnormalities in carbohydrate metabolism and arteriosclerotic changes.[102] There does therefore appear to be a series of linkages whereby high sucrose intake produces surges in insulin production and eventual insulin resistance with its adverse cardiovascular consequences.

Glycosylated haemoglobin is a compound formed by glucose combining with haemoglobin, the carrier of oxygen in the blood. It reflects a tendency for glucose to combine with proteins generally, and in excess the combination is associated with a propensity to development of pathological changes in arteries. The percentage of haemoglobin that is glycosylated constitutes an integrated measure of the fluctuant blood glucose levels over the preceding six to twelve weeks. It is therefore to some extent an indicator of the long-term effects of sugar and complex carbohydrate intake and of the surges in blood glucose that they induce. Gerald Reaven has found that these surges are greater when carbohydrate is taken as cane sugar, i.e. as sucrose, than when a complex form is ingested, on average 137 as against 104 mg/100 mL respectively.[103] In another investigation involving a male cohort of the European Prospective Investigation into Cancer and Nutrition, it was found that among men aged forty-five to seventy-nine, 95 per cent of whom were free of diabetes, glycosylated haemoglobin levels were positively correlated with the subsequent four-year risk of death from ischaemic heart disease. This correlation held even though the levels ranged below the 7 per cent upper limit of normal. Thus the age adjusted relative risk for men with a glycosylated haemoglobin level in the range of 5.0 to 5.4 per cent was 2.74 times that of men in whom it was below 5 per cent. A further

[100] J P Després *et al.*, 'Hyperinsulinemia as an independent risk factor for ischemic heart disease', *N Engl J Med*, 1996, **334**: 952–7, pp. 954–5.

[101] Pyörälä, op. cit., note 99 above, p. 36.

[102] Peter J Savage and Mohammed F Saad, 'Insulin and atherosclerosis: villain, accomplice, or innocent bystander?', *Br Heart J*, 1993, **69**: 473–5, p. 474.

[103] Gerald M Reaven, 'Effects of differences in amount and kind of dietary carbohydrate on plasma glucose and insulin responses in man', *Am J Clin Nutr*, 1979, **32**: 2568–78, p. 2572.

connection between intake of sugar and liability to ischaemic heart disease with its clinical manifestations is thereby established.[104]

Of greater importance in connection with a possible link between sugar and CHD are the effects of its consumption when considered in association with other dietary risk factors. Kevin Grant and his co-workers gave volunteers a single meal of either whipping cream, sucrose or both together. They found that addition of sucrose to a meal with cream amplified both the extent and the duration of the post-prandial elevation of serum triglycerides. There was no short-term deviation of serum cholesterol levels from baseline with either sugar or cream alone, but when taken together an initial mean fasting serum cholesterol of 4.36 rose to 4.52 mmol/L after two hours. This difference, although slight, was significant (P<0.01) and persisted for eight hours.[105] These results could explain the absence of a relationship between elevation of blood insulin and incidence of coronary heart disease in populations such as Pima Indians and West Indians who enjoy a diet high in sugar but very low in animal fat. Conversely, they could implicate sugar as a risk factor for CHD in subjects on fat rich "western" diets with attendant serum cholesterol elevation.

The interactions between sugar and fats do not depend exclusively on complex biochemical relationships. Sugar has a direct positive effect on the palatability of many fat rich foods, notably as a result of the successes of the pastry-cook. When sucrose is added to the ingredients, including fats, used in the baking of cakes, pies and pastries, it raises the temperature at which white of egg solidifies and delays conversion of starch into a gel, thereby allowing cake to rise more effectively. The hydroscopic effect of sugar prevents undue drying during the course of baking and slows the chemical changes that predispose to later staleness. The overall consequence of these actions is to give baked goods that incorporate eggs or butter a longer shelf life and to make them lighter, more attractive and more palatable, qualities that make for increased consumption with an accompanying unavoidable higher animal fat and energy intake with all their undesirable consequences. Observations made by P M Emmett and K W Heaton showed that this is indeed the case. They surveyed 739 men aged forty to sixty-nine years and 976 women aged twenty-five to sixty-nine years. It was found that high sugar consumption with cakes and biscuits was associated with a correspondingly high fat intake. When the highest quartile of consumption was compared with the lowest, baked products provided men and women with an extra daily 12.0 and 13.8 grams of fat respectively.[106] In the late eighteenth century a corresponding increase in consumption would have consisted almost exclusively of animal fats.

Animal fats have for the most part been eaten with meat and poultry, in food cooked with dripping or lard, and in eggs and dairy products. The fat consumed in

[104] Kay-Tee Khaw *et al.*, 'Glycated haemoglobin, diabetes, and mortality in men in Norfolk cohort of European Prospective Investigation of Cancer and Nutrition (EPIC-Norfolk)', *Br Med J*, 2001, **322**: 15–18, pp. 16, 17.

[105] Kevin I Grant, Marielle P Marais and Muhammad A Dhansay, 'Sucrose in a lipid-rich meal amplifies the postprandial excursion of serum and lipoprotein triglyceride and cholesterol concentrations by decreasing triglyceride clearance', *Am J Clin Nutr*, 1994, **59**: 853–60, pp. 855–6.

[106] P M Emmett and K W Heaton, 'Is extrinsic sugar a vehicle for dietary fat?', *Lancet*, 1995, **345**: 1537–40, p. 1539.

baked goods and therefore with sugar has constituted but a small proportion of its total intake, most fat being eaten independently of any sweetening. In contrast, the association of sugar with cream on fruit desserts and with fat in cakes, pies and similar foods results in an overwhelming proportion of the sugar that is consumed being eaten together with fat. Even when sugar is used to sweeten tea or coffee, the addition of milk or cream results in some association. It is consequently possible to dissociate the effects of fat consumption from those of sugar, but virtually impossible to dissociate the effects of sugar consumption from those of fat. This would readily help to explain the negative findings of the Keys multivariate analysis. Keys drew attention to the rising incidence of coronary heart disease in both the United Kingdom and the United States during the first half of the twentieth century when fat consumption in both countries rose considerably but sugar consumption changed very little. This does not exonerate sugar as a risk factor. Theoretically, if both sugar and animal fats were risk factors and sugar consumption held constant while fat consumption increased, the incidence of CHD would rise. Longitudinal studies of food consumption would only exonerate sugar if a society could be found in which fat intake was constant, sugar consumption rose but coronary heart disease incidence did not change. Such a society is unlikely ever to exist. The observations of Keys therefore, while not implicating sugar as a risk factor, certainly do not exclude it.[107]

In conclusion, excessive sugar intake is conducive to obesity and results in surges in serum insulin levels with an eventual increase in insulin resistance. The results of experimental dietary studies suggest that, particularly in the context of a coincidental liberal saturated fat intake, high sugar consumption is followed by elevation of serum cholesterol as well as triglyceride levels. The relation of high cholesterol levels to increasing incidence of coronary heart disease is well established and recent studies have implicated liberal sugar consumption with serum triglyceride elevation, insulin resistance and rising glycosylated levels as well. All of these are established risk factors for CHD. The great increase in English sugar consumption during the Georgian era has been shown to coincide with a sharp increase in consumption of animal fats and reasons for a direct linkage between the effects of these two dietary changes have been demonstrated. The evidence therefore suggests that the dramatic rise in sugar usage in eighteenth-century England could be implicated as an ancillary factor contributing to the initial emergence of angina pectoris and its increasing prevalence thereafter.

## Coffee

The original home of coffee bushes growing in the wild was probably Ethiopia and it was there that they were first cultivated. The necessary knowledge spread initially through Persia and the medieval Arab world. The stimulating properties of the bean were recognized in antiquity and were the subject of many legends. One that originated in Arabia concerned herdsmen who observed that goats grazing on the berries of certain bushes became exceedingly frisky and gambolled the night

---

[107] Keys, op. cit., note 88 above, pp. 194–5.

through. This unusual behaviour was reported to the local clerics who had an infusion prepared from the berries, the drinking of which enabled them to forego sleep totally and to extend their religious devotions throughout the nights as well as the days.[108] Coffee eventually reached Europe by land routes, largely in association with Turkish conquests in the Balkans during the late Middle Ages. In 1683, after the siege of Vienna was raised, the liberated Austrian garrison found and took possession of supplies of coffee in the abandoned baggage trains of the formerly encircling Turkish armies. The subsequent re-occupation of once held Turkish conquests hastened its widespread dissemination throughout Christian Europe.[109] The process had already begun earlier in the seventeenth century, the first coffee house in England having been opened in 1652.[110] Production for the European markets surged with the development of colonial Spanish and Portuguese plantations in Central and South America that utilized slave labour.

The use of coffee was frowned upon by the Cromwellian government as part of the Puritans' opposition to anything undertaken for pleasure alone. There was a surge in its popularity with the 1660 restoration of the monarchy, but the government of Charles II viewed the newly opening coffee houses with some disapproval, suspecting, not without justification, that many were centres of subversion. An attempt was made to close them in 1675 but enforcement proved impracticable and did little to slow their growing popularity.[111] By the beginning of the eighteenth century there were over 2,000 coffee houses in London alone and their number continued to grow thereafter. Some moral disapproval continued notwithstanding the eclipse of Puritan influences in England, but this disapprobation was blunted by the growing recognition that coffee provided a popular non-intoxicating alternative to alcoholic drinks.

The coffee houses were almost exclusively a male preserve. They were frequented extensively not only by the nobility and the gentry but also by businessmen and professionals, writers and to some extent by working men. Some coffee houses were patronized predominantly by members of a single profession, such as physicians, clergymen or lawyers. Others were the meeting places of men engaged in a particular line of business, insurance brokers for example. They were post office collection and delivery centres, locations for dissemination of news and commercial information as well as for major business transactions.[112] Insurance schemes were operating out of coffee houses by the mid-seventeenth century. The best known subsequently was the one devoted to the arranging of shipping insurance and associated with Edward Lloyd, whose surname has remained synonymous with marine coverage to this day.[113] For aspiring but poverty stricken newcomers to London they provided a presentable address and contacts that could lead to gainful employment. The coffee houses often served as departure points for travel both by land and sea and as sources of

[108] E Robinson, *The early English coffee house*, 2nd ed., Christchurch, Dolphin Press, 1972, pp. 6, 7.
[109] Ibid., p. 5.
[110] Bryant Lillywhite, *London coffee houses*, London, George Allen and Unwin, 1963, p. 17.
[111] Robinson, op. cit., note 108 above, pp. 150, 166.
[112] Lillywhite, op. cit., note 110 above, p. 19.
[113] Ibid., p. 24.

information about the arrivals and departures of stage-coaches and ships. They were centres of literary activity, including readings of newly written plays, prose and poetry. Joseph Addison's contributions to the *Spectator* were penned for the most part in coffee houses. Some of their functions however were less salutary. There were ones which were centres for disposal of stolen goods, and outbreaks of violence within coffee house walls were not unknown.[114]

The multitude of activities associated with the coffee houses resulted in their being patronized, especially in London, by large numbers of men whose visits were frequent and often extended for a great part of the day. The coffee was continuously on the boil in eight to ten gallon pots and the cups or mugs of the patrons were constantly replenished. As a result, consumption was very much higher than is customary nowadays, ten or even more cups a day being not infrequent. Dr Johnson would drink a dozen cups of coffee at a time, and in this respect he was by no means exceptional. The coffee that was drunk was almost invariably black, very strong and taken with large amounts of sugar cut from a loaf. Coffee houses were associated with the smoking of pipes and the atmosphere was usually laden with tobacco smoke. Early in the nineteenth century, Lord Macaulay commented unfavourably on this. When its use spread to private houses, coffee was taken by ladies as well as gentlemen. Invitations to light refreshment, either in late morning or mid-afternoon, became popular. The addition of cream became usual and the jugs used for this purpose became known as creamers.

From 1697 to 1780 data concerning the coffee trade were compiled in the office of the government Inspector General of Imports and Exports. The Inspector obtained returns of both the quantities and the values of all merchandise brought into or sent out from each port and these were combined into annual totals for England and Wales. The data were assembled and tabulated by Elizabeth Schumpeter in a monumental work that embraced trade figures for almost all commodities used in the eighteenth century. The tables that she compiled give both the values and the amounts of coffee imported and re-exported during the eighteenth century, the difference between these two being a presumed measure of domestic consumption. Schumpeter's figures show a more than doubling of domestic coffee consumption between the first and fourth decades of the eighteenth century, net imports (imports minus re-exports) rising from 2,335 to 5,688 cwt, but with a subsequent decline, with retained imports fluctuating between 2,721 and 1,458 cwt during the following four decades. There are, however, cogent reasons for questioning these figures. Her tabulations showed considerable fluctuations from year to year, an extreme example being an excess of imports over re-exports of 11,402 cwt recorded for 1757 and an almost identical figure, 11,173 cwt, for excess of exports over imports for the following year. During the period 1774 to 1780 the numbers show an excess of re-exports over imports of some 12,300 cwt. This would imply that stocks of at least this magnitude were available in 1773 in order to meet these subsequent re-export requirements, a most unlikely possibility. In addition, there was a very dramatic rise in both imports and re-exports during this century. Any errors in these figures, even if minor, would

---

[114] Robinson, op. cit., note 108 above, p. 190.

affect the comparatively small differences between them in a highly significant way. It is hardly credible that the tenfold increase in the documented coffee imports would be unassociated with some corresponding rise in domestic consumption.[115] Smuggling was rampant at the time and the quantities of goods imported illegally very large. The highest in the land were not averse to purchasing the products of such landings.[116] It is therefore likely that the amount of coffee brought into England during the eighteenth century increased to a much greater extent than the Inspector General's figures suggest. Statistics for the whole country would also have failed to reflect changes in consumption by a part of the population such as the middle and upper classes. It was their members who provided most of the coffee house patronage. Their per capita coffee consumption probably exceeded the national average.

An assessment of the possible contribution of increased coffee consumption to the eighteenth-century emergence of symptomatic coronary heart disease requires, *inter alia*, consideration of the effects of caffeine and possibly of other constituents of coffee on cardiovascular haemodynamics and serum lipids. Caffeine increases blood pressure moderately, although with some attenuation of effect with continued use. It raises adrenalin and noradrenaline production, and activates the sympathetic nervous system.[117] In a review, Dag S Thelle and his colleagues noted that twenty-two investigator groups reported a significant positive association between coffee consumption and elevation of serum total cholesterol levels. In seven there was either no relationship or one that was demonstrated only in a subgroup.[118] The discrepancies reflect the difficulty in separating the effects of coffee from those of cream, sugar and tobacco, with all of which drinking coffee is closely associated.

Epidemiologic studies of the relationship between coffee consumption and incidence of CHD in its various clinical manifestations have been bedeviled by several additional difficulties. Estimates of coffee consumption depend on personal recollection of both the recent and the remote past and are therefore liable to be inaccurate. Retrospective investigations based on comparison of the coffee consumption of groups with and without known coronary heart disease are particularly liable to error. Apart from memory lapses, there may be a tendency for patients to understate coffee consumption because they think of it as a beverage of which the investigator disapproves. Individuals with a history of CHD may have reduced their intake of coffee when symptoms first became manifest. As discussed later, differing methods of preparation may have differing consequences. Cups of filtered or instant coffee contain less caffeine than cups made by adding boiling water to the ground beans, which was the eighteenth-century method of preparation. The relationship between the amount of coffee consumed and the caffeine intake can therefore be quite variable. An association between consumption of decaffeinated coffee with elevation of serum cholesterol suggests that one or more ingredients of coffee other than caffeine may

---

[115] Elizabeth Schumpeter, *English overseas trade statistics, 1697–1808*, Oxford, Clarendon Press, 1960, pp. 60–1.

[116] Ramsay, op. cit., note 82 above, p. 132.

[117] J L Izzo Jr *et al.*, 'Age and prior caffeine use alter the cardiovascular and adrenomedullary responses to oral caffeine', *Am J Cardiol*, 1983, **52**: 769–73, pp. 770–1.

[118] Dag S Thelle, S Heyden and J George Fodor, 'Coffee and cholesterol in epidemiological and experimental studies', *Atherosclerosis*, 1987, **67**: 97–103, p. 98.

be culprits.[119] Attempts to establish any connection between coffee consumption and incidence of coronary heart disease have unsurprisingly been inconsistent, yielding variably positive or negative results. Further review of the literature suggests, however, that coffee can under certain circumstances be a risk factor in its own right and contribute to a rise in CHD incidence. In the following discussion some concluding emphasis is placed on the consequences of many years of drinking of large amounts of strong coffee prepared by boiling, this having been the customary eighteenth-century practice.

The Framingham investigators were unable to find any overall association between reported coffee consumption and incidence of angina pectoris during a twelve-year follow-up. However, the results were confounded by a direct relationship between the amount of coffee drunk daily and the number of cigarettes smoked, and only a small minority of the subjects drank six or more cups per day.[120] In contrast, the Boston collaborative investigation did show a significant increase in the standardized mortality ratio particularly when subjects consuming six or more cups of coffee daily were compared with abstainers. In this study, the significance remained even after allowing for traditional risk factors.[121] Andrea Z LaCroix and her colleagues studied 1,130 white males who were followed for periods ranging from nineteen to thirty-five years. Subjects were questioned every five years about the amount of coffee drunk in the recent past. The investigators found only a non-significant association between coffee consumption in excess of two cups daily and the incidence of coronary heart disease. Seven per cent of the study population who drank more than four cups of coffee daily had a relative risk of 2.77 (CL 1.37–5.59) when corrected for smoking habits and 2.49 when corrected for hypertension. The confidence limits were wide and, with multivariate analysis, the relative risk no longer reached significance, having declined to 1.77.[122] On the other hand, the results of a meta-analysis reported by Kawachi and co-workers yielded more positive results. The pooled relative risk of case controlled subjects drinking five or more cups of coffee a day was 1.63 (CL 1.50–1.78) as opposed to 1.00 (by definition) among abstainers.[123]

There is evidence to suggest that apparent inconsistencies can be explained by changes over time in the way coffee was prepared being introduced during the period covered by the studies and the differing methods having differing consequences. In this respect, Michael J Klag and his co-workers' findings were confirmatory. They initiated a study of the relationship between coffee intake and coronary heart disease in 1947 with an entry cut-off in 1964. 1,160 males and 111 females were enrolled and followed until 1986, with a median follow-up time of some thirty-two years.

---

[119] D J Naismith *et al.*, 'The effect, in volunteers, of coffee and decaffeinated coffee on blood glucose, insulin, plasma lipids and some factors involved in blood clotting', *Nutr Metab*, 1970, **12**: 144–51, p. 147.

[120] Thomas R Dawber, William B Kannel and Tavia Gordon, 'Coffee and cardiovascular disease, observations from the Framingham study', *N Engl J Med*, 1974, **291**: 871–4, pp. 872, 873.

[121] Hershel Jick *et al.*, 'Coffee and myocardial infarction. A report from the Boston Collaborative Drug Surveillance Program', *N Engl J Med*, 1973, **289**: 63–7, p. 65.

[122] Andrea Z LaCroix *et al.*, 'Coffee consumption and the incidence of coronary heart disease', *N Engl J Med*, 1986, **315**: 977–82, p. 979.

[123] Ichiro Kawachi, G A Colditz, C B Stone, 'Does coffee drinking increase the risk of coronary heart disease? Results from a meta-analysis', *Br Heart J*, 1994, **72**: 269–75, p. 270.

## Chapter V

### Table V.11
Coffee consumption, serum cholesterol and CHD mortality.
4–6 year follow-up
Norwegian men aged 35–54 at entry

| | <1 | 1–2 | 3–4 | 5–6 | 7–8 | ≥9 |
|---|---|---|---|---|---|---|
| Number of cups of coffee per day | <1 | 1–2 | 3–4 | 5–6 | 7–8 | ≥9 |
| Number of subjects | 870 | 1,651 | 4,995 | 5,845 | 3,481 | 2,556 |
| Mean total serum cholesterol (mmol/L). Adjusted for age | 5.80 | 5.96 | 6.15 | 6.25 | 6.37 | 6.56 |
| Deaths. Number | 3 | 6 | 29 | 45 | 42 | 43 |
| Deaths/100,000 observed years. Adjusted for age | 62 | 61 | 92 | 119 | 186 | 244 |
| Adjusted for age and cigarettes per day | 100 | 83 | 111 | 121 | 158 | 179 |
| Adjusted for age and serum cholesterol | 81 | 73 | 96 | 121 | 177 | 203 |

Adapted from Aage Tverdal et al., 'Coffee consumption and death from coronary heart disease in middle aged Norwegian men and women', *Br Med J*, 1990, **300**: 566–9, p. 567. (With permission from the BMJ Publishing Group.)

Consumption estimates were based on periodic questionnaires. Overall there was a significant stepwise positive relationship between coffee consumption and CHD incidence in all of its manifestations, the extent being directly related to the amount consumed. The results were not affected significantly by correction for traditional risk factors. Of particular importance, in view of the association of coffee with cigarettes, the relationship was significant among non-smokers. Most striking, however, was the impact of temporal factors. The risk associated with coffee drinking before 1975 was markedly higher than in later time periods and could not be attributed to changes in the amount being drunk. Consumption of subjects enlisted in their twenties rose till their early forties and then declined, but not below the level of their twenties. The declining risk coincided with changes in method of preparation with instant, percolating and filtering replacing simple boiling.[124]

The results of Scandinavian studies were similar. A survey in Norway involved 19,398 men and 19,166 women aged from thirty-five to fifty-four years and with no cardiovascular disease at entry. The study extended for a mean of about six years. Comparisons were based on the sixty-eight men and sixteen women who died from this cause during the follow-up period. The relative risk was corrected for age, serum total and HDL cholesterol concentrations, systolic blood pressure and smoking. The CHD mortality rate rose progressively and systematically with each step up in the number of cups drunk each day (Table V.11). Although not proven for women whose numbers were low, the increase in coronary heart disease mortality rates among men was significant.[125] However, the same investigating group found that six further years

[124] Michael J Klag et al., 'Coffee intake and coronary heart disease', *Ann Epidemiol*, 1994, **4**: 425–33, pp. 427–9.
[125] Aage Tverdal et al., 'Coffee consumption and death from coronary heart disease in middle aged Norwegian men and women', *Br Med J*, 1990, **300**: 566–9, p. 567.

Table V.12

Relative risks of death from coronary heart disease according to coffee consumption: 6 and 12 year follow-up

| | 6 Years | | 12 Years | |
|---|---|---|---|---|
| No. of Cups/Day | Relative risk* | Relative risk** | Relative risk* | Relative risk** |
| <1 | 1.0 | 1.0 | 1.0 | 1.0 |
| 1–2 | 1.8 | 1.7 | 0.8 | 0.9 |
| 3–4 | 1.8 | 1.6 | 0.9 | 0.9 |
| 5–6 | 2.2 | 1.8 | 1.1 | 1.0 |
| 7–8 | 3.0 | 2.5 | 1.1 | 1.1 |
| ≥9 | 3.3 | 2.6 | 1.4 | 1.3 |

* Adjusted for age, systolic, B.P., no. of cigarettes per day and HDL level.
** Adjusted additionally for total cholesterol level.

Adapted from I Stensvold, A Tverdal and B K Jacobsen, 'Cohort study of coffee intake and death from coronary heart disease over 12 years', *Br Med J*, 1996, **312**: 544–5, p. 545. (With permission from the BMJ Publishing Group.)

of follow-up greatly weakened the association between coffee consumption and CHD mortality (Table V.12). During the twelve years encompassed by the two studies, there had been a considerable change in Norwegian ways of preparing the drink. Straightforward boiling had been supplemented in large measure by filtering.[126] This raised the possibility that of all possible methods of preparation, boiled coffee has the closest association with increase in risk of CHD. The direct relationship between the quantity consumed and the total serum cholesterol level shown in the earlier Norwegian study was found to be an effect of boiled coffee that could be countered by filtration.[127] In a Finnish cross-over investigation with twenty-one healthy volunteers, I Ahola and colleagues found similarly that a minimum of six cups of boiled coffee daily for four weeks resulted in significant increases in total serum and LDL cholesterol and triglyceride levels, but there were virtually no changes in the lipid profile if the coffee was filtered as well (Table V.13).[128] The differences suggest that one or more potentially triglyceride and cholesterol-elevating constituents present in a cup of the boiled preparation are removed by filtration. It was in fact possible to identify fatty acids in the material retained in the filter. The findings with respect to serum lipids were subsequently confirmed in a study conducted in Holland by Rob Urgert and his associates.[129] Peter Zock and his co-workers also reported that the

[126] Inger Stensvold, Aage Tverdal and Bjarne K Jacobsen, 'Cohort study of coffee intake and death from coronary heart disease over 12 years', *Br Med J*, 1996, **312**: 544–5.

[127] Tverdal *et al.*, op. cit., note 125 above, p. 567.

[128] I Ahola, M Jauhiainen and A Aro, 'The hypercholesterolaemic factor in boiled coffee is retained by a paper filter', *J Intern Med*, 1991, **230**: 293–7, p. 295.

[129] Rob Urgert *et al.*, 'Comparison of the effect of cafetière and filtered coffee on serum concentrations of liver aminotransferases and lipids: six month randomised controlled trial', *Br Med J*, 1996, **313**: 1362–6, p. 1364.

*Table V.13*

Comparative effects of 4 week consumption of boiled and unfiltered or boiled and filtered coffee on serum lipid profile (mmol/L). Mean values $\pm$ standard error of means

|  | Baseline | After 4 weeks | | P value (comparison at 4 weeks) |
|  |  | Unfiltered | Filtered |  |
| --- | --- | --- | --- | --- |
| Total cholesterol | 5.6 $\pm$ 0.9 | 5.93 $\pm$ 0.24 | 5.57 $\pm$ 0.18 | 0.027 |
| LDL cholesterol | 3.8 $\pm$ 0.9 | 4.01 $\pm$ 0.19 | 3.68 $\pm$ 0.16 | 0.014 |
| HDL cholesterol | 1.4 $\pm$ 0.9 | 1.40 $\pm$ 0.08 | 1.46 $\pm$ 0.09 | 0.180 |
| Triglycerides | 0.9 $\pm$ 0.3 | 1.38 $\pm$ 0.22 | 1.12 $\pm$ 0.17 | 0.008 |

Source: I Ahola, M Jauhiainen and A Aro, 'The hypercholesterolaemic factor in boiled coffee is retained by a paper filter', *J Intern Med*, 1991, **230**: 293–7. (With permission Blackwell Sciences Ltd).

material retained on the filter paper includes lipids and its administration results in elevation of the serum total cholesterol and LDL levels (Figure V.4).[130] Other studies have implicated fatty acids esterified with the diterpenes cafestol and kahweol as the offending constituents, present in a variety of coffee beans and removed by filtration. H Heckers and his colleagues, for example, showed that when diterpenes were given orally to healthy volunteers their serum cholesterol levels rose.[131] Urgert and his colleagues found that the concentration of cafestol in percolated coffee was maximally 0.5 mg per cup and in instant coffee 0.2 mg, in contrast with a much higher average of 3.4 mg per cup of the boiled preparation.[132] These differences may account in some part for a negative association between coffee consumption and CHD incidence found in the United States where filtered coffee as well as instant preparations have largely replaced the boiled form.[133]

When assessing a possible relationship between coffee consumption and CHD incidence, the length of follow-up too may be of critical importance. Positive associations found in several relatively long-term studies have been described in previous pages. Table V.14 shows the results of a meta-analysis undertaken by Martin

*Figure V.4: (opposite)* Mean levels of serum total cholesterol, LDL, HDL and triglycerides before, during and after supplementation with lipid-rich coffee filtration fraction. Reproduced from P L Zock *et al.*, 'Effect of a lipid-rich fraction from boiled coffee on serum cholesterol', *Lancet*, 1990, **335**: 1235–7, p. 1236. (Permission granted by The *Lancet* Ltd.)

[130] Peter L Zock *et al.*, 'Effect of a lipid-rich fraction from boiled coffee on serum cholesterol', *Lancet*, 1990, **335**: 1235–7, p. 1236.

[131] H Heckers, U Göbel and U Kleppel, 'End of the coffee mystery: diterpene alcohols raise serum low-density lipoprotein cholesterol and triglyceride levels' (letter), *J Intern Med*, 1994, **235**: 192–3.

[132] Rob Urgert *et al.*, 'Levels of the cholesterol elevating diterpenes cafestol and kahweol in various coffee brews', *J Agric Food Chem*, 1995, **43**: 2167–72, pp. 2169–70.

[133] D E Grobbee *et al.*, 'Coffee, caffeine, and cardiovascular disease in men', *N Engl J Med*, 1990, **323**: 1026–32, pp. 1030–1.

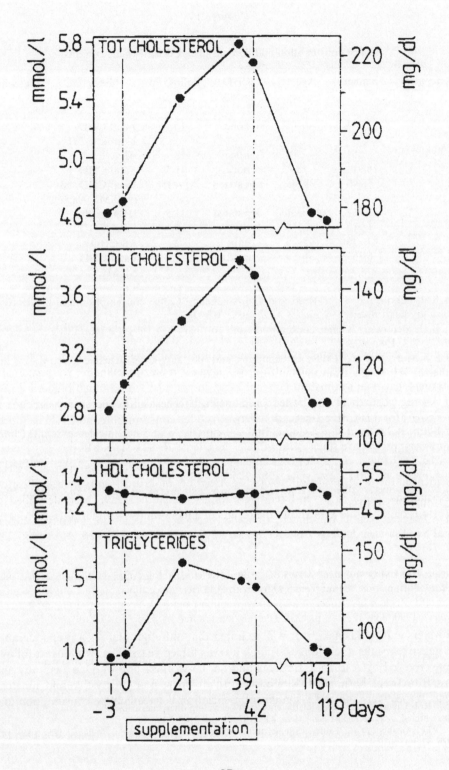

*Table V.14*
Coffee consumption and coronary heart disease: male subjects

| References | Numbers | Age at entry | CHD history | Follow-up (years) | Endpoint | Outcome |
|---|---|---|---|---|---|---|
| a | 7,194 | 46–65 | none | 15 | Fatal CHD Non-fatal MI | + |
| b | 851 | 50 | none | 12 | All MI | — |
| c | 16,911 | >35 | none | 11.5 | Fatal CHD | — |
| d | 1,040 | 19–49 | not stated | 19–35 | Fatal CHD, Non-fatal MI, Angina | + |
| e | 13,664 | not stated | not stated | 11.5 | IHD death | — |
| f | 1,910 | 40–56 | none | 19 | Fatal CHD | + |
| g | 44,736 | 40–75 | none | 2 | All CHD | — |
| h | 6,765 | 51–59 | no MI | 7.1 | Fatal CHD All MI | — |

a) Katsuhiko Yano, D M Reed and C J MacLean, 'Coffee consumption and incidence of coronary heart disease', *N Engl J Med*, 1987, **316**: 946.

b) S Heyden *et al.*, 'Coffee consumption and coronary heart disease mortality', *Arch Intern Med*, 1978, **138**: 1472–5.

c) S S Murray *et al.*, 'Coffee consumption and mortality from ischemic heart disease and other causes: results from the Lutheran Brotherhood Study 1966–1978', *Am J Epidemiol*, 1981, **113**: 661–7, p. 664.

d) Andrea Z LaCroix *et al.*, 'Coffee consumption and the incidence of coronary heart disease', *N Engl J Med*, 1986, **315**: 977–82, p. 979.

e) Bjarne K Jacobsen *et al.*, 'Coffee drinking, mortality and cancer incidence: results from a Norwegian prospective study', *J Nat Cancer Inst*, 1986, **76**: 823–31, p. 825.

f) Dan LeGrady *et al.*, 'Coffee consumption and mortality in the Chicago Western Electric Company study', *Am J Epidemiol*, 1987, **126**: 803–12, p. 807.

g) D E Grobbee, 'Coffee, caffeine, and cardiovascular disease in men', *N Engl J Med*, 1990, **323**: 1026–32, p. 1028.

h) A Rosengren and L Wilhelmsen, 'Coffee, coronary heart disease and mortality in middle-aged Swedish men: findings from the Primary Prevention Study', *J Intern Med*, 1991, **230**: 67–71.

Adapted from M G Myers and A Basinski, 'Coffee and coronary heart disease', *Arch Intern Med*, 1992, **152**: 1767–72, p. 1768. (Copyrighted (1992) American Medical Association.)

G Myers and A Basinski.[134] It will be noted that although there is a preponderance of negative results, their longest follow-up was fifteen years. The two longest follow-ups, reported by Andrea Z LaCroix and her co-workers and by Dan LeGrady and associates were both positive. Follow-ups of nineteen to thirty-five and nineteen years respectively showed a significant association between coffee consumption and

---

[134] Martin G Myers and A Basinski, 'Coffee and coronary heart disease', *Arch Intern Med*, 1992, **152**: 1767–72, p. 1768.

the incidence of CHD.[135] This all suggests that such untoward effects of coffee consumption may take very many years to become manifest. Shorter studies could well fail to show a positive association, however many subjects are entered into the trial. An example is provided by the negative results reported by Grobbee and his co-workers, who followed a cohort of 45,589 men but for only two years.[136]

In conclusion, the introduction of coffee into England in the seventeenth century was followed by a considerable increase in its consumption, especially by male members of the upper and middle classes. The evidence implicating coffee as a risk factor for development of coronary heart disease only appears to be inconclusive if it is considered without regard to other risk factors, method of preparation, duration and extent of consumption. Review of the recent literature suggests that drinking strong boiled coffee has an untoward effect on the serum lipid profile and its consumption in large amounts over a very long period, as was usual in the eighteenth century, is associated with increased risk of developing coronary heart disease. Moreover, the contribution of increasing coffee consumption during the Georgian era to the emergence of angina pectoris must be assessed not in isolation but rather in association with other risk factors. In this connection, any statistical consequences of dissociating the effects of coffee consumption from liberal indulgence in cream and sugar and exposure to tobacco smoke are not strictly relevant to the present postulate. What *is* relevant is the consequence of the eighteenth-century male consumption of very large amounts of concentrated boiled coffee over many years, usually in a smoke-filled atmosphere and in conjunction with excessive sugar intake and occasional use of cream. The evidence from the studies cited suggests that with this combination of factors coffee could have contributed to the emergence of angina pectoris upon the medical scene of Georgian England.

## Menus and Meals

Thus far, eighteenth-century changes in agricultural practice and their effects on the availability and composition of food have been reviewed. In the final analysis, however, the impact on cardiac health in Georgian England was determined by the meals that were actually eaten. Fortunately, data about this are readily available in cookery books of the time, in lists of food ordered for special occasions, records completed by diarists and descriptions of eating habits by foreign observers of the English scene.

Gargantuan meals that included large amounts and great varieties of animal foods had been usual among the nobility and gentry during many centuries preceding the Georgian era. The well recognized frequency of gouty arthritis may well have had among its causes grossly excessive consumption of high protein animal foods. It was observed of Charles V, the sixteenth-century King of Spain and Emperor of the Holy Roman Empire, that his inability to control either his appetite or the resulting

[135] LaCroix *et al.*, op. cit. note 122 above, pp. 979; Dan LeGrady *et al.*, 'Coffee consumption and mortality in the Chicago Western Electric Company study', *Am J Epidemiol*, 1987, **126**: 803–12, pp. 806–7.
[136] Grobbee *et al.*, op. cit., note 133 above, pp. 1030–1.

corpulence contributed in large measure to his final illness.[137] On 13 January 1663, Samuel Pepys recorded in his diary that at a dinner party which he gave, the guests partook of "a hash of rabbits and lamb, a rare chine of beef . . . [and] a great dish of roasted fowl".[138] On April 4th of the same year his visitors were provided with a meal that included, amongst other foods, rabbits and chickens, a boiled leg of mutton, a great dish of a side of lamb, and roasted pigeons.[139] Samuel Pepys and his guests were probably not exceptional in their eating habits, but only in the detail with which they were documented.

In 1688 Gregory King calculated that the yearly meat consumption of the population of England averaged about 72 lbs a year. He estimated, however, that the meat consumption of the more affluent members of society was more than double this, averaging $147\frac{1}{2}$ lbs per year. King defined the affluent as being members of a family whose head had an annual income of £12.18.0 or more.[140] The meat in all probability had the low fat content and composition characteristic of animals reared prior to the Agricultural Revolution.

When the present work was approaching completion, I had occasion to see in consultation a lady of forty with a complaint of chest pain, ultimately diagnosed as being of musculoskeletal, i.e. non-cardiac, origin. The patient lived in a heavily forested and remote part of the Canadian mid-west. She bought a package of frozen chicken parts about three times a year, but with this exception she was entirely dependent on venison for meat. Her husband would shoot a deer in the wild when occasion demanded and the family would have a couple of meat meals a week without having to stint themselves. She drank only 1 per cent milk, usually less than a litre a week, and had cheese no more than once a month. She rarely fried foods and used a soft margarine. Her carbohydrate consumption was very high; she ate half a loaf of bread every day and large quantities of noodles.

She was enormously obese. Her height was only 161 cm, her weight 154.2 kg and her body mass index 59.5. The blood pressure, measured with a wide cuff, was 130/70. Her total serum cholesterol was 5.2, HDL 1.59, LDL 3.16 and triglycerides 2.18 mmol/L. The total/HDL ratio was 3.27 and a random blood sugar 7.2 mmol/L.

In many respects the patient's diet resembled the eating patterns of wealthy people who lived unstintingly prior to the Agricultural Revolution. It shows that consumption grossly in excess of energy requirements and with a plentiful supply of meat obtained from animals grazing in the wild is compatible with a lipid profile that is completely normal, even by current stringent standards. It is illustrative of findings reported by Kevin O'Dea and his colleagues who studied ten volunteers for whom animal protein was provided by beef from which all visible fat was very carefully trimmed. "Ordinary" beef in identical amounts was allowed during a

---

[137] William Robertson, *History of the reign of Charles the Fifth*, 3 vols, London, George Routledge and Sons, 1896, vol. 2, p. 531.

[138] *The diary of Samuel Pepys. Volume IV, 1663*, ed. R C Latham and W Matthews, University of California Press, 1971, p. 14.

[139] Ibid., p. 95.

[140] Gregory King, *Natural and political observations and conclusions upon the state and condition of England 1696*, ed. George E Barnett, Baltimore, Johns Hopkins Press, 1936, p. 38.

control period. In two weeks the substitution of low fat beef resulted in a reduction of serum total cholesterol from 5.84 ± 0.36 to 4.84 ± 0.31 mmol/L, and the LDL from 3.88 ± 0.44 to 2.82. The HDL rose minimally from 1.71 ± 0.18 to 1.60 ± 0.15 mmol/L. The total and LDL changes were significant, the HDL not so.[141] My patient's incidentally normal blood pressure and sugar add to the favourable prognostic implications.

Seventeenth-century eating habits were continued into the eighteenth, but with advantage taken of the greatly increased availability of animal foods. The changes in food characteristics that accompanied the Agricultural Revolution were welcomed with enthusiasm by the consumer, especially when costs were not a concern. B A Holderness calculated that by 1760 per capita meat consumption in England averaged 100.8 lbs a year.[142] Compared to Gregory King's 1696 estimate it was half as much again. It is probable that the consumption by the affluent, as earlier defined by King, increased proportionally to at least the same extent. In absolute amounts it would have been to a greater extent. Not uncommonly, an entire chicken was consumed at a meal by one person. The amount of meat and poultry eaten was proportional to a family's position in the social scale. In the eighteenth century gluttony was regarded as "honourable" and "handsome eating", a measure of the status of the host. A contemporary historian, commenting on Elisabeth Ayrton's 1765 recipes in *The cookery of England* (1974) refers to "the heroic days of English cattle when carnivorous gusto was virtually a condition of patriotism".[143]

The evidence in Chapters IV and V indicated that the changes from the seventeenth to the eighteenth century resulted not only in increasing availability, but, more importantly, in marked differences in the characteristics of the animal food that became available. In the earlier period eating to excess resulted for the most part in a surfeit in energy and protein intake. In contrast, the evidence reviewed earlier suggests that the food consumed in ever greater amounts during the course of the eighteenth century also contained ever increasingly large quantities of animal and therefore predominantly saturated fat. The changes were regarded by consumers as highly desirable, fatty meat for example being considered more succulent and tasty. William Cobbett, famed for his descriptions of English rural life in a slightly later period, remarked in 1828 that, "Lean bacon is the most wasteful thing that a family can use"[144] and he was by no means alone in his opinion. Even today, a greater appeal of fatty meat to the palate often dictates consumer preference, despite current knowledge of its potentially harmful effects on the heart and circulation.[145] With adequate means, the middle and upper classes were probably able to increase their intake of animal foods to at least the extent that is suggested by the reported rise in consumption in England as a whole. Meals taken by the affluent during the late eighteenth century frequently included a late breakfast and a substantial midday

[141] Kevin O'Dea *et al.*, 'Cholesterol-lowering effect of a low-fat diet containing lean beef is reversed by the addition of beef fat', *Am J Clin Nutr*, 1990, **52**: 491–4, p. 493.

[142] Holderness, op. cit., note 64 above, p. 155.

[143] Simon Schama, 'Mad cows and Englishmen', *New Yorker*, 8 April 1996, pp. 61–3.

[144] Julian Wiseman, *A history of the British pig*, London, Duckworth, 1986, p. 18.

[145] Adam Drewnowski, 'Sensory properties of fats and fat replacements', *Nutr Rev*, 1992, **50** (4, Part 2): 17–20, p. 18.

*Chapter V*

meal, possibly accompanied by some entertainment. After this there was often a dinner at four in the afternoon that would usually last a couple of hours or more and be followed by some late evening refreshment to conclude the day. The length of time spent at table contributed to excessive consumption. Meat in one form or an other was often a mainstay of every meal of the day and of many individual courses. Fridays were no longer different in this regard. Because of their fatty nature, the high proportion of lamb, duck and goose in the diet contributed in a specific way to increases in fat consumption, as did the greater availability and richness of dairy products. Hannah Glasse, writing in the mid-eighteenth century, mentioned a cook who used six pounds of butter to fry twelve eggs and commented, with what she must have thought to be relative austerity, that even half a pound would have been more than necessary.[146] Egg yolks were frequently used to enrich bread, butter, biscuits, cakes and pastries. Added sugar improved the palatability of cakes, biscuits and pastries, and if more were eaten there was inevitably a rise in consumption of sucrose as well as fats.

The eighteenth-century changes in the relative availability of different cereals were reflected in the new eating habits as recorded by contemporary writers. As dietary staples, wheaten loaves replaced oatmeal, oat cakes and rye bread. However, the cart must not be put before the horse, even if eating oats. The agricultural innovations were to a large extent driven by changing tastes and fashions in food. The increasing demand for wheaten loaves was accompanied by an expectation that they should be as light in colour as possible. White bread was considered more attractive in appearance, more palatable and digestible, less flatugenic and of greater food value. In contrast, because of the bulkier stools associated with high intake of coarse grains, they were thought to have poorer nutritional qualities.[147] Eating white bread was considered a mark of refinement and gentility, while dark breads were "common". With improvements in milling techniques the demand was being met by removal of the husks to an ever increasing extent.[148] Wheat ground in this way replaced coarse grains in the flour used for making biscuits, cakes and pastries as well as bread. The changes were earlier and greater among the prosperous than among the poor who could only follow the example of their "betters" if and when they could afford so to do.[149] These eighteenth-century dieting innovations suggest that in all probability there was at that time a reduction in the consumption of fibre, particularly among the upper and middle classes.

Country gentry were reportedly prodigious meat eaters. In 1731 Lord Hervey partook of a dinner that included beef, venison, geese and turkeys.[150] The Reverend

---

[146] Hannah Glasse, *The art of cookery made plain and easy*, facsimile reprint of 1796 ed., Hamden, CT, Archon Books, 1971.

[147] J C Drummond and Anne Wilbraham, *The Englishman's food*, London, Readers Union and Jonathan Cape, 1959, p. 212.

[148] W A Armstrong and J P Huzel, 'Food, shelter and self help', in G E Mingay (ed.) *The agrarian history of England and Wales, Volume VI: 1750–1850*, Cambridge University Press, 1989, pp. 731–2.

[149] Jennifer Tann, 'Corn milling', in G E Mingay (ed.) *The agrarian history of England and Wales, Volume VI: 1750–1850*, Cambridge University Press, 1989, pp. 404–9.

[150] H J Habbakuk, 'England's nobility', in Daniel A Baugh (ed.), *Aristocratic government and society in England*, New York, Francis Watts, 1975, p. 100.

Woodforde kept an eighteenth-century diary in which meals figured prominently. He described an weekday dinner in which he was served boiled chicken and tongue, bacon, stewed beef and roasted venison. Roasted duck and leveret were part of a second course. Another time, he partook of a dinner which included a boiled turkey, roasted saddle of lamb, beef steak pie, slices of veal and roast chicken. On an occasion when he entertained neighbours to a dinner, it included ham, boiled chickens, a leg of mutton and a goose.[151] Like Samuel Pepys, Parson Woodforde was probably not exceptional in his daily eating habits, but only in the detail with which he documented them. His niece Nancy could not only rival him at the table but showed the not uncommon eighteenth-century ability to overcome speedily any temporary indisposition that might have interfered with gluttonous eating habits. She once developed abdominal pains and vomiting after a meal that included beef that was rather fat, a good deal of roast duck and a dessert that included raspberries with cream. Nancy recovered after being treated by her Reverend uncle with large quantities of rum. By the next day she was partaking of roast neck of mutton.[152]

Pastor Woodforde's "ordinary" meals pale into insignificance in comparison with celebratory repasts. The Duke of Marlborough commemorated the birth of his fourth son with a supper that included roast beef, mutton, pork, veal, pork and mutton pies, chicken, ducks, geese and tongue. Without knowledge of the number of guests, the amounts consumed by each person cannot be ascertained. However, the list gives an excellent idea of the relative importance of the various foods. Not listed above but noteworthy, apart from the large variety of meat and poultry, is the limited amount of fish and the low proportion of green vegetables on the menu.

Green vegetables constituted only a relatively small part of the ingredients of the meals described in books of the era such as that of Hannah Glasse, published in 1796.[153] The newly urbanized affluent classes could no longer depend exclusively on vegetables grown in their own gardens. They had to rely largely on market gardens and there was some aversion to use of their produce because of the conditions under which they were transported. The wagons that brought vegetables into the towns were utilized on the return journey for carrying night soil from the cesspools and privies of London back to the country for use as fertilizer. Despite washing, knowledge of this practice reduced the attractiveness of greens as food and heightened health concerns. Vegetables in the diet were associated with flatulence and their tendency to produce bulky stools was thought to indicate a lack of nutritive value. For all of these reasons they were not held in high regard by the more "refined" members of society and were "distrusted" by most medical experts of the day.[154] Appreciation of vegetables for their nutritive value only began to come late in the Georgian era. Green vegetables also had to compete for space on the plate with the newly introduced

---

[151] *The diary of a country parson 1788–1792, The Reverend James Woodforde*, ed. John Beresford, 3 vols, Oxford University Press, 1927, vol. 3, pp. 208, 242, 279.

[152] Ibid., p. 217.

[153] Glasse, op. cit., note 146 above.

[154] Vincent J Knapp, 'The coming of vegetables, fruits and key nutrients to the European diet', *Nutr Health*, 1996, **10**: 313–21, pp. 314–15.

potato and with foods such as rice and sago that were arriving from faraway countries for the first time. As a consequence a mild form of "land scurvy" became recognized among members of the middle and upper classes during the eighteenth century. Low and possibly decreasing green vegetable consumption may also have been significant in view of what is now known about the resulting dietary low folic acid intake and consequent elevation of serum homocysteine levels. One can speculate too that the latter would also have been aggravated by the high consumption of meat and therefore of methionine of which it is a constituent. Taken in excess, this amino-acid can cause increase in blood levels of homocysteine, currently recognized as a cause of damage to the endothelium of blood vessels and a significant risk factor for coronary heart disease.[155]

Recipes of the period depict in detail numerous examples of evolving traditional tastes that took full advantage of the now readily available animal fats and the abundance of sugar. Some examples from Hannah Glasse's 1796 publication *The art of cookery made plain and easy* serve as illustrations.

### Different Sorts of Sauce for a Hare
Take for sauce, a pint of cream and half a pound of fresh butter; put them in a saucepan, and keep stirring it with a spoon till the butter is melted and the sauce is thick; then take out the hare, and pour the sauce into the dish.

### Sauce for a Boiled Turkey
Take as many oysters as you want ... in a stew pan ... some butter rolled in flour ... boil them up, and then put in cream in proportion ...

### To Fry Cold Veal
Cut it in pieces about as thick as half-a-crown ... dip them in the yolk of an egg ... and fry them in fresh butter ...[156]

Similar lavishness characterized the use of dairy products. In Hannah Glasse's 1796 recipes butter was a common ingredient of stuffing for a pig, used for basting rabbits and when preparing "ragoos" of beef. After being dipped in egg yolk, sheep's rumps were commonly fried in butter. Ever lavish, the eighteenth century can be described with justification as "the age of cream". It was used extensively in sauces, with meats and chicken, in entrées, with vegetables and desserts and with coffee.[157] Hannah Glasse, when giving instructions for preparation of a drink to accompany meals, advised using the thickest and sweetest cream obtainable together with double refined sugar. Her recommendations for making a butter cake are equally lavish. "You must take a dish of butter and beat like cream with your hands, two pounds of fine sugar well beat, three pounds of flour well dried and mix them in with the butter, 24 eggs, leave out half the whites and then beat all together for an hour."[158] The modern reader can almost sense the coronary arteries of eighteenth-century diners narrowing even as they ate.

[155] Douglas R Murphy-Chutorian *et al.,* 'Methionine intolerance: a possible risk factor for coronary artery disease', *J Am Coll Cardiol*, 1985, **6**: 725–30, p. 728.

[156] Glasse, op. cit., note 146 above, pp. 35, 142.

[157] Sara Paston-Williams, *The art of dining: a history of cooking and eating*, London, National Trust, 1993, p. 177.

[158] Glasse, op. cit., note 146 above, p. 310.

Table V.15

Relationship between relative weight and cardiovascular disease incidence. Non-diabetic, non-smokers, total serum cholesterol <250 mg/dl

| Relative weight* | Cardiovascular disease 26 year incidence/1000 | | | |
| | Men | | Women | |
| | No. | Incidence | No. | Incidence |
| --- | --- | --- | --- | --- |
| <110 | 56 | 125 | 191 | 105 |
| 110–129 | 75 | 200 | 199 | 121 |
| 130+ | 30 | 267 | 78 | 128 |

* Percentage of desirable weight, i.e. midpoint of weight range for persons of medium build at specified heights, based on Metropolitan Life Insurance Co. data.

Source: H Hubert *et al.* 'Obesity as an independent risk factor for cardiovascular disease. A 26-year follow-up of participants in the Framingham heart study', *Circulation*, 1983, **67**: 968–77. (With permission of the publishers (Lippincott Williams & Wilkins) and Dr H Hubert.)

The impact of these dietary practices on the incidence of obesity in Georgian England is discussed in Chapter VII. Here it suffices to note the well-established linkage of obesity with a high incidence of coronary heart disease. It is due in large measure to the association of excessive weight with other risk factors, notably hypertension and abnormalities of lipid and glucose-insulin metabolism. However, the Framingham study and insurance company data (Table V.15) suggest that when marked, obesity is by itself a significant risk factor with a stepwise relation between the extent of weight excess and cardiovascular disease incidence (Figure V.5).[159]

Eating on the scale described was not confined to the nobility, but also became a part of the way of life of the affluent among the growing eighteenth-century middle classes. Successful shopkeepers' tables were as well served as those of rich merchants. The physician and the man of law ate as well as the archbishop, and the landowning gentry as well as the nobleman with his broad acres. In contrast, with the exception of the potato, the newly available foods, and those with a high amount of fat content in particular, were far beyond the reach of labourers and their families. The great majority of them suffered from chronic nutritional deprivation, especially when harvests failed and the price of the bread that was their main staple rose precipitately. They may have even suffered a decline in the adequacy of their diets during the course of the eighteenth century. Many of those who remained on the land ate less well as the practice of having labourers board with the farmers that employed them

[159] Helen H Hubert *et al.*, 'Obesity as an independent risk factor for cardiovascular disease: a 26-year follow-up of participants in the Framingham heart study', *Circulation*, 1983, **67**: 968–77, p. 970.

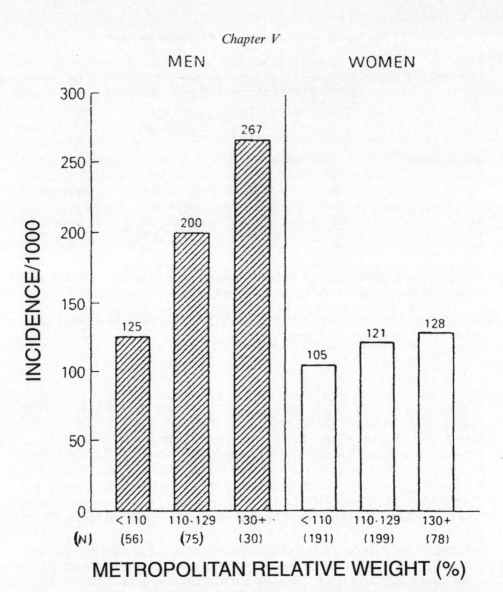

*Figure V.5:* 26-year incidence of cardiovascular disease by Metropolitan Life Insurance Co. relative weight. Framingham men and women below age 50, normotensive, with cholesterol below 250 mg/dl, not using cigarettes, no evidence of glucose intolerance. Number at risk bracketed. Incidence rates/1000 above the bars. Source: Helen B Hubert *et al.*, 'Obesity as an independent risk factor for cardiovascular disease; A 26-year follow-up of participants in the Framingham heart study', *Circulation*, 1983, **67**: 968–77, p. 974. (With permission of the publishers (Lippincott Williams & Wilkins) and Dr H Hubert.)

grew less common.[160] Indigent migrants from the countryside to the towns lost the small plots of land on which some food may have been grown or one or two animals

---

[160] B H Slicher van Bath, *The agrarian history of western Europe* A.D. 500–1800, transl Olive Ordish, London, Edward Arnold, 1965, p. 321.

kept. The plight of the labourer without work was even worse. The consequences of nutritional differences between the upper and lower classes can be gauged by comparison of their heights, a physical feature highly sensitive to any prolonged dietary inadequacies.[161] The stunted and delayed growth of sons of the impoverished working classes has been well documented and is detailed in Chapter III and shown in Table III.4. Their general health suffered, but in so far as a high incidence of angina pectoris is linked with prolonged dietary excess and a surfeit of fats in particular, the absence of this complaint among the labouring classes can be explained readily. The small shopkeepers and the skilled workers, the artisans, and their families ate somewhat better and their nutritional and general physical state and health may well have improved towards the end of the eighteenth century.[162] However, even for these people, eating on the scale of the affluent middle and upper classes was not usually affordable or practicable and they too were apparently spared the untoward cardiac consequences of the dietary excesses of the opulent.

---

[161] Roderick Floud, Annabel Gregory and Kenneth Wachter, *Height, health and history: nutritional status in the United Kingdom 1750–1980*, Cambridge University Press, 1990, p. 17.

[162] Ibid., pp. 140–1, 148.

# VI

# Tobacco

Well before 1492 the use of tobacco and its effects were known to the original inhabitants of what was to become the Americas. Europeans first made its acquaintance during Columbus' first voyage of discovery when two of his sailors observed natives in Cuba smoking the leaf.[1] Columbus was offered a bunch of the leaves, which were subsequently brought back to Europe. By the middle of the sixteenth century tobacco was being grown in Western Europe and had become generally available in countries fronting the Atlantic Ocean. Consumption increased rapidly from the mid-sixteenth century onwards.[2] Its initial introduction into England is traditionally attributed to Sir Walter Raleigh, although the story of his alarmed servant extinguishing the fire in his master's pipe with a bucket of water is probably apocryphal. As with sugar, mercantilist restrictions on trade with foreign countries delayed importation of tobacco into England on any scale until after the 1607 establishment of the Virginia colony, where plantations were developed using West African slave labour. Its popularity was enhanced initially because it was thought by some contemporary medical writers to have medicinal value, for chest diseases in particular.[3] These beliefs were countered to some extent by the classical 1604 *Counterblaste to tobacco* by King James I. Concerned with the physical and mental well-being of his subjects, he denounced smoking as "a custom loathsome to the eye, hateful to the nose, harmful to the brain, dangerous to the lungs".[4] His criticisms were remarkably prescient and today they would be regarded as eminently justified. However, attempts at prohibition having proved ineffective, English governments turned to the obvious alternative. They taxed all tobacco imports at the port of landing. Growing tobacco at home was prohibited and existing plants uprooted in order that revenue from import duties would not be foregone.[5] Yearly government statistics relating to imports are therefore available and reflect consumption. The economic disruptions produced by the Civil War temporarily reduced the availability of tobacco, but after the monarchial restoration of 1660 its importation, distribution and consumption rose very rapidly,[6] notwithstanding the royal censure by the now long dead James I.

Despite some marked year to year fluctuations, the documented net tobacco imports (total imports less re-exports) rose dramatically, from 25,000 lbs in 1603 to

[1] Jordan Goodman, *Tobacco in history*, London, Routledge, 1993, p. 37.

[2] Ibid., pp. 37, 59.

[3] Ibid., pp. 44, 61.

[4] Quoted in David Harley, 'The beginnings of the tobacco controversy: puritanism, James I, and the royal physicians', *Bull Hist Med*, 1993, **67**: 28–50, p. 43.

[5] Stanley Gray and V J Wykott, 'Tobacco trade in the eighteenth century', *Southern Econ J*, 1940–41, **7**: 1–26, p. 15.

[6] Ibid., pp. 19, 20.

over 18,000,000 lbs towards the end of the century.[7] If anything, the official figures are underestimates because smuggling was rampant.[8] By 1670, 25 per cent of the population was smoking at least one pipeful a day, annual consumption per head having risen from 0.01 lbs in the decade 1620–1629 to 2.30 lbs in the period 1698–1702 and then tended to decline slightly, to within the range of 1.56 to 2.00 lbs during the years 1738–52.[9]

Two major problems need to be addressed before possibly accepting the introduction and increasing use of tobacco as a factor that contributed to the initial emergence and subsequent rise in incidence of angina pectoris during the late eighteenth century. Firstly, tobacco was sometimes chewed and, during the reign of Queen Anne, taking it in the form of snuff became quite widespread.[10] Secondly, the twentieth-century association of coronary heart disease with tobacco smoking is associated almost exclusively with the use of cigarettes, whereas pipes alone were used in the eighteenth century. Pipe smoke is inhaled at a lower temperature than that of cigarettes and is alkaline, in contrast to cigarette smoke, which is acidic; the chemical content of the two forms of smoke therefore differ somewhat. Pipe tobacco products are absorbed more readily from the mouth into the bloodstream and the need to draw the smoke into the lungs is less. This could account for differences in localization of their carcinogenic effects. As a cause of death, the ratio of mouth to lung cancers is greater among pipe than among cigarette smokers.[11] Either way, however, nicotine is absorbed and pipe smokers obtain the same mildly stimulating, calming and euphoric effects that cigarette smokers sense. Because of this, pipe smokers might be expected to suffer the same undesirable systemic cardiovascular effects of nicotine as cigarette smokers, notably the sympathetic nervous stimulation and epinephrine release with a rise in heart rate and blood pressure.[12] Pipe smokers also absorb carbon monoxide with its potential for damaging vascular endothelium and inducing hypoxaemia. Noel Hickey and his co-workers found a mean carboxyhaemoglobin level of 3.2 per cent among thirteen pipe smokers, somewhat less than the 4.3 per cent in seventy-nine cigarette smokers who were comparable with regards to the extent of their tobacco consumption, but significantly greater than the 0.56 per cent average among non-smokers.[13]

The differences between the characteristics and the effects of pipe and cigarette smoke are counterbalanced to some extent by their similarities once absorbed into the bloodstream, so that reasons for any differing systemic effects on cardiovascular disease incidence are not readily apparent. Nevertheless, pipe smoking has been

[7] Ibid., pp. 18–23.

[8] Goodman, op. cit., note 1 above, p. 60.

[9] Ibid., pp. 60, 72.

[10] George Macaulay Trevelyan, *English social history*, 3rd ed., London, Longmans, Green, 1947, p. 315.

[11] E Cuyler Hammond, 'Smoking in relation to death rates of one million men and women', *Nat Cancer Inst Monogr*, 1966, **19**: 127–204, p. 151, 158.

[12] Joel G Hardman and Lee E Limbird (eds), *Goodman & Gilman's The pharmacological basis of therapeutics*, 9th ed., New York, McGraw-Hill, 1996, p. 192.

[13] Noel Hickey et al., 'Cigar and pipe smoking related to four year survival of coronary patients', *Br Heart J*, 1983, **49**: 423–6, p. 425.

*Table VI.1*
Male CHD death rates/100,000 person years: non-smokers and pipe smokers
(mortality ratios in parentheses)

| | Number of Subjects | | |
| --- | --- | --- | --- |
| Age | 45–54 | 55–64 | 65–74 |
| Never smoked regularly | 150 (1.00)* | 542 (1.00)* | 1,400 (1.00)* |
| Current pipe smoker | 141 (0.94) | 647 (1.19) | 1,396 (1.00) |

\* By definition.

Source: E Cuyler Hammond, 'Smoking in relation to death rates of one million men and women', *Nat Cancer Inst Monogr*, 1966, **19**: 127–204, p. 145.

implicated only inconsistently as a risk factor for coronary heart disease. Epidemiological studies relating tobacco consumption to any disease, cardiovascular or otherwise, are dependent very largely on information provided by the subjects themselves with all its attendant limitations. More importantly, people who have never smoked anything but a pipe are nowadays few in numbers, so that meaningful statistical studies become difficult and pipe smokers are often grouped together with cigar smokers in epidemiological investigations. Hickey and his colleagues observed the impact of smoking a pipe on the four-year survival of patients who had suffered either a myocardial infarction or an episode of unstable angina prior to entry into the study. During the follow-up 12.3 per cent of the pipe smokers suffered a CHD death, in contrast to 9.4 per cent of the non-smokers. With small and unbalanced numbers, 28 and 299 respectively, the differences show a trend but fail to reach statistical significance.[14] In an extensive study, E Cuyler Hammond was able to incorporate sufficient numbers of exclusive pipe smokers for overall comparison with non-smokers and for subgroup analyses. When compared to men who had never smoked regularly, no statistically significant differences in CHD mortality could be found (Table VI.1). However, in the combination of negative results with adequacy of numbers, this investigation is unique.[15] In contrast, a study involving British civil servants showed that men who were exclusively pipe smokers had a 40 per cent higher coronary heart disease mortality than did "never smokers". Although the pipe smokers numbered only 492 out of a sample of 19,018, these results were statistically significant.[16]

Exposure to secondary smoke was frequent in the eighteenth century. Ventilation of many homes and buildings was poor. Early in the eighteenth century, a tax based on the number of windows in a house had been imposed and as a result many windows were bricked up. Because coal fires heated only adjacent parts of the rooms, the need to keep the remaining windows closed in winter was often compelling. As

[14] Ibid., p. 424.
[15] Hammond, op. cit, note 11 above, p. 145.
[16] Yoav Ben-Shlomo *et al.*, 'What determines mortality risk in male former cigarette smokers?', *Am J Public Health*, 1994, **84**: 1235–42, p. 1237.

## Tobacco

### Table VI.2

Exercise duration to angina. Effect of exposure to tobacco smoke. Patients serving as their own controls

| Room status | Exposure status | Time to angina (seconds) | P value |
| --- | --- | --- | --- |
| Well ventilated | Smoke free | 232.3 ± 68.4″ | <0.001 |
| | Smoke exposure | 181.1 ± 52.4″ | |
| Unventilated | Smoke free | 233.7 ± 64.8″ | <0.001 |
| | Smoke exposure | 145.8 ± 36.9″ | |

Adapted from data published by W S Aronow, 'Effect of passive smoking on angina patients', in *N Engl J Med*, 1978, **299**: 21–4, p. 22.

a consequence air exchange and clearance of atmospheric tobacco smoke were presumably reduced. Exposure to environmental tobacco smoke was also a hazard in places such as coffee and ale houses where men gathered socially.

The differences in characteristics of pipe and cigarette smoke are lessened appreciably when they are inspired secondarily. The two forms are then at similar temperatures and inhaled in the same way. The harmful effects of secondary smoking are now well attested. A Judson Wells noted that the smoke-laden atmosphere in an indoor environment could contain as much as 50 parts per million of carbon monoxide, and commonly result in blood carboxyhaemoglobin concentrations of 2 to 4 per cent.[17] Wilbert S Aronow exercise tested non-smoking patients with stable angina pectoris in a room which was smoke free one time but on a second occasion contained the exhalations of three healthy volunteers, each of whom had smoked five cigarettes during the two hours before the exercising patients began their tests. Aronow found that when the subjects were stress tested in a smoke filled atmosphere they developed angina earlier in the course of the exercise and at a lower heart rate-blood pressure product. The effect of the smoky environment was greater when the room was kept unventilated (Table VI.2).[18]

A United States survey by Dale P Sandler and his co-workers showed that, when compared to male non-smokers living in a smoke-free home, the relative risk of coronary heart disease among non-smoking men living in a smoke-laden home atmosphere was significantly increased, with a risk ratio of 1.31 (CL 1.05-1.64). The results were obtained after adjustment for age, marital status, education and quality of housing.[19] Findings in the Boston Nurses Survey also confirmed an association between secondary smoking and coronary heart disease, both in its incidence and in the mortality. In a ten-year follow-up of 32,046 women aged thirty-two to

---

[17] A Judson Wells, 'Passive smoking as a cause of heart disease', *J Am Coll Cardiol*, 1994, **24**: 546–54, p. 549.

[18] W S Aronow, 'Effect of passive smoking on angina pectoris patients', *N Engl J Med*, 1978, **299**: 21–4, p. 22.

[19] Dale P Sandler *et al.*, 'Deaths from all causes in non-smokers who lived with smokers', *Am J Public Health*, 1989, **79**: 163–7, p. 165.

*Table VI.3*

Relative risks associating ischaemic heart disease morbidity and mortality with passive cigarette smoking. Meta-analysis results.

(95% confidence intervals in parentheses)

|  | Sex | No. of studies | Relative risk* |
|---|---|---|---|
| Morbidity | Women | 6 | 1.51 (1.16–1.97) |
|  | Men | 4 | 1.28 (0.91–1.81) |
| Mortality | Women | 8 | 1.23 (1.11–1.36) |
|  | Men | 5 | 1.25 (1.03–1.51) |

* Relative risk with no exposure 1.0.

From A Judson Wells, 'Passive smoking as a cause of heart disease', reprinted with permission from the American College of Cardiology, *J Am Coll Cardiol*, 1994, **24**: 546–54, pp. 549–50.

sixty-one at entry into the study, the relative risk of contracting any form of CHD was 1.91 (CL 1.113.28) among non-smokers who were regularly exposed either at home or at work. The differences remained significant after adjustment for other traditional risk factors. There was a dose-response gradient between frequency of self-reported passive smoking and cardiovascular risk.[20] A far-reaching review by Wells combined Sandler's study with seven others in a meta-analysis. This too showed secondary smoking to be associated with a significant increase in the relative risk of coronary heart disease morbidity among women and an increase that approached significance among men (Table VI.3). More than the men, the women in that era were in the smoke laden home atmosphere for longer periods. The greater effect of home exposure to tobacco smoke on non-smoking women is thus readily explained. The relative morbidity risk with passive smoking was significantly increased in both sexes.[21] The significantly greater impact of secondary smoking on male mortality as opposed to morbidity may reflect an effect on the severity of the disease as well as on its incidence. There is support from animal studies for this possibility. Karin Przyklenk produced myocardial infarction in dogs by coronary artery ligation. When compared to controls, the myocardial infarcts were larger among the dogs that had been previously exposed to tobacco smoke.[22]

Taking snuff and chewing tobacco are exceedingly rare in the twentieth century and the need to establish their effects on cardiovascular health have been minimal and therefore gone unstudied. Either would spare users the harmful effects of tobacco smoke, but they would still be exposed to the systemic effects of nicotine. The consequences of absorbing nicotine without smoke were shown by Lennart Kaijser and B Berglund who studied the effects of chewing 4 mg pieces of nicotine gum in eight healthy non-smokers aged between twenty-one and fifty-two years. In addition

[20] Ichiro Kawachi *et al.*, 'A prospective study of passive smoking and coronary heart disease', *Circulation*, 1997, **95**: 2374–9, p. 2376.

[21] Wells, op. cit., note 17 above, p. 550.

[22] Karin Przyklenk, 'Nicotine exacerbates postischemic contractile dysfunction of "stunned" myocardium in the canine model. Possible role of free radicals', *Circulation*, 1994, **89**: 1272–81, p. 1277.

to confirming the previously known rise in heart rate and blood pressure, these investigators studied the effects of raising myocardial oxygen demand by pacing the hearts of their subjects at increasing rates, coronary arteriovenous oxygen differences and haemodynamics being recorded throughout. They found that following administration of the gum, myocardial contractility increased and oxygen requirements rose more than would be expected from control observations of a pacemaker induced rise in the rate-pressure product. Additionally, when compared to the control observations, there was a relative increase in coronary circulatory resistance and the coronary arterial blood flow increase with pacing was blunted after chewing of the gum.[23] Because of these haemodynamic effects, smoke-free nicotine usage, as with snuff or chewing tobacco, has the potential to lower the threshold for angina in patients with established coronary heart disease.

In conclusion, there is good historical evidence to indicate that tobacco consumption increased very considerably during the lead time for the eighteenth-century appearance of angina pectoris as a new clinical entity. One suspects that there is some connection between the two and that despite insufficient epidemiological support, grounds exist for incriminating the use of snuff, chewing tobacco and pipe smoking. Recent observations have established that exposure to secondary smoke is a risk factor for coronary heart disease, and this association may be one way in which eighteenth-century pipe smoking and emergence of angina pectoris might have been linked.

[23] Lennart Kaijser and B Berglund, 'Effect of nicotine on coronary blood-flow in man', *Clin Physiol*, 1985, **5**: 541–52, pp. 549–50.

# VII

# High Blood Pressure

In 1733 the Reverend Stephen Hales cannulated a mare's carotid artery using a goose's trachea to which an eleven foot upright glass tube was attached. The blood rose in the tube to a height of eight feet three inches above the level of the left ventricle.[1] No other direct ways of recording blood pressure and no indirect means were devised before the end of the eighteenth century even though a "hard" artery difficult to compress when taking the pulse had long been recognized. The incidence and severity of high blood pressure during the Georgian era will therefore never be known. However, it is possible to garner information about the changing eighteenth-century incidence of factors now known to be associated with blood pressure elevation, notably age, smoking, obesity and some specific aspects of diet. The changing age structure of the population of eighteenth-century England was reviewed in Chapter III where it was shown that there was a rise in the absolute numbers of people living to middle and old age. The growth in tobacco usage at the turn of the eighteenth century has been detailed in the previous chapter where a connection between nicotine absorption and blood pressure elevation was noted. Consideration of other factors conducive to high blood pressure follows.

## Obesity

The gargantuan meals that were consumed by members of eighteenth-century English society have been described above. The resulting obesity did not escape contemporary notice. It received considerable attention in the cartoons of Thomas Rowlandson, the engravings of William Hogarth and the caricatures of James Gillray (Illustrations 6–8). Rowlandson's depiction of feasting aldermen (Illustration 7) and Gillray's caricature of the Prince of Wales (Illustration 8) are exaggerations, but they have a basis in reality. The judge in illustration 3 shows a typical eighteenth-century example of fairly marked truncal obesity. Although gluttony and its consequences were subject to criticism by contemporary moralists, both religious and secular, being overweight was not generally viewed askance in the Georgian era, attitudes towards corpulence contrasting with those of later times. "The boards of the rich remained mountainous and unsubtle."[2]

One detailed record of people's weights in the eighteenth century has been preserved. Messrs Berry Brothers, a firm of wine and coffee merchants founded in 1698, installed a beam scale in their London shop for the exclusive use of their customers (Illustration 9). Beginning in the early eighteenth century their patrons weighed themselves year

---

[1] George Pickering, 'Systemic arterial hypertension', in A P Fishman and D W Richards (eds), *Circulation of the blood: men and ideas*, New York, Oxford University Press, 1964, p. 489.

[2] Roy Porter, *English society in the eighteenth century*, London, Penguin, 1990, p. 216.

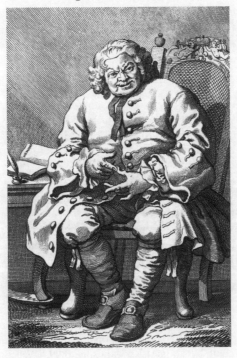

*Illustration 6:* Simon Fraser, Lord Lovat (1667–1747). Etching after W Hogarth (from the collection of Ronald Paulson, reproduced with permission).

by year and the results were duly noted in the firm's records. Note was made of whether the person wore ordinary clothes or an army or navy uniform. The scale is still in use and the firm continues to record the weights of its patrons. Unfortunately, listings prior to 1765 are no longer available and, with few exceptions, there is no information about the ages of the patrons. In 1884, Francis Galton used this source to publish data concerning the weights of 139 members of the greater and lesser nobility who were born in the eighteenth century. They were selected because serial measurements could often be obtained and the age of each subject ascertained readily from other sources. The initial average weights are not necessarily indicative of obesity, especially as the heights were not recorded, but the results indicate an overall considerable gain in weight after early adulthood (Table VII.1).[3] Unless underweight in early adult life, many must have been overweight by middle age.

My own perusal of the records from 1765 to 1780 resulted in a listing of the weights of some 305 men, civilian and military who were patrons of Berry Brothers. If serial weights of any individual had been listed, the first alone was tabulated. Shoes or boots had been worn while the person was weighed and occasionally military accoutrements were not removed. The weights are therefore over-estimates to some extent and they cannot be related to height, which, as noted above, had

[3] Francis Galton, 'The weights of British noblemen during the last three generations', *Nature*, 1884, **29**: 266–8, p. 267.

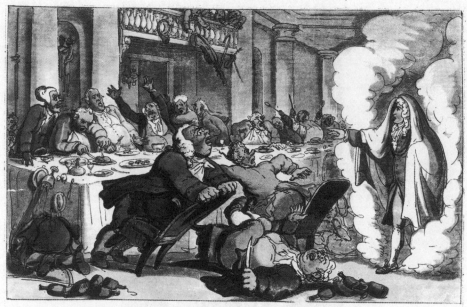

MANSION HOUSE MONIT

*Illustration 7:* A vision of the first of Mayor of London appears to feasting aldermen to warn them against luxury. Etching by Thomas Rowlandson, 1809. (Wellcome Library, London.)

*Table VII.1*
Average weights (lbs) of male members of the English nobility. Cohort born between 1740 and 1769

| Mean age (1st weighing) | Average weight | No. of observations* |
|---|---|---|
| 27 | 166 | 13 |
| 30 | 176 | 18 |
| 40 | 184 | 24 |
| 50 | 181 | 21 |
| 60 | 181 | 18 |
| 70 | 180 | 12 |

* These exceed the number of subjects as serial weights were obtained in some instances.

Source: Francis Galton, 'The weights of British noblemen during the last three generations', *Nature*, 1884, **29**: 266–8, p. 267.

not been measured. However, even with these limitations, the records indicate that obesity was certainly not uncommon. Forty-two of the 305 men weighed 200 pounds or more and four were in excess of 250 pounds (Table VII.2).

Examination of the association of hypertension with obesity has to take account of cuff artefact: apparently high blood pressure readings are observed when a cuff

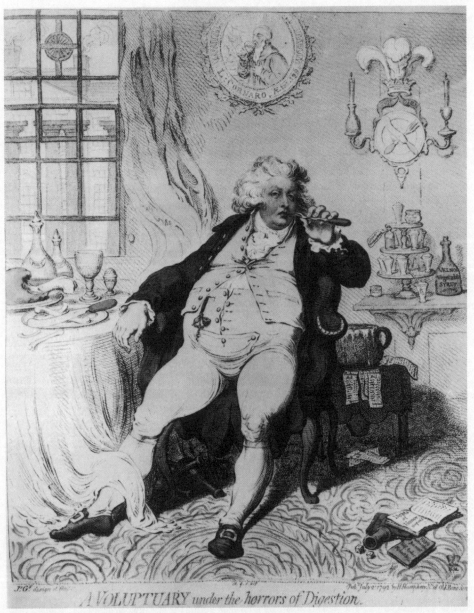

*Illustration 8:* 'A Voluptuary under the horrors of Digestion'. The Prince of Wales lingers over a meal at Carlton House. Caricature by James Gillray, 1792. (© Copyright The British Museum.)

of standard width is wrapped around an "outsize" arm. The pressure to which the cuff has to be inflated in order to compress the main artery in the upper arm is increased in this circumstance. However, the falsely high readings thus obtained can

*Table VII.2*
Weights of male wine store patrons, 1765–80

| Weight (lbs) | Number | % of total |
|---|---|---|
| <150 | 87 | 28.5 |
| 150–174 | 117 | 38.4 |
| 175–199 | 59 | 19.3 |
| 200–224 | 28 | 9.2 |
| 225–249 | 10 | 3.3 |
| >250 | 4 | 1.4 |

Based on author's perusal of Messrs Berry Brothers' and Rudd's records. (Permission for abstracting records given and facilitated.)

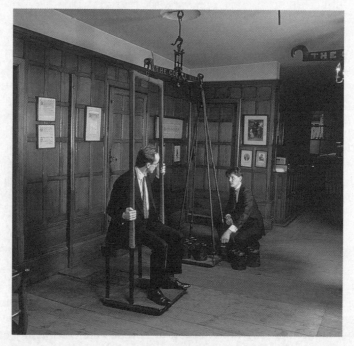

*Illustration 9:* The beam scale at Berry Brothers and Rudd Ltd. (Reproduced with permission.)

be avoided quite simply by use of a special wide cuff. With this measure an association of obesity with high blood pressure has been found to be independent of cuff artefact. As examples, this relationship was found in insurance company data (Table V.15) and in the Framingham study in which blood pressure was reported to be, among various risk factors, the "strongest correlate" with weight. Jeremiah Stamler and his colleagues recorded very highly significant positive correlations between weight and blood pressure, systolic and diastolic, in both sexes and at various ages.[4] A direct

[4] Jeremiah Stamler, R Stamler and T N Pullman (eds), *The epidemiology of hypertension: proceedings of an international symposium . . . Chicago, Illinois*, London, Grune and Stratton, 1967, p. 113.

causative relationship is suggested by the findings of Efrain Reisin and his colleagues who showed that even if salt intake is kept constant, overweight hypertensive subjects who diet successfully have significant reductions in blood pressure.[5] More specifically, Pirjo Pietinen and fellow workers undertook a comprehensive review of studies relating animal fat intake to blood pressure elevation. It was found that in populations as disparate as those of Finland and the United States there was a positive relationship between a diet high in saturated and low in polyunsaturated fat on the one hand and blood pressure levels on the other.[6] Conversely, other studies reviewed by these authors showed that increasing the P/S ratio was followed by a fall in blood pressure even if the total fat intake remained the same. The decline in systolic blood pressure ranged from 1 to 13 mmHg and up to 8 mmHg in the case of the diastolic. Switchback observations with reduction in P/S ratio were made in nine studies. In seven they resulted in an increase in systolic and diastolic pressures when the ratio was low.[7] The findings of J M Iacono and co-workers were confirmatory. They found that a six-week reduction in dietary fat content from 42 to 25 per cent with an *increase* in the polyunsaturated–saturated ratio resulted in a reduction in both the systolic and the diastolic pressures of normotensive healthy adult volunteers. The total energy intake was unchanged during the observation period.[8] Quantitatively, linoleic acid was the commonest polyunsaturated fatty acid in these diets. In experimental rats its administration has been found to have a diuretic effect, increasing sodium excretion, a precursor of blood pressure fall.[9] In contrast, Pietinen and colleagues have reported animal studies indicating that diets *deficient* in linoleic acid are associated with blood pressure *elevation*.[10] In combination these observations indicate a linkage of hypertension with diets conducive to obesity and either high in saturated or low in unsaturated fats.

### Fibre

The evidence for a decline in consumption of fibre by the middle and upper classes during the course of the eighteenth century was presented in Chapter V. A considerable body of evidence is indicative of an inverse relationship between fibre intake and blood pressure levels. Angela Wright and her colleagues compared the blood pressures of ninety-four subjects taking experimental diets that were consistently either high or low in fibre. At the end of four weeks the mean systolic and diastolic pressures

---

[5] Efrain Reisin *et al.*, 'Effect of weight loss without salt restriction on the reduction of blood pressure in overweight hypertensive patients', *N Engl J Med*, 1978, **298**: 1–6, pp. 2–4.

[6] Pirjo Pietinen *et al.*, 'Dietary fat and blood pressure—a review', *Eur Heart J*, 1987, **8**: Suppl B 9–17, p. 11.

[7] Ibid., p. 12.

[8] J M Iacono *et al.*, 'Reduction in blood pressure associated with high polyunsaturated fat diets that reduce blood cholesterol in man', *Prev Med*, 1975, **4**: 426–43, p. 443.

[9] J Rosenthal, P G Simone and A Silbergleit, 'Effects of prostaglandin deficiency natriuresis, diuresis and blood pressure', *Prostaglandins*, 1974, **5**: 435–40, p. 440.

[10] Pietinen *et al.*, op. cit., note 6 above, p. 13.

*Table VII.3*
Relationship between fibre intake and blood pressure

| | Number of subjects | Blood pressure (mmHg) | |
|---|---|---|---|
| | | Systolic | Diastolic |
| High fibre | 45 | 116 ± 1.5* | 75.2 ± 1.0** |
| Low fibre | 49 | 123 ± 1.3* | 78.5 ± 0.8** |

* P<.001 ** P<.02

Source: Angela Wright, P G Burstyn and M J Gibney, 'Dietary fibre and blood pressure', *Br Med J*, 1979, **ii**: 1541–3, p. 1542. (With permission of the BMJ Publishing Group.)

were slightly but significantly higher in the low fibre group (Table VII.3).[11] Their findings were subsequently confirmed in a study conducted by Lawrence Appel and his co-workers. At the end of a three week run in and eight weeks of controlled diets, volunteer subjects whose blood pressures were initially comparable diverged. The control subjects who were continued on a typical North American diet ended with mean blood pressures higher than those of the subjects whose diet was enriched in fibre.[12] Together the two studies indicate that a diet lacking in fibre is conducive to blood pressure elevation, both systolic and diastolic.

## Salt

Salt is the only condiment which is a physiological necessity. Concern about harmful effects of high consumption arose only in the twentieth century. Salt as a supplement had been deemed invaluable as a preservative and esteemed from the early days of recorded history.[13] It was included in sacrifices in early biblical times when inviolable obligations were designated salt covenants.[14] Homer considered the salt with which the meat of celebratory feasts was sprinkled to be divine.[15] Its commercial importance in Roman times is attested by the designation of money given to soldiers for salt (*sal*) as *salarium* from which the word salary is derived. Until recently a person in authority visiting a community would often be offered bread and salt as a ceremonial expression of welcome and a form of homage.

In medieval and Tudor times salt was produced exclusively by evaporation of sea water in maritime basins.[16] In England the climate prevented this from occurring naturally to a reliable extent as in Mediterranean countries, and evaporation depended

[11] Angela Wright, P G Burstyn and M J Gibney, 'Dietary fibre and blood pressure', *Br Med J*, 1979, **ii**: 1541–3, p. 1542.
[12] Lawrence J Appel *et al.*, 'A clinical trial of the effects of dietary patterns on blood pressure', *N Engl J Med*, 1997, **336**: 1117–24, p. 1122.
[13] S A M Adshead, *Salt and civilization*, New York, St Martin's Press, 1992, pp. 25, 27.
[14] Leviticus, 2:13; Numbers 18:19.
[15] Homer, *Iliad*, 9.214.
[16] Adshead, op. cit., note 13 above, p. 86.

on heating sea water with charcoal. The salt pans were made of lead, which limited the temperatures that could be attained. Charcoal was relatively inefficient as a fuel and its use contributed to the denudation of forests, resulting in a growing scarcity by the start of the eighteenth century. However, coal was then substituted for charcoal, the change being facilitated by improvement in mining methods and in transport facilities, both by sea and through inland waterways. At about the same time there was a considerable improvement in evaporative techniques with construction of larger iron salt pans that could withstand higher temperatures. More important, however, was the discovery of rock salt in Cheshire in 1670 with exploitation of the deposits in that county and subsequently, and to a somewhat lesser extent, in nearby Worcestershire. The salt was either mined directly or extracted by pouring water into the mines in order to produce a brine which was then pumped up to the surface, a process facilitated by the newly invented steam powered pumps.[17] Transport of the final product became easier with improvements in waterway management, notably the changes which made the River Weaver navigable so that Cheshire's salt could be shipped to Liverpool and thence by sea to other parts of the country and points beyond.[18]

Records of eighteenth-century salt production are based largely on figures documented by excise officers. These, however, were subject to considerable error. Scales were not always accurate, excise officers were inefficient, the desire of merchants to evade taxes great and weight checks inaccurate, especially when dealing with salt imports. When ships were loaded or unloaded it was often difficult to distinguish between coastal and foreign traffic.[19] Despite the resulting underestimation of salt production in official statistics, the numbers indicate a dramatic increase in output during the eighteenth century. Total English salt production in 1700 was estimated at 500,000 cwt. It rose eightfold during the eighteenth century. By 1796, 2 million cwt of Cheshire salt alone was being shipped through the River Weaver outlet.[20] Its importance to the national economy can be gauged by the fact that in 1696 a £2,500,000 government loan from the Bank of England was secured by the anticipated salt duties.[21]

The dramatic rise in salt production during the eighteenth century is indicative of a considerable rise in individual consumption. In addition to being used as a condiment, it was utilized extensively as the only means of preserving meat, fish and dairy products such as butter and cheese. A rise in salt intake was consequently an inevitable accompaniment to the increasing consumption of these foods. The eightfold eighteenth-century growth in production calculated by Adshead far exceeded the rate of population growth and therefore indicated a doubling of average daily intake per head, from about 14 grams of salt in 1700 to 28 grams by 1800.[22] The overall impression is of a very considerable rise in salt consumption during the eighteenth

[17] Ibid., pp. 378, 385, 398.
[18] Ibid., pp. 105–6.
[19] Edward Hughes, *Studies in administration and finance 1558–1825*, Philadelphia, Porcupine Press, 1934, pp. 308, 364–5.
[20] Ibid., p. 114.
[21] Ibid., p. 171.
[22] Adshead, op. cit., note 13 above, p. 21.

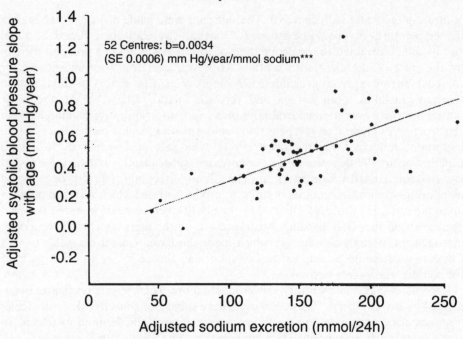

*Figure VII.1a*

century, with some subsequent levelling off, at amounts that would now be considered excessive.

The relationship of hypertension to salt consumption is complex. Studies of pre-industrial populations with low salt consumption have shown that sodium intake averaging below 30 mEq per person per day is compatible with good health and in such communities blood pressure does not rise with age. In striking contrast were the results of a study of the Lau, a people living on very small Solomon Islands in the Western Pacific. They were fishermen who differed from neighbouring islanders by using salty coastal water to prepare meals, and their daily intake of sodium of 150 to 230 mmol/day was in consequence much the greater. The Lau as a group had systolic and diastolic pressures that were higher than those of the adjacent islanders, consistent with an association of generous salt intake with elevation of blood pressure.[23] A comparative interstate study of westernized countries that included all continents except Australasia showed that both systolic and diastolic blood pressures, were positively correlated with salt excretion, the latter being a good indirect measure of intake (Figures VII.1a and 1b).[24] Lillian Gleibermann's conclusions were similar.

[23] Lot B Page, Albert Damon and Robert Moellering Jr, 'Antecedents of cardiovascular disease in six Solomon Islands societies', *Circulation*, 1974, **49**: 1132–46, p. 1136.
[24] Interstate Cooperative Research Group, 'Intersalt: an international study of electrolyte excretion and blood pressure. Results for 24-hour urinary sodium and potassium excretion', *Br Med J*, 1988, **297**: 319–28, p. 323.

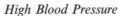

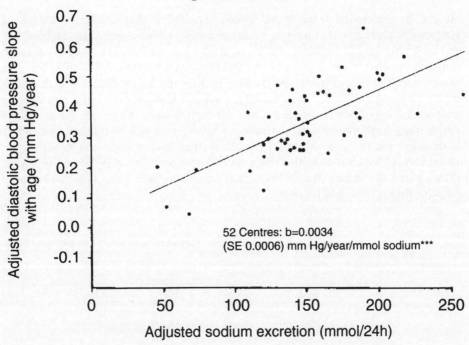

*Figures VII.1a and 1b:* Relation of age changes in blood pressure to daily sodium excretion as a reflection of salt intake. Adjusted for body mass index, age, sex and alcohol intake. Source: Interstate Cooperative Research Group, 'Intersalt: an international study of electrolyte excretion and blood pressure. Results for 24-hour urinary sodium and potassium excretion', *Br Med J*, 1988, **297**: 319–28, p. 323. (With permission from the BMJ Publishing Group.)

In a review of twenty-seven worldwide populations she found that, with few exceptions, salt excretion and hence intake correlated positively with blood pressure levels.[25]

In a comprehensive review, Martin Muntzel and Tilman Drüeke reported considerable individual variability in blood pressure responses following dietary salt restriction. Depending on variation in compensation mechanisms, the mean arterial pressure could increase, decrease or remain more or less unchanged but with decrease being the most frequent.[26] Overall, the evidence indicates that in communities with a high average salt consumption there will be considerable variations in blood pressure levels, but some part of the population will be salt sensitive and become hypertensive, the tendency increasing with age, as is usual in developed societies. Muntzel and Drüeke noted that the sensitivity is greater in elderly subjects and in the obese.[27]

[25] Lillian Gleibermann, 'Blood pressure and dietary salt in human populations', *Ecol Food Nutr*, 1973, **2**: 143–56, p. 144.
[26] Martin Muntzel and Tilman Drüeke, 'A comprehensive review of the salt and blood pressure relationship', *Am J Hypertens*, 1992, **5**: Suppl 4, 1S–42S, p. 7.
[27] Ibid., 26S.

It can be concluded from twentieth-century studies that a high incidence of hypertension characterizes an aging and increasingly obese community, especially if combined with liberal consumption of saturated animal fats, low polyunsaturated fat intake, increasing use of salt and reduced fibre consumption. All of these features characterized the way of life of the growing middle and upper classes of eighteenth-century England and raise the possibility, even if not measurable, of a rise in their incidence of hypertension at that time. Its significance relates to the status of hypertension, both systolic and diastolic, as a long and well-established risk factor for development of coronary heart disease in men and women and in all of the clinical ways in which it presents.[28] We cannot know what blood pressure levels were in the eighteenth century. We do know that much was then being done unwittingly to ensure that they would be raised.

[28] William Kannel, 'Role of blood pressure in cardiovascular disease: the Framingham study', *Angiology*, 1975, **26**: 1–14, p. 5.

# VIII

# Stress

A 1794 biographer commenting on the angina pectoris suffered by John Hunter, the distinguished experimentalist, surgeon and pathologist, wrote, "It is a curious circumstance that the first attack of these complaints was produced by an affection of the mind and every future return of any consequence arose from the same cause". John Hunter himself remarked prophetically that his life was in the hands of any rascal who chose to annoy him, and in this matter he was indeed prescient. His death occurred suddenly in 1793 during a violent altercation during which he was trying to control his anger.[1] The importance of mental stress as a coronary heart disease risk factor has continued to be recognized.[2] However, the extent to which increasing societal stresses may have played a significant part in the eighteenth-century evolution of coronary heart disease is not easily determined. The risk factors that have been considered so far lend themselves to measurement, even if Georgian era data are imprecise by present day standards or have to be deduced. In contrast, even today, assessment of the possible causes of stresses and their severity remain largely subjective and difficult to quantify. Notwithstanding these difficulties, the importance of stress (individual types of which are considered presently) as a factor conducive to development of CHD is strongly suggested by late-twentieth-century studies and the pathophysiological mechanisms have been elucidated.[3] For the most part these investigations have been conducted at a time when high animal fat consumption in the western world not only characterized the eating habits of the prosperous, but had recently become the norm among classes who were less well off, but enjoying a recent rise in living standards. During the eighteenth and nineteenth centuries, however, the poor had subsisted on diets lacking in animal fats and deficient enough generally to have affected their physical status in obvious ways, such as rate of growth and final height.[4] Despite their inadequacies, the low fat diets appeared to confer upon the labouring classes some immunity to symptomatic coronary heart disease as discussed earlier. It was a peculiarity of angina pectoris noted by Black as early as 1819,[5] by Osler as late as 1910,[6] and others in between. Other adverse health consequences of the stresses and strains to which the labouring

---

[1] E Home, 'A short account of the author's life', in J Hunter, *A treatise on the blood, inflammation and gunshot wounds*, London, John Richardson, 1794, p. lxi.

[2] Stewart G Wolf, 'History of the study of stress and heart disease', in Robert E Beamish, Pawalk Singal and Naranjan S Dhalla (eds), *Stress and heart disease*, Boston, Martinus Nijhoff Publishing, 1985, pp. 3–14.

[3] Ibid., pp. 7–14.

[4] Roderick Floud, A Gregory and K Watcher, *Height, health and history: nutritional status in the United Kingdom 1750–1980*, Cambridge University Press, 1990, pp. 140–1, 148.

[5] Samuel Black, *Clinical and pathological reports*, Newry, Alexander Wilkinson, 1819, p. 8.

[6] William Osler, 'The Lumleian lectures on angina pectoris, Lecture I', *Lancet*, 1910, i: 697–702, p. 698.

classes were then undoubtedly subject are therefore outside the purview of the present inquiry, however important in themselves. What is relevant here and therefore needs consideration is an examination of, firstly, the impact of the stresses to which the eighteenth-century middle and upper classes were subject along with the population in general and, secondly, the consequences of the strains to which they may have been uniquely subject.

The only eighteenth-century effect of stress that lends itself to direct measurement is the suicide rate. London deaths attributed to suicide were recorded weekly in the parish Bills of Mortality and summarized for the whole of the metropolis at the end of each year. The means of self-destruction included hanging, cutting the throat, jumping from a height, drowning, use of a firearm and poisoning. The numbers listed in the Bills are of necessity less than accurate. Unless the suicide was witnessed there could be difficulty in distinguishing it from murder, accident, or even natural causes. Families often felt a sense of shame and attempted to conceal the possibility that death was self-inflicted. There is, however, no evidence of any systematic change in the way deaths were recorded that would have affected the early- and late-eighteenth-century listings differently. The territory covered by the London Bills of Mortality changed very little between late Stuart and mid-Georgian times. There were 134 parishes included in 1690 and just 14 more by 1770. A transient surge in suicide rates during the 1750s has been reported.[7] On the other hand, my own perusal of the Bills, whilst revealing an increase in numbers in line with population growth, uncovered very little change in suicide rates between the late seventeenth and eighteenth centuries. During the periods 1691–95 and 1771–79 they numbered 16.9 and 15.8 per 10,000 deaths respectively.

Eighteenth-century factors that caused stress with outcomes less dramatic than suicide involved far greater numbers of people, and therefore warrant detailed review despite the difficulties to which reference has been made. The factors considered here are urbanization, emotional strains associated with upward mobility, financial worries, work insecurity, subordinate status, wartime worries and separation, bereavement and health concerns.

Twentieth-century studies in the United Kingdom, Norway and the United States (Tables VIII.1–3) showed that in the years before effective treatment, preventive and therapeutic, became available ischaemic heart disease mortality was greater among urban as opposed to rural populations.[8] The excess of urban over rural coronary heart disease death rates has been found not only among people born in the cities for whom town living did not represent any major change in their way of life, but among migrants from the countryside into the towns and residents of village

---

[7] Paul Langford, *A polite and commercial people: England 1727–1783*, Oxford University Press, 1992, p. 479.

[8] G M Howe, *National atlas of disease mortality in the United Kingdom*, London, Butler and Tanner, 1970, Appendix 2, p. 184; Øystein Krüger, A Aase and W Steinar, 'Ischaemic heart disease mortality among men in Norway: reversal of urban–rural difference between 1966 and 1989', *J Epidemiol Community Health*, 1995, **49**: 271–6, pp. 272–3; H H Hechter and N O Borhani, 'Mortality and geographic distribution of arteriosclerotic heart disease', *Public Health Rep*, 1965, **80**: 11–24, p. 22.

*Table VIII.1*

Ischaemic heart disease average annual mortality/100,000: male residents of S.E. English counties, 1959–63. Greater urban mortality indicated in bold type

| County | Mortality | |
|---|---|---|
| | Rural | Urban |
| Bedfordshire | 205 | **209** |
| Berkshire | 191 | **237** |
| Buckinghamshire | 221 | 218 |
| Cambridgeshire | 240 | 198 |
| Essex | 275 | 240 |
| Hampshire | 244 | **259** |
| Hertfordshire | 195 | **201** |
| Kent | 244 | **272** |
| Norfolk | 226 | **297** |
| Oxfordshire | 215 | **270** |
| Suffolk | 246 | **312** |
| Surrey | 234 | **268** |
| Sussex | 324 | **342** |

Source: G M Howe, *National atlas of disease mortality in the United Kingdom*, London, Butler and Tanner, 1970, Appendix 2, p. 184.

communities that were engulfed by growth of neighbouring cities.[9] During the eighteenth-century, English town dwellers grew both in absolute numbers and as a proportion of the general population, Londoners numbered 575,000 in 1700 and 960,000 by 1801.[10] In 1700, 13.3 per cent of the population lived in towns with 10,000 or more inhabitants. By 1800 the percentage had risen to 20.3.[11] However, it is difficult to apply the results of twentieth-century studies to eighteenth-century circumstances in the expanding towns. The differences are too great and in any case the upper and middle classes would have escaped the worst consequences of urbanization. Living as they did for the most part in the newly developed suburbs, they were well away from the areas of greatest crowding, noise and violence. They were also to some extent sheltered from the bustle and faster pace of life in the older and more central parts of the cities. Their sense of security was increased by distancing themselves from the areas of most violence and by improvements in street lighting.[12] Many retained country homes in which they spent part of the year. Irrespective of any factors that may now contribute to the higher incidence of coronary heart disease among town as opposed to country dwellers, there is no clear evidence of

[9] H A Tyroler and John Cassel, 'Health consequences of culture change, II. The effect of urbanization on coronary heart mortality in rural residents', *J Chronic Dis*, 1964, **17**: 167–77, p. 169.

[10] E Anthony Wrigley, 'Urban growth and agricultural change: England and the continent in the early modern period', *J Interdis Hist*, 1985, **15**: 683–728, p. 688.

[11] R A Houston, *Population history of Britain and Ireland, 1500–1750*, London, Macmillan Education, 1992, p. 32.

[12] Dorothy George, *London life in the eighteenth century*, New York, Harper and Row, 1965, pp. 95–6.

*Table VIII.2*

Ischaemic heart disease mortality among Norwegian men, 1966–70

| | Mortality/100,000/year | |
|---|---|---|
| Age | Rural | Urban |
| 40–49 | 121 | 141 |
| 50–59 | 350 | 455 |
| 60–69 | 918 | 1,221 |

Adapted from Ø Krüger, A Aase and W Steiner, 'Ischaemic heart disease mortality among men in Norway: reversal of urban–rural difference between 1968 and 1989', *J Epidemiol Community Health*, 1995, **49**: 271–6. (With permission from the BMJ Publishing Group.)

*Table VIII.3*

USA male urban and rural mortality. Age adjusted (No./100,000/year, 1959–61)

| | Mortality |
|---|---|
| 1. Rural | 349 ± 33 |
| 2. Lesser Metropolitan | 359 ± 28 |
| 3. Greater Metropolitan | 365 ± 28 |

$\chi^2 = 2.33$ P $= 0.52$ (comparing 2 & 3).

Source: H H Hechter and N O Borhani, 'Mortality and geographic distribution of arteriosclerotic heart disease', *Public Health Rep*, 1965, **80**: 11–24, p. 22. (With permission from Oxford University Press.)

any overall eighteenth-century impact of urbanization on upper- and middle-class liability to stress. Furthermore, as judged by twentieth-century studies, the heightened incidence of the urban coronary heart disease mortality rates was modest. In the United Kingdom it was only about 13 per cent in mid-century and unevenly distributed from county to county. Although in Norway the differences were fairly substantial, in the United States they were slight and not significant.[13] The three studies were selected because they were initiated, and in two instances completed, before medical management, prophylactic or therapeutic, had begun to have any impact on coronary heart disease incidence and mortality and they were therefore unaffected by any differences between rural and urban availability and quality of treatment. All in all, there is insufficient evidence to warrant incriminating the growing urbanization of the Georgian era as a factor contributing to middle class stress and thereby to the emergence of angina pectoris.

The middle class, although not designated as such in early mid-eighteenth-century writings, grew during the Georgian era both in absolute numbers and as a proportion of the total population of England and Wales. The extent of the increase can be gauged by comparing the numbers of the "middling sort" reported by occupation

[13] Howe, op. cit., note 8 above; Krüger *et al.*, op. cit., note 8 above, pp. 272–3; Hechter and Borhani, op. cit., note 8 above, p. 22.

by Gregory King in 1688[14] with the findings of Joseph Massie for 1759–60[15] (see Tables III.8–9). Between them the tabulations show that over a seventy-year period there was more than a doubling of the number of families that, based on either status or occupation, could be considered middle-class. Natural increase played some part in this growth, but much was the result of increasing prosperity among the higher ranks of the labouring population and their entry into the middle class, with consequent changes in values and lifestyles. Unlike the Continent where classes were frequently defined by law, there were no legal impediments to upward mobility in England. The artisan, after years of working for a master, often struck out on his own and prospered. The shop assistant went into business for himself. The successful small-scale tenant farmer became a landowner, enlarged his acreage and perhaps subsequently became an employer of farm labour. Some entered the middle class by engaging in occupations unknown in previous centuries, such as insurance brokers and distribution agents. Samuel Johnson remarked that "there was never from the earliest ages a time in which trade so much engaged the attention of mankind or commercial gain was sought with such general emulation".[16] The personality traits of the men who successfully rose from the labouring to the middle classes were likely to have been the ones which have been characterized by Ray Rosenman and his colleagues as Type A and found by them to predispose to development of coronary heart disease.[17] An association between upward mobility and liability to develop ischaemic heart disease has been demonstrated. William N Christensen and Lawrence E Hinkle Jr compared two groups of Bell System young executives for differences in the amount of illness in general and cardiovascular problems including angina in particular. These were less frequent among the college graduates who were hired as managers and more common among the high school graduates who had started work on the factory floor and worked their way up to managerial positions.[18] These differences in CHD incidence between the two groups were greater when reported at follow-up seven years later (Table VIII.4).[19]

Movement into the business, manufacturing and land-owning classes was accompanied by the need for credit with consequent increase in indebtedness, often with usurious interest rates. The associated insecurity was compounded by the dire consequences of bankruptcy and the penalties for indebtedness. Creditors had the power to have defaulters punished by indefinite incarceration in the Fleet or other equally disagreeable prisons. This fate was not rare. Of the 4,084 prisoners that the prison reformer John Howard counted on his 1770s tours, 2,437 were debtors. The incarceration was a civil process with the state merely providing a place of

[14] Gregory King, *Natural and political observations and conclusions upon the state and condition of England 1696*, ed. George E Barnett, Baltimore, Johns Hopkins Press, 1936, p. 31.

[15] Langford, op. cit., note 7 above, p. 64.

[16] Quoted in Roy Porter, *English society in the eighteenth century*, Harmondsworth, Penguin, 1990, p. 186.

[17] Ray H Rosenman *et al.*, 'A predictive study of coronary heart disease', *JAMA*, 1964, **189**: 15–22, p. 21.

[18] William N Christensen and Lawrence E Hinkle Jr, 'Differences in illness and prognostic signs in two groups of young men', *JAMA*, 1961, **177**: 247–53, p. 241.

[19] Lawrence E Hinkle Jr *et al.*, 'Occupation, education, and coronary heart disease', *Science*, 1968, **161**: 238–46, p. 241.

*Table VIII.4*

First disabling CHD event. Bell System staff aged 30–59 at entry to study. Annual rates/1000, 1963–5. College and non-college educated

| | Rate/1000/year | |
| --- | --- | --- |
| Category | Non-college | College |
| Executive | 2.46 | 1.65 |
| General area managers | 5.14 | 2.07 |
| Local area managers | 4.28 | 3.68 |

Abstracted with permission from Lawrence E Hinkle Jr *et al.*, 'Occupation, education, and coronary heart disease', *Science*, 1968, **61**: 238–46, p. 241. (American Association for the Advancement of Science.)

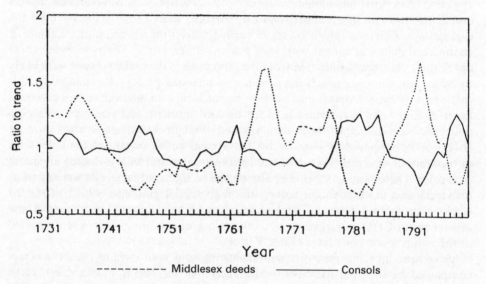

Figure VIII.1: Variations in Middlesex land registry deed values and yields on consols, 1731–1800. Source: J Landers, *Death and the metropolis*, Cambridge University Press, 1993, p. 79. (Reproduced by permission of Cambridge University Press.)

confinement. Where the prisoner's well being and even his food and drink depended entirely on his own inadequate means.[20] The risks were compounded by the considerable economic upswings and downturns that occurred throughout the eighteenth century (Figure VIII.1),[21] starting with the most dramatic of all, the crisis and ongoing sense of investment insecurity that followed the expansion and subsequent bursting of the South Sea Bubble in 1720.[22] The eighteenth-century merchant was

[20] N Morris and D J Rothman (eds), *The Oxford history of the prison: the practice of punishment in western society*, Oxford University Press, 1996, pp. 79–81.

[21] J Landers, *Death and the metropolis: studies in the demographic history of London 1670–1830*, Cambridge University Press, 1993, p. 79.

[22] Langford, op. cit., note 7 above, p. 198.

also subject to the vicissitudes of the economy caused by the disruptions that resulted from the numerous wars that were then fought.[23] The return of peace could also produce dislocations in trade as government procurements were reduced and competition from former enemy countries resumed. Peggy McDonough and her colleagues have found that falls in income, even if followed by upswings, are associated with an increase in mortality odds ratio. This was observed particularly in basically middle income groups.[24] During the Georgian era, employed persons in middle-class occupations, such as teachers or the lower level parish clergymen, enjoyed no work security. They were at constant risk of arbitrary dismissal at the whim of a superior and with little or no notice, possible loss of a work-related home and often with no severance compensation whatsoever. The landowner was subject to the consequences of cattle plague, drought and harvest failure with resulting loss of either direct or rental income. He suffered the consequences of falling agricultural prices and wartime rises in the land tax.[25] Persons whose livelihood depended on overseas commerce and who had an interest in the major trading associations such as the East India Company could face potential ruin due to losses at sea. Besides the hazards of nature, piracy and seizure of vessels by privateers from belligerent countries were ever present dangers. The merchant community also suffered from a continuous sense of insecurity because of the length of time without news that would elapse between the departure and the return of ships engaged in trade with ever more distant lands. The maritime insurance market was then fragmented and underwriters covered only part of the insured value, the extent reflecting the high risks involved.[26] All of these causes for anxiety became greater as commerce became worldwide during the Georgian era. The impact of the commercial stresses increased with expansion of maritime trade and the members of the moneyed classes who were at risk grew more numerous. They all had ever more to lose and the consequences of loss were horrendous. All in all, the eighteenth-century social and economic changes were causes of stress that were greater than had existed in earlier times and involved more people. Untoward consequences of the increasing prosperity did not go unnoticed by physicians of the time. Dr George Cheyne, for example, writing in 1733, designated the nervous diseases affecting the growing élite as "the English malady".[27] It could well have contributed to the "British disease" that became manifest thirty-five years later.[28]

Eighteenth-century society was very much a hierarchical one. It was an age of bowing, scraping and touching of forelocks. All but the highest strata of society had

[23] Ibid., pp. 631ff.

[24] Peggy McDonough *et al.*, 'Income dynamics and adult mortality in the United States, 1972 through 1989', *Am J Public Health*, 1997, **87**: 1476–83, p. 1480.

[25] Frank O'Gorman, *The long eighteenth century: British political and social history 1688–1832*, London, Arnold, 1997, p. 103.

[26] H A L Cockerell and E Green, *The British insurance business, 1547–1970*, London, Heinemann Educational Books, 1976, p. 13.

[27] George Cheyne, *The English malady; or, A treatise of nervous diseases of all kinds, as spleen, vapours, lowness of spirits, hypochondriacal and hysterical distempers*, Dublin, S Powell, 1733, p. i.

[28] William L Proudfit, 'Origin of concept of ischaemic heart disease', *Br Heart J*, 1983, **50**: 209–12, p. 209.

*Table VIII.5*

Ten-year CHD mortality percentage: British civil servants

| Age at entry (1967–9) | Percentage mortality | |
|---|---|---|
| | Grade | |
| | Administrative | Professional and executive |
| 40–49 | 0 | 1.4 |
| 50–59 | 3.3 | 4.5 |
| 60–64 | 4.2 | 7.2 |
| Age adjusted | 2.2 SE 0.5 | 3.6 SE 0.5 |

Source: M G Marmot, M J Shipley and G Rose, 'Contribution of job control and other risk factors to social variation in coronary heart disease incidence', *Lancet*, 1997, **i**: 235–9, p. 238. (Permission granted by The *Lancet* Ltd.)

to maintain constantly a deferential attitude to persons categorized as their superiors or in positions of authority.[29] It was a constraint that the "middling sort" resented increasingly and ultimately sought to change in the years leading to their enfranchisement with passage of the 1832 Reform Act.[30] In the meantime they had to suffer continuously an accompanying loss of self-esteem and the mental strains associated with the suppression of resentment and anger, now recognized as factors contributing to an increase in incidence of coronary heart disease. Thus in the Whitehall study of British civil servants Michael G Marmot and his colleagues found that the ten-year mortality at all ages was greater among staff in the relatively lower professional/executive grades when compared to those at the highest and decision-making administrative level (Table VIII.5). The lifestyles of persons at each of these two levels were comparable with respect to all other traditional risk factors, and both grades had mortality rates below those of personnel at still lower levels. The comparison indicates therefore that subordinate status and inability to exert personal control of workaday activities constitutes a cardiac risk factor.[31] The authors' conclusions received subsequent confirmation in a prospective cohort study of all grades in the same population among whom the effects of high versus low job control were compared with respect to coronary heart disease incidence in all of its forms. The attack rates in the lowest grades where there was the least job control were higher than among personnel in the topmost ranks, even after correction for significant differences in other lifestyle risk factors.[32]

[29] O'Gorman, op. cit., note 25 above, p. 12.

[30] Ibid., p. 368.

[31] Michael G Marmot *et al.*, 'Contribution of job control and other risk factors to social variations in coronary heart disease incidence', *Lancet*, 1997, **350**: 235–9, p. 238.

[32] Hans Bosma *et al.*, 'Low job control and risk of coronary heart disease in Whitehall II (prospective cohort) study', *Br Med J*, 1997, **314**: 558–65, p. 562.

Parenthetically, members of the eighteenth-century English middle classes who had worked their way up from humbler origins were possibly at high risk for reasons other than any social and economic stress occurring after the improvement in their lot. D J P Barker and C Osmond's studies have shown a significant correlation between nutritional deprivation early in life and increased liability to coronary heart disease mortality in middle and later years. Areas of England and Wales that were characterized by high infant mortality rates in the years 1921 to 1925 suffered high ischaemic heart disease death rates during the period 1968–78. By these later dates the people concerned had long ceased to suffer deprivation. The linkage persisted when allowance was made for the impact of other cardiac risk factors.[33] George A Kaplan and Jukkat T Salonen reported confirmatory findings in the Kuopio study in Eastern Finland. Poor socioeconomic conditions in childhood were associated in middle life with a significantly raised incidence of electrocardiographic ischaemic changes on stress testing (RR 1.44, CI 1.171.78). The significance remained after adjustment for traditional risk factors.[34] Similarly, A Forsdahl found that counties in Norway characterized by high infant mortality in the years 1896 to 1925 had correspondingly higher death rates from arteriosclerotic conditions during the 1964–67 period and that were also above the Norwegian national average (Figures VIII.2a and 2b). The one-time infants were by then aged from about forty to seventy years and by the 1960s county to county adult nutritional differences had largely disappeared. There was very little in or out migration to confound the findings. Forsdahl too concluded that deprivation in childhood, even if corrected during adult life, resulted in a heightened likelihood of ischaemic heart disease developing in middle and later life.[35] The labouring classes in eighteenth-century England suffered from chronic nutritional deprivation, particularly in winter and during years when the harvests were bad. It is possible, therefore, that members of the eighteenth-century middle class who were of humble origin became especially liable to suffer the pains of angina pectoris in their later years when, having moved into the middle class, affluence enabled them to adopt dietary and other lifestyle features conducive to development of coronary heart disease.

Eighteenth-century stresses due to armed conflict at home were significantly less than in the seventeenth century when England had suffered the ravages of the Civil War, the 1715 abortive rebellion staged on behalf of the Old Pretender had virtually no effect on the country and, except during the short-lived uprising led by Bonny Prince Charlie in 1745–6, the country remained internally at peace throughout the Georgian era.[36] However, foreign wars were frequent, prolonged and fought in faraway places to an extent unknown previously. England was engaged in major conflicts for forty-two years of the eighteenth century. People then, as always, worried about their loved ones fighting in distant lands, symbolized by the mother whose

---

[33] D J P Barker and C Osmond, 'Infant mortality, childhood nutrition and ischaemic heart disease in England and Wales', *Lancet*, 1986, **i**: 1077–81, p. 1078.

[34] George A Kaplan and Jukkat T Salonen, 'Socioeconomic conditions in childhood and ischaemic heart disease during middle age', *Br Med J*, 1990, **301**: 1121–23, p. 1122.

[35] A Forsdahl, 'Are poor living conditions in childhood and adolescence an important risk factor for arterosclerotic heart disease?', *Br J Prev Soc Med*, 1977, **31**: 91–5, p. 92.

[36] George Macaulay Trevelyan, *History of England*, London, Longmans, Green, 1947, p. 529–36.

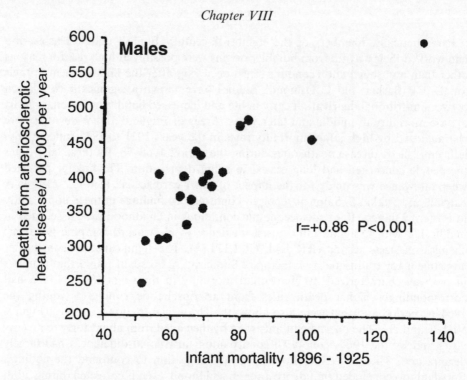

*Figure VIII.2a:* Correlation between mortality from arteriosclerotic heart disease, 1964–67, in men aged 40 to 69 years (standardized rates/100,000 population) and infant mortality rates, 1896–1925. Source: A Forsdahl, 'Are poor living conditions in childhood and adolescence an important risk factor for atherosclerotic heart disease?', *Br J Prev Soc Med*, 1977, **31**: 91–5, p. 92. (With permission from the BMJ Publishing Group.)

son had, "Gone to fight the French, for King George upon the throne," sighing, "And it's Oh! in my heart, how I wish him safe at home!"[37] They grieved at the deaths of their lovers, husbands, brothers and sons whether in battle or, more often, from exotic diseases to which their men-folk had never been exposed in peacetime and to which they consequently lacked immunity. Those who remained at home to worry and grieve grew in the eighteenth century both in absolute numbers and as a proportion of the total population as the size of the army and the navy engaged in war became ever greater over the long haul. The number of men serving rose from 120,000 in 1746 during the War of the Austrian Succession to a peak of 150,000 during the Seven Years' War, 230,000 by 1783 at the end of the War of American Independence, and 482,000 in 1802 when the Treaty of Amiens terminated the French Revolutionary War. By the mid-eighteenth century large overseas garrisons were being maintained even in peacetime.[38]

[37] Dorothea Jordan (1762–1816), *The blue bell of Scotland.: a favourite ballad, as composed and sung by Mrs Jordan at the Theatre Royal, Drury Lane*, London, Longman, Clementi, [1800].

[38] J Landers, *Death and the metropolis: studies in the demographic history of London 1670–1830*, Cambridge University Press, 1993, p. 287–8.

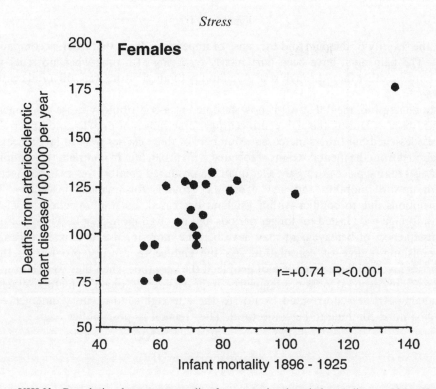

*Figure VIII.2b:* Correlation between mortality from arteriosclerotic heart disease, 1964–67, in women aged 40 to 69 years (standardized rates/100,000 population) and infant mortality rates, 1896–1925. Source: A Forsdahl, 'Are poor living conditions in childhood and adolescence an important risk factor for atherosclerotic heart disease?', *Br J Prev Soc Med*, 1977, **31**: 91–5, p. 92. (With permission from the BMJ Publishing Group.)

The psychological trauma associated with death of children must of necessity have been endured with greater equanimity in Georgian times than is now the case as infant, childhood and early adult mortality rates were then incomparably higher. However, the pain of bereavement may have become greater during the eighteenth century as the solace afforded by religion became less with declining belief in its consolations in general and in an afterlife in particular. Rationalism was receiving growing emphasis even within the church.[39] The fear of illness must have been an additional potent cause for anxiety in an era in which means of obtaining symptomatic relief were limited and curative procedures for all practical purposes not only non-existent but known by most sufferers to be so. In general this fear may not have been any worse than in earlier times. However, in the late eighteenth century the severity of the recently manifest angina pectoris could in itself have been a new cause of anxiety, both for the patient and for those in his immediate circle who became familiar with the condition secondarily. William Heberden himself commented

[39] John Walsh and Stephen Taylor, 'The Church and Anglicanism in the "long" eighteenth century', in John Walsh, Colin Haydon and Stephen Taylor (eds), *The Church of England* c. *1689–c. 1833: from toleration to tractarianism*, Cambridge University Press, 1993, p. 42.

on the severity of the pain and the sense of impending death that often accompanied it.[40] The pain must have been particularly terrifying at a time when no relief was obtainable other than through rest. Availability of amyl nitrite was still a full century away.

In conclusion, mental stress is now accepted as a contributory cause of ischaemic heart disease. During the eighteenth century some causes of middle- and upper-class stress lessened but others increased. Members of these classes were in large measure sheltered from the mental strains associated with urban life. In contrast, the economic changes taking place during the Georgian era produced greater stresses in connection with upward mobility and new economic grounds for financial insecurity. The disruptions due to conflict within England decreased, but the anxieties associated with foreign wars lasted for longer periods and involved more people. The emotional consequences of bereavement may have become more intense as religion became a diminishing source of consolation. As the eighteenth century progressed, these worries involved larger numbers of people at the very time when they were becoming increasingly exposed to the consequences of the other traditional risk factors. Whether changing stresses contributed or not to the late eighteenth-century emergence of angina must continue to be conjectural. They remain as possibilities.

[40] William Heberden, *Commentaries on the history and cure of diseases*, 2nd ed., London, T Payne, 1802, p. 364.

# IX

# Exercise

The greater coronary heart disease morbidity of sedentary as opposed to physically active workers was demonstrated many years ago by J N Morris and his colleagues in a comparison of London bus drivers and conductors. These two groups of transport workers belonged to the same social class and had similar lifestyles. They differed principally in the amount of physical activity in which they engaged when at work. The drivers were confined to a small enclosed driving compartment which rendered them almost completely immobile, whilst the conductors were continuously active, especially as they constantly had to run up and down the stairs of the double-decker London buses. During the five-year follow-up the drivers had a CHD incidence almost double that of the conductors. The differences between the two groups became greater as their members grew older (Table IX.1).[1] The finding of this untoward accompaniment of physical inactivity has been confirmed by the results of the Framingham study[2] and a 27 cohort based rigorous meta-analysis reported by Jesse Berlin and Graham Colditz. These authors found a relative risk of death from coronary heart disease of 1.9 (CL 1.6-2.2) for sedentary as opposed to high physical activity groups, and the benefits were shown to be greater in the studies that the authors judged to be methodologically stronger.[3] Conversely, in the Whitehall study of British civil servants leisure-time physical activity has been found to have cardiovascular health benefits similar to those apparently conferred on the London bus conductors by their workaday exertions. Vigorous weekend exercise apparently protected the middle-aged men from fatal heart attacks and non-fatal first episodes of coronary heart disease.[4]

It is probable that a randomized and controlled prospective study of the cardio-vascular consequences of prolonged inactivity will never be undertaken. It would be both unethical and impractical to enforce a long-term sedentary lifestyle on a control group. However, the physiological means by which regular exercise has cardioprotective effects are now well defined. Animal studies have shown that the coronary arterial capacity becomes greater relative to the cardiac muscle mass and an increase in coronary artery diameter has been demonstrated angiographically. Capillary growth is induced and increase in coronary blood flow in response to need

[1] J N Morris et al., 'Incidence and prediction of ischaemic heart-disease in London busmen', Lancet, 1966, ii: 553–9, p. 553.

[2] T R Dawber, The Framingham study: the epidemiology of atherosclerotic disease, Cambridge, MA, Harvard University Press, 1980, p. 161.

[3] J A Berlin and G A Colditz, 'A meta-analysis of physical activity in the prevention of coronary heart disease', Am J Epidemiol, 1990, 132: 612–28, p. 621.

[4] J N Morris et al., 'Vigorous exercise in leisure-time and incidence of coronary heart-disease', Lancet, 1973, i: 333–9, p. 337.

## Chapter IX

### Table IX.1
Five-year incidence/100 of CHD in London bus crews

| | Conductors | | | Drivers | | |
| | Numbers | | | Numbers | | |
| Age at entry | In study | CHD | Incidence | In study | CHD | Incidence |
|---|---|---|---|---|---|---|
| 40–49 | 62 | 1 | 1.6 | 66 | 5 | 7.6 |
| 50–59 | 117 | 6 | 5.1 | 183 | 18 | 9.8 |
| 60–69 | 68 | 5 | 7.4 | 139 | 11 | 7.9 |
| TOTAL | 247 | 12 | 4.7 | 388 | 34 | 8.5 |

Source: J N Morris et al., 'Incidence and prediction of heart disease in London busmen', *Lancet*, 1966, ii: 553–9, p. 553. (Permission granted by The *Lancet* Ltd.)

is enhanced.[5] When compared to inactive controls, ligation of the left coronary artery in rats results in smaller myocardial infarcts among animals preconditioned by exercise.[6] The beneficial consequences of human physical exertion have been summarized by Albert Oberman. By increasing energy expenditure, exercise conditioning has been shown to reduce body weight and excess fat preferentially. Physical training reduces insulin secretion while improving glucose tolerance. It improves the lipid profile by increasing levels of serum HDL and apolipoprotein A1 while reducing those of LDL cholesterol and serum triglycerides. There is an inverse correlation between intensity of physical activity and blood pressure level at rest and with submaximal exercise. The heart rate at rest and during submaximal exertion decreases with training, parasympathetic activity being increased at rest.[7] An increase in heart muscle mass with exercise has been shown by echocardiography.[8] Training has the potential for mitigating the undesirable left ventricular remodelling and loss of contractile function that often follows an infarct, should one occur. The benefits of exercise having been shown, the opposite and untoward cardiac consequences of an inactive life pattern can be inferred.

Occasional favourable comments on the value of physical activity were made by eighteenth-century physicians. George Cheyne for one advocated walking and horseback riding.[9] On the whole though, the medical community made little general impression in this regard. Gymnasia for "Medicinal Exercises" were located in spas such as Bath, but the concept of exertion in order to attain physical fitness, for the

[5] Thomas F Schaible and James Scheuer, 'Cardiac adaptations to chronic exercise', *Prog Cardiovasc Dis*, 1985, **27**: 297–324, p. 310.

[6] C L McElroy, S A Gissen and M C Fishbein, 'Exercise-induced reduction in myocardial infarct size after coronary artery occlusion in the rat', *Circulation*, 1978, **57**: 958–62, p. 960.

[7] Albert Oberman, 'Exercise and the primary prevention of cardiovascular disease', *Am J Cardiol*, 1985, **55**: 10d–20d, p. 17d.

[8] Schaible and Scheuer, op. cit., note 5 above, p. 299.

[9] Trevor H Howell, 'George Cheyne's essay on health and long life', *Gerentology*, 1969, **9**: 226–8, p. 227.

maintenance of health or just for its own sake, was little known and applied less.[10] The pursuits encouraged in the Middle Ages because of their military value had lost their importance as guns replaced swords and bows and arrows. Archery survived but only as a sport and fencing contests became the sole legacy of medieval jousting tournaments. In an era in which servants were both readily available and easily affordable, physical activity in connection with either work or home was virtually unknown even among people whose means were only moderate. As far as the middle and upper classes were concerned, exercise was confined for the most part to a limited range of participatory sporting activities, and to travel, whether on foot or horseback. All of these activities had to compete with less desirable spectator pursuits such as patronage of cock fighting bouts and bull baiting displays or attendance at public hangings.[11]

Earlier linkage of games with religious holidays such as Easter had declined in popularity by the eighteenth century. On the other hand, the restrictions on sporting events and games imposed by the Puritans during the Commonwealth era had largely disappeared after the 1660 Stuart restoration. Authorities of the established church accepted and even encouraged Sunday sports, in part as legitimate pastimes in their own right and in part in order to divert their flock from other activities that were considered less desirable. Fields for sports were often available on the outskirts of towns. Some events, such as horse-racing, wrestling and boxing, were essentially spectator pursuits. The choice of participatory activities reflected the class divisions of the time. There were sports such as football in which the common folk took part and other activities that engaged all strata of society, such as foot races, whether on level ground or including hurdles. Hunting, as a "courtly" exercise and "gentlemanly" pastime, was reserved largely for the nobility and the gentry. It involved participation but provided exercise infrequently and less intensively than today. Hunting hares was common and for the hunter less taxing than the current pursuit of foxes. Neither horses nor hounds had been bred selectively to any extent and both were slower than they are now. Among the middle class, early forms of golf, cricket and tennis were played and enjoyed some limited popularity. Water events such as swimming, rowing and yachting had enthusiastic participants and the primitive forms of exercise machines that were available were occasionally used at home.[12] With the exception of horse riding, these activities were exclusively masculine, their pursuit was less intense than now and far from universal, and they were usually discontinued in middle life. That George Osbaldeston and Assheton Smith still hunted to hounds, the former when nearly forty-five, the latter at age fifty-four, was remarked upon by contemporaries as highly exceptional.[13] There is, however, no evidence to indicate any change in the extent to which these sporting activities were pursued as Stuart times were succeeded by Georgian.

[10] L Picard, *Dr. Johnson's London*, London, Weidenfeld and Nicolson, 2000, pp. 126, 129.

[11] A S Turberville (ed.), *Johnson's England*, 2 vols, Oxford, Clarendon Press, 1952, vol. 1, p. 366.

[12] W J Baker, *Sports in the western world*, Urbana and Chicago, University of Illinois Press, 1988, pp. 66, 67.

[13] G M Young (ed.), *Early Victorian England*, 2 vols, London, Oxford University Press, 1934, vol. 1, p. 266.

## Chapter IX

During the eighteenth century there were significant developments in travel patterns and in their impact on levels of physical activity. During the Middle Ages, roads, even between important cities, had been little more than muddy potholed tracks. The old Roman roads had been neglected and had deteriorated badly. The construction of medieval roads consisted for the most part of removal of trees and undergrowth and the clearing of obvious obstructions such as boulders. The road surfaces were little more than beaten earth so that they were dusty in summer, muddy in winter and deeply rutted at all times. Even the most luxurious of coaches, available only to the wealthy and then used almost exclusively by ladies, were heavy, clumsy and exceedingly uncomfortable. The wheels were solid and neither the body of the coach nor the seating had springs. Every jolt in the uneven and potholed tracks was transmitted to the unfortunate passengers. Because roads were narrow, passage of vehicles travelling in opposite directions was hazardous. Horse litters were used by the wealthy but had the added disadvantage of close confinement for their passengers.[14] For the less affluent travel was even more uncomfortable; for them there were only wagons which were often without cover. Travel was exceedingly slow. In 1575 a wagon took two and a half days for the journey from London to Cambridge, averaging about two miles an hour.[15] For young children, the elderly and the infirm, there was no choice. For others, there was the alternative of walking for neighbourhood journeys, and in fact people did walk very considerable distances. For many it was virtually their sole form of exercise, taken because of necessity. For long journeys, horseback was the only other possibility and provided the rider with a measure of physical exertion, currently estimated to average 2.6 METS for walking, 3.0 to 6.5 for trotting and 8.0 METS for galloping.[16] One of Fothergill's patients with angina pectoris developed the typical pain when riding a horse at any speed faster than a trot and he had to stop his mount in order to obtain relief.[17]

There was little improvement in either the roads or the means of travelling on them during Tudor and early Stuart times, but major changes followed passage of the first Turnpike Act in 1663. This transferred responsibility for maintenance of roads from local authorities to Turnpike Trusts which were able to recoup the money spent on improvements by charging tolls. The system worked only imperfectly as many trusts were underfunded or maladministered. Payment of tolls was sometimes evaded, frequently with the connivance of tollgate keepers who were less than totally incorruptible.[18] Nevertheless, the late seventeenth century saw a beginning of road improvement and the pace of change accelerated greatly during the eighteenth with the development by mid-century of what has been described as "turnpike mania". Although the greatest changes in road surfacing awaited the efforts of Thomas Telford and John Macadam in a later period, the improvements during the early

[14] J Joyce, *The story of passenger transport in Britain*, London, I Allen, 1967, p. 28.

[15] Ibid., p. 3.

[16] William Haskell *et al.*, 'Task force II: Determination of occupational working capacity in patients with ischemic heart disease', *J Am Coll Cardiol*, 1989, **14**: 1025–34, p. 1028.

[17] John Fothergill, 'Case of an angina pectoris with remarks', *Medical Observations and Inquiries*, 1776, **5**: 233–51, p. 245.

[18] William Albert, *The turnpike road system in England 1663–1840*, Cambridge University Press, 1972, p. 19.

eighteenth century were considerable. Foundations of faggots or brush were laid and stones, gravel and sand were used for surfacing and packed down for hardness. Road surfaces were cambered for drainage, which was further improved by ditching along the sides. Wear was reduced by penalizing owners of exceptionally heavy vehicles and controlling wheel width. Ferries were replaced increasingly by bridges. By 1750 towns throughout the length and breadth of England were linked by a network of the new roads and served by scheduled stage-coach services.[19]

The same period saw considerable improvements in vehicle design. Steel springing was introduced to reduce jolting and seating became more comfortable. Greater strength and stability of construction made it possible to seat passengers outside as well as inside the coach. Increased wheel width gave added stability. The pulling power became greater as selective breeding and improved feeding resulted in stronger horses. The harnesses and traces were improved so that it became possible to link four or even six horse teams to the coach. The coachman no longer walked with the horses. He now sat in a special box in the front of the carriage so that for the first time the capacity of the horses rather than the walking pace of the man determined the speed which could be maintained. It increased from about two miles an hour in the sixteenth century to ten by the end of the eighteenth. The journey from London to Manchester, which took four and a half days in 1754, required only three in 1760 and two by 1776.[20] Travel times between other cities became correspondingly less.

The improvement in transport did not impact on the physical energy expended by passengers who had always ridden long distances by coach. It simply increased their comfort, speed and convenience and perhaps diminished the danger of hold-ups by highwaymen. However, for others, it did encourage the use of stage-coaches or post-coaches in place of riding on horseback. More importantly, for short distances it encouraged travelling by carriage rather than walking. The children and grandchildren of people who had journeyed by coach from London to York in the seventeenth century would have used the same means in the eighteenth. However, someone whose forebears had walked the twelve miles from Bath to Bristol in Stuart times might well have taken a coach a century later. Excursions by carriage replaced some walks undertaken for pleasure and without a specific destination. Even before the end of the seventeenth century, the antiquarian John Aubrey had remarked that gentlemen were travelling in carriages instead of on horseback as previously. A 1779 observer complained of "indolence ever worsening among civilized society with the neglect of going on foot; the encrease of carriages, the high finishing of roads".[21] Short journeys were facilitated by a great variety of new vehicles that became available for the purpose, especially for travel within towns. They were owned in ever larger numbers by the lesser gentry and the commercial classes and included the gig, the barouche and, for the adventurous, the phaeton. There were also vehicles for hire, notably the post-chaise and the hackney carriage. The increase in their number during the Georgian era is well documented as many types of carriage had

---

[19] Ibid., pp. 133ff.

[20] Joyce, op. cit., note 14 above, p. 197.

[21] W Grant, *Some observations on the origins, progress, and method of treating the atrabilious temperament and gout*, London, T Cadell, 1779, p. 4.

to be licensed because they were subject to taxation. In eighteenth-century London sedan chairs too were available for hire. They had first come into use in France in the mid-seventeenth century, were introduced into England shortly afterwards and became very popular during the next hundred years. They spared their patrons fatigue and the porters who furnished the motive power also provided protection against assault and robbery. The attraction of all the new forms of transportation was further increased by the tendency for streets in the better parts of the larger cities to be paved to an ever greater extent during the course of the eighteenth century.[22] Towns were growing in population and area, and in London fashionable new suburbs such as Bloomsbury and Marylebone were extending to the north and west of the city.[23] The resulting dispersion added to the distances that had to be travelled for local purposes, whether social or business, and thereby increased the attraction of riding as compared to walking. The combined impact of all these changes on regular physical exertion was not far removed from that which resulted two centuries later from the growing use of the motor car. In the eighteenth century, as in the twentieth, riding replaced walking.

In conclusion, historical evidence suggests that during the eighteenth century the intensity of exercise associated with formal sports probably continued at a low level, and their popularity remained more or less unchanged. Growth in the size of the middle classes resulted in an increase in the number of people who could replace their own exertions with the labours of their servants and substitute the ease of a conveyance for the effort of either walking or riding on horseback. In light of the evidence now linking lack of exercise to predisposition to coronary heart disease, a decline in middle- and upper-class physical activity during the Georgian era could well have been a factor, not perhaps the greatest, but contributing in some measure to the emergence and subsequent increase in incidence of angina pectoris observed at the time.

[22] Joyce, op. cit., note 14 above, pp. 114ff.
[23] George Macaulay Trevelyan, *English social history*, 3rd ed., London, Longmans, 1947, p. 592.

# X

# Susceptibility and Resistance

The Capitoline Museum in Rome contains an extensive collection of busts of Roman Emperors, carved during their lifetimes. These sculptures constitute a veritable portrait gallery of the Imperial Era and the depiction of their subjects reflects the pursuit of realism rather than idealism by Roman artists. The busts of three of the Emperors, Tiberius, Vespasian and Trajan (Illustration 10), depict earlobe clefts, now known to be an epiphenomenon that marks a predisposition to the development of coronary heart disease.[1] None of the three Emperors suffered or died from anything that could be interpreted as a direct manifestation of heart disease. Vespasian reputedly passed away after suffering from a stomach chill and Trajan after a paralytic stroke.[2] Gaius Suetonius recorded a belief that at the age of seventy-seven Tiberius was the victim of a debilitating poison administered by his designated successor Caligula and finally smothered.[3] Whilst therefore something of a curiosity, the earlobe clefts portrayed in three sculptures suggest that many centuries before William Heberden made his historic presentation to the Royal College of Physicians of London, an inborn predisposition to coronary heart disease may have existed, awaiting the impact of the risk factors to which people were subsequently to become exposed for the first time. It is consequently worth considering whether, by analogy with infectious diseases, populations newly exposed to lifestyle changes and the associated risk factors could initially have had a heightened susceptibility to coronary heart disease that was innate. Would this susceptibility have lessened subsequently as a result of natural selection during continued exposure to lifestyle risk factors over many generations? Specifically, could vulnerability to the changed diets and their consequences have been greater among eighteenth-century Englishmen than among their twentieth-century descendants? It is necessary, therefore, to examine relationships between some genetic factors predisposing to coronary heart disease and their interplay with lifestyle changes. Finally, consideration must be given to possible evolution of these relationships over many generations.

There is epidemiological evidence to indicate that some communities of recent migrants from the developing to the western world have an incidence of CHD that is not just equal to but greater than that of the indigenous populations, South Asian migrants to the UK constituting an example. R Balarajan and colleagues calculated the 1975–77 circulatory mortality ratios of Indian immigrants from the subcontinent

---

[1] Edgar Lichtstein et al., 'Diagonal ear-lobe crease and coronary artery sclerosis', letter in *Ann Intern Med*, 1976, **85**: 337–8.
[2] M Grant, *History of Rome*, New York, Charles Scribner and Sons, 1978, pp. 291, 297.
[3] Gaius Suetonius Tranquillus, *Lives of the Caesars*, transl. C Edwards, New York, Oxford University Press, 2000, pp. 133–4.

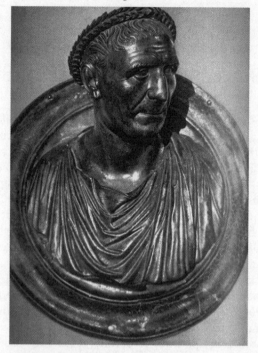

*Illustration 10:* Emperor Trajan (*c.* 53–117), from a sculpture in the Museum of Anatolian Civilisation, Ankara, Turkey. The earlobe cleft is clearly visible. (Photograph by Professor James Russell, reproduced with permission.)

using overall 1975–77 deaths in England and Wales as a basis for comparison. The South Asians suffered an excess of circulatory (notably ischaemic heart disease) deaths of 20 and 17 per cent among men and women respectively. The excess was evident among both Hindus and Moslems, as well involving groups with differing places of origin within the subcontinent.[4] P M McKeigue and M G Marmot's findings revealed even greater differences. They reported that among South Asian immigrant residents in various parts of London the 1979–83 coronary heart disease death rate excess was 50 per cent. Whether the Asians were located in areas of affluence or deprivation made no difference and the findings constituted a worsening over the previous decade.[5] The blood pressures of the Asians were on average slightly lower than those of the whites. The Asian mortality cannot be explained by changing living patterns and adoption to excess of the undesirable health practices of the western world, specifically limited physical activity, excessive consumption of animal fats, energy intake in excess of needs and cigarette smoking. Immigrants do indeed adopt these lifestyles, but comprehensive reviews by Jatinder Dhawan and co-workers

[4] R Balarajan *et al.*, 'Patterns of mortality among migrants to England and Wales from the Indian subcontinent', *Br Med J*, 1984, **289**: 1185–7.
[5] P M McKeigue and J G M Marmot, 'Mortality from coronary heart disease in Asian communities in London', *Br Med J*, 1988, **297**: 903.

*Table X.1*
Risk factors: British white and Asian patients. Mean SD ( ) or confidence limits [ ]

| Risk factor | | White (n = 87) | Asian (n = 83) |
|---|---|---|---|
| Age (years) | | 56.7 (8.7) | 51.9 (7.1) |
| Social Class | I | 11 | 12 |
| | II | 38 | 34 |
| | III | 44 | 47 |
| | IV | 7 | 7 |
| BMI (kg/m$^2$) | | 25.7 (3.2) | 25.5 (9.9) |
| Waist/hip ratio | | 0.97 (0.06) | 1.02 (0.05) |
| % Physically Active | | 37 | 23 |
| Mean lifetime cigarette consumption (1000s) Ex and current smokers | | 212 [164–267] | 159 [121–203] |
| BP (mmHg) | Systolic | 137.8 (24.4) | 130.2 (20.6) |
| | Diastolic | 81.8 (10.5) | 79.1 (8.3) |

Adapted from Jatinder Dhawan *et al.*, 'Insulin resistance, high prevalence of diabetes and cardiovascular risk in immigrant Asians. Genetic or environmental effect?', *Br Heart J*, 1994, **72**: 413–21, p. 415. (With permission from the BMJ Publishing Group.)

(Table X.1) and by McKeigue and colleagues (Table X.2) suggest that, in the case of South Asian immigrants to the United Kingdom, this adoption is not excessive by overall English standards. Compared to the general population, the immigrants' energy intake was not excessive, and their mean body mass index virtually the same. Their consumption of animal fats was low, their fibre intake high, and their carbohydrate consumption only marginally greater. They were less active physically, but on the other hand they smoked less.[6] It is therefore possible that these immigrants had an innately high degree of vulnerability to the coronary risk factors to which they had become exposed for the first time. These considerations also raise the possibility that the heightened susceptibility to coronary heart disease among recent migrants to the western world could have had a parallel in the population of late eighteenth-century England. In both groups this vulnerability would have become manifest with their first exposure to the same unhealthy lifestyles, the one with change of location, the other with passage of time. Twentieth-century geographical and eighteenth-century historical developments would have been obverse and reverse sides of the same coin. Evolutionary adaptation to the new risk factors over the course of many generations might therefore account for twentieth-century native English having gradually become less vulnerable and consequently having a lower incidence of CHD than the recent unadapted immigrants to the UK. The evidence for this will be discussed later in some detail.

[6] Jatinder Dhawan *et al.*, 'Insulin resistance, high prevalence of diabetes, and cardiovascular risk in immigrant Asians. Genetic or environmental effect?', *Br Heart J*, 1994, **72**: 413–21, pp. 415–16; P M McKeigue *et al.*, 'Diet and risk factors for coronary heart disease in Asians in northwest London', *Lancet*, 1985, **ii**: 1086–90, p. 1087.

*Table X.2*

Nutrient intakes in Asian households compared with national food survey

| | Asian (184 households) Mean ± SE | UK national food survey |
|---|---|---|
| *Consumption per person per day* | | |
| Energy (Kcal) | 2415 ± 83 | 2210 |
| Fat (g) | 106.1 ± 4.4 | 104 |
| Fatty Acids: | | |
|   Saturated (g) | 36.8 ± 1.8 | 45.6 |
|   Monosaturated (g) | 38.8 ± 1.4 | 38.9 |
|   Polyunsaturated (g) | 27.2 ± 1.2 | 11.4 |
|   Linoleic Acid (g) | 25.6 ± 1.2 | 9.8 |
| Cholesterol (mg) | 200 ± 15 | 405.0 |
| Carbohydrate (g) | 284 ± 9 | 264.0 |
| Dietary fibre | | |
|   Cereal fibre (g) | 10.4 ± 0.4 | 8.7 |
|   Vegetable fibre (g) | 18.7 ± 1.1 | 9.2 |
| *Source of energy (per cent of total)* | | |
| Fat | 38.8 ± 0.6 | 42.2 |
| Carbohydrate | 48.6 ± 0.6 | 44.9 |
| P/S ratio | 0.85 ± 0.04 | 0.28 |

Source: P M McKeigue *et al.*, 'Diet and risk factors for coronary heart disease in Asians in northwest London', *Lancet*, 1985, **ii**: 1086–90, p. 1087. (Permission granted by The *Lancet* Ltd.)

A suggestion of such adaptation is provided by comparative studies of the relationship between fat intake and serum lipid levels among males of Japanese ancestry resident in either Japan or the USA. Not surprisingly, it was found that the higher intake of fat among people of Japanese origin living in California was reflected in abnormal lipid profiles (Table X.3). Particularly noteworthy, however, was a finding that the degree of significance of the positive correlations between saturated fat intake and serum cholesterol levels was greater among the residents in Japan whose intake of animal fats was customarily low, and weaker in the Japanese men who were living in either Hawaii or the Continental United States and habituated to a higher intake (Table X.4). An apparent ability to compensate biochemically for the changes in dietary practices that followed emigration had become evident within a generation or two.[7]

As noted earlier, the incidence of coronary heart disease mortality among Asian immigrants to the United Kingdom exceeds the national rates, and differing exposure to lifestyle risk factors could not explain the excess.[8] When patients from both

[7] Hiroo Kato *et al.*, 'Epidemiological studies of coronary heart disease and stroke in Japanese men living in Japan, Hawaii and California. Serum lipids and diet', *Am J Epidemiol*, 1973, **97**: 372–85, pp. 375, 378.

[8] Dhawan *et al.*, op. cit, note 6 above, pp. 415–16.

*Table X.3*

Nutrient intake (24 hour recall) and serum lipid levels of Japanese resident in Japan or California

| Intake/day | Japan | | California | |
|---|---|---|---|---|
| | Mean | SD | Mean | SD |
| Total calories | 2164 | 619 | 2262 | 695 |
| Total fat (g) | 36.6 | 20.4 | 94.8 | 36.4 |
| Saturated fat (g) | 16.0 | 13.3 | 66.3 | 30.5 |
| Unsaturated fat (g) | 20.6 | 13.7 | 28.5 | 20.4 |
| Cholesterol (mg) | 464.1 | 324.4 | 533.2 | 297.8 |
| Weight (kg) | 55.2 | 9.0 | 65.9 | 9.2 |
| Serum cholesterol (mg/dl) | 181.1 | 38.5 | 228.2 | 42.2 |
| Serum triglycerides (mg/dl) | 133.8 | 87.1 | 233.7 | 144.4 |

Source: Hiroo Kato *et al.*, 'Epidemiological studies of coronary heart disease and stroke in Japanese men living in Japan, Hawaii and California. Serum lipids and diet', *Am J Epidemiol*, 1973, **97**: 372–85, p. 375. (By permission of Oxford University Press and Dr J L Tillotson (co-author)).

*Table X.4*

Regression coefficient between saturated fat intake and serum cholesterol.* Subjects of Japanese origin

| Place of residence | Number of subjects | Regression coefficient |
|---|---|---|
| Japan | 1717 | 0.434** |
| Hawaii | 7949 | 0.0766** |
| California | 178 | 0.0965 |

* Adjusted for age and relative body weight.
** Significant at 1% level.

Source: Hiroo Kato *et al.*, 'Epidemiological studies of coronary heart disease and stroke in Japanese men living in Japan, Hawaii and California. Serum lipids and diet', *Am J Epidemiol*, 1973, **97**: 372–85, p. 378. (By permission of Oxford University Press and Dr J L Tillotson (co-author)).

populations who had angiographically proven coronary arterial disease were compared, their lipid profiles were almost identical, but the South Asian patients had somewhat higher blood sugar levels when fasting and significantly higher levels after a glucose load. Their insulin levels were significantly and strikingly higher (Table X.5), and their incidence of diabetes mellitus greater. These findings indicate that the South Asians were characterized by differences in carbohydrate metabolism and above all by greatly heightened insulin resistance. Comparisons of subgroups of white and Asian patients who exercised regularly yielded similar differences in glucose/insulin metabolism (Table X.6) despite nearly identical mean body mass indices (24.55 and 24.32 respectively). The serum insulin, both fasting and after a glucose load, was significantly higher in the exercising Asian group and indicative

*Table X.5*
Biochemical risk factor profile: British Asian and white patients* (SD 95% confidence limits otherwise)

|  |  | British Asian | White |
|---|---|---|---|
| No. of patients |  | 83 | 87 |
| Total cholesterol (mmol/L) |  | 6.16 (1.09) | 6.32 (1.14) |
| HDL cholesterol (mmol/L) |  | 1.02 (0.97–1.07) | 1.08 (1.20–1.14) |
| Glucose (mmol/L) | fasting | 5.34 (4.97–5.74) | 4.77 (4.5–5.0) |
|  | 2 hr after glucose | 7.37 (6.64–8.19)** | 6.13 (5.61–6.70)** |
| Insulin (µU/ml) | fasting | 122.0 (104.8–142.0) | 12.7 (10.8–14.9)** |
|  | 2 hr after glucose | 90.0 (79.3–102.3)** | 43.5 (36.5–51.9)** |

* Angiographically proven CHD ** P<0.05

Adapted from Jatinder Dhawan *et al.*, 'Insulin resistance, high prevalence of diabetes and cardiovascular risk in immigrant Asians. Genetic or environmental effect?', *Br Heart J*, 1994, **72**: 413–21, pp. 416–17. (With permission from the BMJ Publishing Group.)

*Table X.6*
Comparison of aspects of risk factor profile. Exercising British Asian and white coronary heart disease patients

|  |  | British Asian | White |
|---|---|---|---|
| Body mass index |  | 24.32 (0.71)* | 24.55 (0.52)** |
| Total serum cholesterol (mmol/L) |  | 5.96 (1.8)* | 6.56 (0.23)** |
| Log insulin (µU/ml) fasting |  | 18.9 (15.1–21.7) | 8.41 (7.1–9.8)** |
|  | 1 hr after glucose | 125.2 (77.4–135.6) | 54.9 (43.8–68.1)** |
|  | 2 hr after glucose | 50.9 (37.7–68.7) | 27.66 (22.1–34.4)** |

SD singly starred. Numbers in brackets are confidence limits. ** P<0.05

Adapted from Jatinder Dhawan *et al.*, 'Insulin resistance, high prevalence of diabetes and cardiovascular risk in immigrant Asians. Genetic or environmental effect?', *Br Heart J*, 1994, **72**: 413–21, p. 417. (With permission from the BMJ Publishing Group.)

of their greater insulin resistance.[9] As the differences between the white and Asian patients could not be explained by differences in diet, physical activity or incidence of obesity, a possible genetic basis suggests itself.

N Shaukat, D P de Bono and D R Jones compared the biochemical profiles of eighty-nine healthy sons of South Asian cardiac patients and eighty-two healthy sons of comparable North European cardiac patients. The two parent groups were matched for age and symptom duration, and all had been investigated by coronary

[9] Ibid., pp. 416–17.

Table X.7

Biochemical physical features. South Asian and North European patients and their sons free of CHD. Means and 95% probability intervals ( )

| | Patients | | Sons | |
|---|---|---|---|---|
| | Asian | N. European | Asian | N. European |
| Total cholesterol (mmol/L) | 6.0 (5.8–6.2) | 5.9 (5.7–6.2) | 4.2 (4.0–4.4) | 4.1 (4.0–4.2) |
| HDL cholesterol | 1.1 (1.0–1.1) | 1.1 (1.0–1.3) | 1.2 (1.2–1.3) | 1.3 (1.2–1.3) |
| Lp(a) (mg/dl) | 27.2 (25.8–28.5) | 19.5 (18.3–20.4) | 19.1 (16.8–21.8) | 10.5 (8.3–12.8) |
| Fasting glucose (mmol/L) | 4.6 (4.2–5.1) | 4.1 (3.7–4.6) | 4.4 (4.1–4.6) | 4.2 (3.9–4.5) |
| Insulin (fasting) (μmol/L) | 17.6 (16.4–19.0) | 13.5 (12.4–14.8) | 14.3 (12.9–15.8) | 8.43 (7.29–9.60) |
| Waist/hip ratio | 0.94 (0.92–0.96) | 0.89 (0.87–0.91) | 0.87 (0.85–0.89) | 0.83 (0.81–0.85) |
| Body mass index (kg/m²) | 25.4 (24.5–26.3) | 26.3 (25.7–26.9) | 24.1 (23.6–24.6) | 24.0 (23.6–24.8) |

Adapted from N Shaukat, D P de Bono and D R Jones, 'Like father like son? Sons of patients of European or Indian origin with coronary heart disease reflect their parents' risk factor patterns', *Br Heart J*, 1995, **72**: 318–23, pp. 320, 322. (With permission from the BMJ Publishing Group.)

angiography. The sons ranged in age from fifteen to thirty years (Table X.7). Comparison of the two groups showed that the European and Asian sons had almost identical fasting blood sugars but the latter had significantly higher serum insulin levels, indicating that the young overtly healthy Asians already had greater insulin resistance.[10] This is a recognized risk factor for arteriosclerosis, which could account in some measure at least for the excess South Asian incidence of coronary heart disease.[11] As it manifested itself early in life and in the absence of either higher young Asian energy intake or reduced energy needs, a genetic basis is here too a distinct possibility.

Finally, N Shaukat and colleagues compared cardiac patients of South Asian and North European origin and their sons with respect to serum Lp(a) levels, elevations of which are associated with heightened susceptibility to CHD. All the diagnoses of ischaemic heart disease had been confirmed by coronary angiography. The Lp(a) levels were almost 50 per cent higher among the Asian patients, 27.2 as opposed to 19.5 mg/dl, a highly significant difference. When the biochemical profiles of the healthy sons of these two patient groups were studied, there was found to be a very high correlation between fathers and sons with respect to Lp(a) concentrations, the sons of Asian patients having serum Lp(a) levels significantly higher than those of

[10] N Shaukat, D P de Bono and D R Jones, 'Like father like son? Sons of patients of European or Indian origin with coronary artery disease reflect their parents' risk factor patterns', *Br Heart J*, 1995, **74**: 318–23, p. 321.

[11] P J Savage and M F Saad, 'Insulin and atherosclerosis: villain, accomplice, or innocent bystander?', *Br Heart J*, 1993, **69**: 473–5.

their North European counterparts.[12] As Lp(a) levels are largely independent of diet, the combination of the differences between the two communities and the similarities between the two generations of each suggests a genetic basis for Lp(a) abnormalities and their cardiac consequences.

The South Asian groups in the various studies were made up almost exclusively of Punjabis or Gujeratis whose ancestors had originated in Central Asia in the distant past and subsequently migrated to North West India. They therefore had the same remote prehistoric Indo-European ethnic origins as the white English subjects. However, the forebears of the South Asian patients had not been exposed to high animal fat and energy intake until their migration to Britain in the mid-twentieth century. The differences between the two populations that have been described are therefore compatible with the white English population alone of the two groups having undergone some favourable evolutionary adaptive changes. These would have occurred during the two centuries and more during which their forefathers had been eating a diet changed permanently by the Agricultural Revolution and high in its animal fat content.

Any favourable influences of natural selection on vulnerability to CHD risk factors may be diminished but are certainly not nullified by the tendency for the disease to become manifest late in male reproductive life. Reasons for this conclusion have their bases in the demographics of eighteenth-century England. E Anthony Wrigley and Roger Schofield's early studies have shown that, in general, marriage in the eighteenth century took place when men were in their late twenties. Marriage tended to be later still among the middle and upper classes as it was commonly delayed until a man had the means to support a wife, and it may even have had to wait upon an inheritance.[13] Thomas H Hollingsworth reported that throughout the eighteenth century the age of marriage of 35 to 40 per cent of male members of the nobility was above thirty years.[14] The tendency for men to father some children relatively late in life was increased by the large numbers of their progeny and also by the high maternal mortality rates, with subsequent second marriages of men, often to younger women. The average age of widowers marrying spinsters in the late eighteenth century was estimated by the Cambridge Group to be between thirty-nine and forty years.[15] This frequently brought the age of a second round of fathering into the fifth decade of life, if not later still. William Heberden himself was a typical example. Of the three sons by his second marriage who survived to adult life, the oldest was born when their father was fifty-six, the second three years and the youngest five years later.[16] Before the late twentieth-century adoption of risk factor control measures, symptoms of ischaemic heart disease not infrequently became

---

[12] Shaukat, de Bono and Jones, op. cit., note 10 above, p. 320.

[13] E Anthony Wrigley and R S Schofield, *The population history of England 1541–1871: a reconstruction*, Cambridge, MA, Harvard University Press, 1981, p. 255.

[14] T H Hollingsworth, *Demography of the British peerage*, *Population studies*, **18**: Supplement No. 2, London, Population Investigation Committee, London School of Economics, 1964, pp. i–iv, 3–108.

[15] E Anthony Wrigley *et al.*, *English population history from family reconstitution, 1580–1837*, Cambridge University Press, 1997, p. 149.

[16] Ernest Heberden, *William Heberden: physician of the age of reason*, London, Royal Society of Medicine Services, 1989, p. 80.

manifest as early as the fifth decade of life. They were so reported by Heberden and subsequent eighteenth-century English medical writers. One of John Fothergill's two documented patients with angina pectoris was only thirty years old.[17] John Ryle and W T Russell, writing in 1949, reported that 39 of their 149 male patients developed angina pectoris below the age of fifty and in 16 it was below forty years.[18] It follows that despite a tendency for ischaemic heart disease to occur somewhat late in male reproductive life, there was an opportunity for the forces of natural selection to effect evolutionary changes in the successive generations born in England after the mid-eighteenth century.

In conclusion, there are possible genetic factors that predispose to development of coronary heart disease and manifest themselves, *inter alia*, as abnormalities in the serum cholesterol response to dietary fats, glucose/insulin metabolism and serum Lp(a) levels. Evidence has been adduced to suggest that, because of these presumed genetic factors, a population first exposed to a diet high in animal fats and to other lifestyle risk factors may be particularly vulnerable to the cardiovascular consequences. The population of England was thus exposed during the course of the eighteenth century, when heightened susceptibility could have then contributed to the emergence and subsequent increasing prevalence of coronary heart disease with natural selection playing some part in lessening predisposition during the subsequent two centuries.

---

[17] John Fothergill, 'Case of an angina pectoris with remarks', *Medical Observations and Inquiries*, 1776, **5**: 233–51, p. 241.
[18] John A Ryle and W T Russell, 'The natural history of coronary heart disease', *Br Heart J*, 1949, **11**: 370–89, p. 381.

# XI

# The Interplay of Risk Factors

The risk factors that might have contributed to the eighteenth-century English emergence of recognizable angina pectoris and its subsequent increase in frequency have hitherto been considered individually. Age, dietary factors, obesity, limited physical activity, use of tobacco, stress and genetic factors have all been examined in isolation. Of necessity, epidemiologists have to follow this course in order to establish whether or not any one suspected risk factor is or is not associated with an increase in the incidence of coronary heart disease. Multivariate analysis is therefore always used in order to eliminate the impact of any factor *not* under immediate study.

In the real world one or more, or even all of the traditional risk factors often co-exist, either in any one individual or in clearly defined groups of people, and they do so with a frequency greater than would be expected by chance alone. In some cases an individual may have adopted a life pattern that involved more than one risk factor. Often, for example, a diet is unhealthy in several respects. High fat and carbohydrate consumption tend to go together and both are associated with low fibre intake. An inverse relationship tends to govern consumption of fish on the one hand and animal foods including fats on the other. Coffee is frequently taken with both cream and sugar, and in the eighteenth century the patrons of coffee houses suffered secondary exposure to tobacco smoke for long periods and in high concentrations. A high fat diet is often associated with heavy smoking. Obesity is linked with low physical activity and low physical activity is conducive to obesity.

Some risk factors, even if adopted singly by an individual, lead inexorably to others. Excessive consumption of fat, and of saturated fats in particular, is associated with both systolic and diastolic hypertension,[1] as are high coffee, salt and energy intake, and diets low in fibre. Sucrose (cane sugar) elevates the total serum cholesterol level for up to eight hours when it is taken in conjunction with a high fat diet.[2] When compared to people on a high fibre diet, those with relatively low fibre intake tend to have not only higher blood pressures, but also elevated serum total cholesterol and lower HDL levels, i.e. they show adverse trends in their lipid profiles.[3] The latter are also associated with smoking and mental stress, and these two are often associated. An extreme example of risk factors being combined is seen in the patient with syndrome X, a combination of truncal obesity, hypertension, elevated serum

[1] Pirjo Pietinen *et al.*, 'Dietary fat and blood pressure—a review', *Eur Heart J*, 1987, **8**: Suppl B9-17, p. 11.

[2] Kevin I Grant, Martelle P Marais and Muhammad A Dhansay, 'Sucrose in a lipid-rich meal amplifies the postprandial excursion of serum and lipoprotein triglyceride and cholesterol concentrations by decreasing triglyceride clearance', *Am J Clin Nutr*, 1994, **59**: 853–60, p. 856.

[3] Angela Wright, P G Burstyn and M J Gibney, 'Dietary fibre and blood pressure', *Br Med J*, 1979, ii: 1541–3, p. 1542.

triglycerides, raised blood sugar, and insulin resistance.[4] Increasing age impacts unfavourably on all other risk factors.

There is now good evidence to show that when more than one risk factor is present, either in an individual or in a population, the impact on the likelihood of coronary heart disease developing is often characterized not only by an additive, but also by a multiplicative effect. John Muir and David Mant summarized the MRFIT findings concerning the impact of three risk factors on male coronary heart disease rates. In the absence of any of these risk factors as defined by the authors, the six-year "basic" mortality rate was 3.0/1000. By themselves, smoking, serum total cholesterol elevation and a high diastolic blood pressure were associated with increases above the "basic" in six-year death rates of 5.9, 6.9 and 4.7 per thousand respectively. On a simple additive basis, the three factors together would have accounted for an excess cardiac mortality rate of 17.5 per thousand. In fact, the subgroup in which all three were present suffered an excess six-year death rate per thousand of 30.5. In a small population, these conclusions might have been invalidated by failure of the investigators to stratify by the actual number of cigarettes smoked or the degree of elevation of the serum cholesterol and diastolic blood pressure levels. However, this study involved a total of about one-third of a million men, so that any such variations in risk factor "intensity" would have averaged out. The increase in relative risk produced by smoking was shown clearly to be greater when either the diastolic blood pressure, the total serum cholesterol or both were in the higher category. Figure XI.1 shows that the effects of elevated serum triglycerides on CHD incidence are greatly magnified when the total serum cholesterol is also elevated. All of these findings indicate that there is a multiplicative effect when two or more traditional risk factors co-exist in any one patient.[5]

There is increasing evidence to suggest that blood levels of some of the more recently recognized CHD risk factors, although genetically determined in varying degree, are of more serious consequence when also associated with presence of traditional factors. Those newly recognized include elevation of serum lipoprotein (a) and homocysteine levels and a variety of plasma clotting factors, notably fibrinogen and factor VII. A five-year prospective study of 2,156 men free of clinical CHD and aged forty-seven to sixty-four years at entry showed that the association of an elevated Lp(a) level with a high risk of subsequent CHD is significantly increased when the serum LDL cholesterol is in the highest tertile (RR 2.15, CL 1.34–3.44).[6] Serum concentrations of the amino-acid homocysteine rise with age and are higher in men and in smokers.[7] Platelet aggregation, which initiates blood

---

[4] Syndrome X, American Heart Association internet posting, http://www.americanheart.org/.

[5] John Muir and David Mant, 'Multiple risk', in Martin Lawrence *et al.* (eds), *Prevention of cardiovascular disease: an evidence-based approach*, Oxford University Press, 1996, p. 187; G Assmann and J H Schulte, 'Relation of high-density lipoprotein cholesterol and triglycerides to incidence of atherosclerotic coronary artery disease (the PROCAM experience)', *Am J Cardiol*, 1992, **70**: 733–7, p. 736.

[6] Bernard Cantin *et al.*, 'Is lipoprotein (a) an independent risk factor for ischemic heart disease in men? The Quebec cardiovascular study', *J Am Coll Cardiol*, 1998, **31**: 519–25, pp. 521–2.

[7] Ottar Nygård *et al.*, 'Total plasma homocysteine and cardiovascular risk profile. The Hordaland homocysteine study', *JAMA*, 1995, **274**: 1526–33, pp. 1526–7.

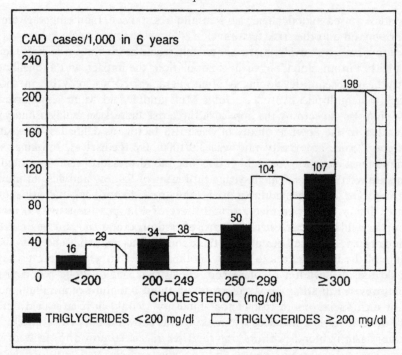

*Figure XI.1:* Incidence of CHD/1000 subjects over a 6-year follow-up in relation to triglyceride and cholesterol levels. Reproduced from G Assmann and H Schulte, 'Relation of high-density lipoprotein cholesterol and triglycerides to incidence of atherosclerotic coronary artery disease (the PROCAM experience)', *Am J Cardiol*, 1992, **70**: 733–7, p. 736. (With permission from Excerpta Medica Inc.)

coagulation, is enhanced when the lipid profile is abnormal and clot formation is promoted as a consequence.[8] Clotting factor VII activity correlates positively with both total and serum HDL cholesterol levels.[9] In men the plasma levels of the clot precursor fibrinogen are positively correlated with physical inactivity, smoking and with total serum cholesterol, triglyceride and LDL levels.[10] In the PROCAM study it was found that the impact of plasma fibrinogen levels on the combined incidence of sudden cardiac death and myocardial infarction was more than doubled when the serum cholesterol level was in the highest tertile.[11] The Whitehall health study of British civil servants showed plasma fibrinogen levels to be significantly higher

[8] Angelina C A Carvalho, Robert W Colman and Robert S Lees, 'Platelet function in hyper-lipoproteinemia', *N Engl J Med*, 1974, **290**: 434–8, p. 435.
[9] Carol J Hoffman, Robin H Miller and Mae B Hultin, 'Correlation of factor VII activity and antigen with cholesterol and triglycerides in healthy young adults', *Arterioscler Thromb*, 1992, **12**: 267–70, p. 269.
[10] Edzard Ernst and Karl L Resch, 'Fibrinogen as a cardiovascular risk factor: a meta-analysis and review of the literature', *Ann Intern Med*, 1993, **118**: 956–63, p. 959.
[11] Jürgen Heinrich *et al.*, 'Fibrinogen and factor VII in the prediction of coronary risk. Results from the PROCAM study in healthy men', *Arterioscler Thromb*, 1994, **14**: 54–9, p. 56.

among smokers when compared to non-smokers.[12] Similar differences were also observed when the job-stressed personnel in the lowest employment categories were compared with the relatively unstressed members of the highest civil service grades. The plasma fibrinogen levels of the former were the higher and the differences significant.[13]

During the eighteenth century there was, as pointed out in earlier chapters, an increase in both the relative and the absolute numbers of the English middle and upper classes and a growing tendency for them to live to a greater age than the general population. These relatively privileged members of society embraced a pattern of living that included low intake of fibre, but consumption of increasing amounts of animal fats, coffee, sugar and salt and a tendency to become obese in later life. Tobacco products were being used more extensively. Upward mobility with adoption of affluent living styles was associated with a decrease in physical activity as servants became affordable. The middle classes probably walked and rode on horseback less during the course of the eighteenth century as roads became better and horse-drawn vehicles improved in availability, speed, comfort and efficiency. Some causes of the mental stresses to which the commercial classes were uniquely subject appear to have increased during the Georgian era. In England, therefore, the multiplicative effects of the various risk factors in combination could well have accentuated the contribution of the individual elements to the late eighteenth-century development of coronary heart disease with its overt clinical manifestations, notably angina of effort.

[12] Eric Brunner *et al.*, 'Childhood social circumstances and psychosocial behavioural factors as determinants of plasma fibrinogen', *Lancet*, 1996, **347**: 1008–13, p. 1011.

[13] H L Markowe *et al.*, 'Fibrinogen: a possible link between social class and coronary heart disease', *Br Med J*, 1985, **291**: 1312–14, p. 1313.

# XII

# The Aftermath

## Angina Pectoris Comes of Age

By the start of the nineteenth century, case reports of either individual or small numbers of patients with angina pectoris were becoming less common. They had ceased to be "newsworthy" as a new generation of physicians became able to recognize the characteristic features of the pain. As early as 1809 "syncope angiosa" was being described by Allan Burns as "frequent",[1] and in later nineteenth-century general medical textbooks, such as one compiled by G B Wood in the United States in 1852, there was no longer a suggestion of anything novel about angina pectoris.[2] Authors of textbooks were able to combine composite descriptions with a tally of patients in their own practices. P M Latham, writing in 1876, referred to his last 13 cases,[3] whilst in France, H Huchard had by 1889 drawn upon his experience of 78 of his own patients (excluding syphilitics)[4] and he quoted M Gauthier as having seen 172.[5] In 1901 William Osler, then practising in the United States, reported 40 cases of his own.[6] Set against the close to 100 patients with angina pectoris seen by William Heberden a century earlier,[7] the numbers seen by any one of these physicians of the Victorian era are not particularly striking. However, the total number of doctors in the western world had greatly increased since the mid-eighteenth century. There were 15,116 physicians and surgeons practising in England in 1881[8] in contrast to 363 physicians and 89 surgeons when the first comprehensive register was established in 1783.[9] Cardiology did not have any formal status as a speciality in the nineteenth century and with treatment limited to amyl nitrite and glyceryl trinitrate, which any doctor could prescribe, there were no compelling reasons for referrals to specialists in internal medicine. There are therefore grounds for presuming that the average practitioner saw as many patients with angina pectoris as did the academic physicians who compiled the textbooks. With the greater number of the

[1] Allan Burns, *Observations on some of the most frequent and important diseases of the heart*, Edinburgh, T Bryce, 1809, p. 137.

[2] G B Wood, *A treatise on the practice of medicine*, Philadelphia, Lippincott, Grambo, 1852, Part II, p. 202.

[3] P M Latham, *Collected works*, vol. 1, *Diseases of the heart*, London, New Sydenham Society, 1876, pp. 445ff.

[4] H Huchard, *Maladies du coeur et des vaisseaux*, Paris, Octave Doin, 1889, p. 400.

[5] Ibid., p. 394.

[6] William Osler, *The principles and practice of medicine*, 4th ed., Edinburgh and London, Y J Pentland, 1901, p. 761.

[7] William Heberden, *Commentaries on the history and cure of diseases*, Boston, Wells and Lilly, 1818, p. 295.

[8] W J Reader, *Professional men: the rise of the professional classes in nineteenth-century England*, London, Weidenfeld and Nicolson, 1966, p. 211.

[9] Joan Lane, 'The medical practitioners of provincial England in 1783', *Med Hist*, 1984, **28**: 353–71, p. 353.

*Table XII.1*

Annual mortality per million from diseases of the circulatory system and dropsy

| Age | Annual mortality | | | |
| --- | --- | --- | --- | --- |
| | 1851–60 | | 1861–70 | |
| | Male | Female | Male | Female |
| 25–34 | 514 | 603 | 665 | 631 |
| 35–44 | 1,002 | 1,118 | 1,233 | 1,191 |
| 45–54 | 1,898 | 2,664 | 2,187 | 2,176 |
| 55–64 | 4,130 | 4,588 | 4,581 | 4,762 |
| 65–74 | 8,714 | 8,916 | 9,229 | 9,431 |
| 75+ | 12,203 | 11,234 | 12,825 | 12,027 |

Source: *Supplement to the 45th annual report of the registrar-general of births, deaths and marriages in England and Wales*, London, Eyre and Spottiswood, 1885, p. cxv.

former it would be reasonable to conclude that angina pectoris was becoming more prevalent in England during the nineteenth century. Clinical accounts, examples of which have been given, indicate that it was also becoming more widespread in the western world and no longer exclusively "a British disease".[10] It still involved males predominantly and remained an affliction of the affluent. Samuel Black had noted in 1819 that there was "none in the poor and laborious".[11] Half a century later, G W Balfour commented that it was "not a very common disease amongst the lower classes and we very rarely have it in the infirmary".[12] This characteristic was confirmed by Osler, who reported in 1910 that, in all his years of practice, he had record of only one patient with angina pectoris in his hospital clinics. All the others were private paying patients.[13]

From 1837 onwards, vital statistics were tabulated nationally in England and Wales. They show an increase in death rates from cardiac and circulatory causes during the Victorian era. An example is given in Table XII.1 which compares the annual circulatory disease death rates per million population at ages twenty-five and upwards during two consecutive mid-century decades and shows an increase even in this short time.[14] The rise in the actual numbers in each age category is somewhat greater because from 1856 to 1866, mid-years of the two decades being compared, the population as a whole rose by about 12 per cent. A D Morgan has compiled data from the Registrar General's reports to indicate that deaths attributed to angina

[10] William Proudfit, 'Origin of concept of ischaemic heart disease', *Br Heart J*, 1983, **50**: 209–12, p. 209.

[11] Samuel Black, *Clinical and pathological reports*, Newry, Alexander Wilkinson, 1819, p. 8.

[12] G W Balfour, *Clinical lectures on diseases of the heart and aorta*, London, Churchill, 1876, Lecture xii, p. 279.

[13] William Osler, 'The Lumleian lectures on angina pectoris, Lecture I', *Lancet*, 1910, i: 697–702, p. 698.

[14] *Supplement to the 45th annual report of the registrar-general of births, deaths and marriages in England and Wales*, London, Eyre and Spottiswood, 1885, Table 5, p. cxv.

pectoris increased from about 250 in 1855 to 600 annually by the end of the century.[15] Unfortunately, with the exception of these suspiciously small numbers, it is impossible in nineteenth-century official statistics to distinguish coronary heart disease mortality from other cardiac or even some general causes. On occasion, deaths due to heart disease were tabulated as such. At other times they were combined with dropsy and diseases of the circulatory system in general. A preponderance of male deaths at younger ages would have been expected if coronary heart disease was then a major cause, as before the age of fifty-five it has been very largely an affliction of males. In fact the government statistics indicate that mid-century male and female death rates were almost identical at all ages.[16] It is unlikely that many deaths after, say, the age of sixty were due to rheumatic heart disease as such patients rarely survived that long. The remainder, however, would not necessarily have been CHD deaths. The then undiagnosable hypertension may have contributed to the rising total of deaths late in life and their number is unknowable. One suspects that, although indeterminate in its extent, some rise in CHD death rates did contribute to the documented overall nineteenth-century increase in all causes of cardiovascular disease mortality, and consideration of possible reasons is warranted.

Demographic changes during the century that followed the first recognition of angina pectoris exceeded the sum of all that had gone before. Between 1771 and 1871 the population of England rose threefold, from 6,623,000 to 21,501,000, all the more remarkable as emigrants vastly outnumbered immigrants.[17] Fertility may have continued to increase modestly during the early nineteenth century as the age of spinsters at marriage continued to decline slightly.[18] Mortality at all ages decreased. In particular, deaths due to infectious diseases lessened with improvements in sanitation and in the quality of the water supply, notably as a result of the reforms instigated by Edwin Chadwick.[19] As the country's inhabitants grew more numerous, they also tended to live longer. Male life expectancy at birth increased from 40.4 years in the period 1838–44 to 44.1 in the last ten years of the nineteenth century. For women the corresponding rise was from 42.0 to 47.8 years. There was even a modest increase in the expectation of life at age 45. In the period 1838–44 it was 23.1 and 24.2 years for men and women respectively. By 1870 it had risen to 27.5 and 32.7 years respectively. The absolute number of persons who lived not only to middle age but even beyond increased considerably. There were 629,000 people over 60 in England in 1801; by 1871 they numbered 1,515,000.[20]

During the Victorian era the middle classes increased in number at an even faster rate than the general population, a rise well documented by W J Reader in the case of family heads in professional occupations. These included clergymen and persons engaged in finance, the arts, medicine, law and teaching. Between 1841 and 1881,

---

[15] A D Morgan, 'Some forms of undiagnosed coronary disease in nineteenth-century England', *Med Hist*, 1968, **12**: 344–58, p. 356.

[16] *Supplement to the 45th annual report of the registrar-general*, op. cit., note 14 above, p. cxv.

[17] E Anthony Wrigley *et al.*, *English population history from family reconstitution 1580–1837*, Cambridge University Press, 1997, p. 614.

[18] Ibid., p. 134.

[19] Roy Porter, *The greatest benefit to mankind*, London, HarperCollins, 1997, p. 410.

[20] Wrigley, *et al.*, op. cit., note 17 above, p. 614.

for example, their numbers rose by 125,000 to 315,000,[21] while, in contrast, the general population of England and Wales grew by only 63 per cent. The total number of middle-class heads of family was even larger than indicated by these figures; to them must be added army and navy officers, large numbers of small-scale entrepreneurs engaged in manufacturing and distribution and the mechanical engineers and technicians needed to keep the growing number of factories in operation. The middle classes' rise in number was in part a reflection of the general increase in population, but they also gained recruits from the working classes. As an example, artisans employed in expanding sections of the economy were often able to set up in business on their own and eventually become employers of labour. J Seed estimated that about 20 per cent of such people eventually moved into the middle class, defined as possession of capital credentials and/or property and with emancipation from manual labour.[22] Seed drew particular attention to the small farmers and semi-independent craftsmen from among whom an emergent middle class could be traced.[23] Finally, there were aspects of middle-class life that would have resulted in mortality rates below the national average and the proportion reaching middle and later life being higher. It is doubtful if greater access to doctors and medical advances made much of a contribution to this difference, despite developments such as the introduction of general anaesthesia[24] and antiseptic surgery.[25] The middle class may, however, have benefitted the more from medical and surgical treatment at home rather than in hospital where risk of acquiring lethal infections was very high. By and large they had better housing, adequate nutrition and higher standards of personal hygiene. They usually reaped the benefits of public health improvements in the water supply and sewer systems before these became generally available.

Reliable estimates of the incomes of persons in any one middle-class occupation are hard to obtain. There was no income tax during many years of the nineteenth century and calculations of income from the revenue records for years in which it was levied probably result in underestimates. Collection was not very efficient; avoidance and evasion were widespread. Conclusions drawn from probate data are also unreliable because of the not uncommon practice of transferring money and assets to heirs prior to death of the benefactor.[26] It is noteworthy that when the Reform Act of 1832 extended the franchise to some 300,000 male members of the middle class, their status was based on the rental value of their property rather than on income.[27] Membership of the middle class did not guarantee freedom from want. There were certainly wide variations in income within all professions. Some barristers may have enjoyed a five-figure income, others were desperate for a brief. Some manufacturers numbered their employees in the hundreds, others in single digits. It

[21] Reader, op. cit., note 8 above, p. 21.

[22] J Seed, 'From "middling sort" to middle class in late eighteenth- and early nineteenth-century England', in M L Bush (ed.), *Social orders and social classes in Europe since 1500*, London, Longman, 1992, p. 115.

[23] Ibid., p. 117.

[24] Porter, op. cit., note 19 above, p. 367.

[25] Ibid., p. 371.

[26] Seed, op. cit., note 22 above, p. 123.

[27] George Macaulay Trevelyan, *History of England*, London, Longmans, Green, 1947, p. 634.

is therefore difficult to determine for any period the proportion of middle-class persons whose means enabled them to eat without having to consider the cost of food, denoted here as members of the "upper middle class". It would be reasonable, however, to assume that between the eighteenth and nineteenth centuries this more affluent group at minimum did not decline as a proportion of the middle class as a whole, but shared in its rise in numbers and expectation of life. It is likely, therefore, that the overall population growth and increase in the number of over 45s during the period under review was greatly exceeded by the rate of rise in the number of "upper middle class" persons reaching middle age and beyond. These were the people most likely to become victims of coronary heart disease.

It follows that more than in the eighteenth century, demographic changes in the nineteenth could account in large measure for any rise in the incidence of the already prevalent coronary heart disease. However, the part played by changes in lifestyle risk factors needs consideration as well. Evidence was presented earlier to suggest that of all the changes in eighteenth-century life that contributed to the emergence and subsequent increasing incidence of angina pectoris, the most important was the greater production and rising consumption of fatty animal foods. The advances in farming methods that had been introduced in eighteenth-century England were developed further in the nineteenth and adopted ever more widely. Pastures were better drained and improved by being sown with selected grasses of proven value. Manure was used intensively and guano imported as a fertilizer from about 1820 onwards. The breeding techniques introduced by Robert Bakewell continued to be applied and their potential was the more fully realized because of the continued enhancement of the nutrition of farm animals. These changes however were largely quantitative and lacked the revolutionary character of the earlier period.[28] Despite these improvements, there is little evidence of much overall increase in the number of animals farmed in England and Wales. Comparison of 1770 with 1870 estimates indicate a 14 per cent growth in the cattle population[29] and a 38 per cent increase in the number of pigs, whilst that of sheep declined by almost a quarter.[30] Reliable estimates of the poultry population are not available.

For several reasons an increase in the amount of marketable meat and fat was greater than the rise in the number of animals would suggest. Firstly, the proportion of mature animals among those available annually for slaughter rose during the intervening century. The techniques of selective breeding pioneered by Bakewell and improvements in pasturing and stall feeding resulted in early attainment of adult weight of both sheep and cattle.[31] Secondly, as oxen continued to be replaced at the plough by horses,[32] and sheep were raised less for their wool and more for their meat, the proportion of animals available for human consumption increased. Holderness

[28] B A Holderness, 'Prices, production and output', in G E Mingay (ed.), *The agrarian history of England and Wales, Volume VI: 1750–1850*, Cambridge University Press, 1989, p. 334.
[29] G E Fussell, 'The size of English cattle in the eighteenth century', *Agric Hist*, 1929, **3**: 160–81, p. 163.
[30] G E Fussell and L Goodman, 'Eighteenth century estimates of British sheep and wool production', *Agric Hist*, 1930, **4**: 131–51, p. 134.
[31] Holderness, op. cit., note 28 above, pp. 332, 338.
[32] Ibid., p. 289.

estimated that between 1750–70 and 1850 domestic meat production increased slightly over twofold in the case of mutton and lamb, beef and veal, and a little less than twofold for pork and bacon.[33] After the legislative union with Great Britain in 1800, animals from Ireland became available, and, with some supplies from the Continent, meat imports into the United Kingdom reached over one million cwt by 1870, adding perhaps 5 per cent to the domestic supply. However, even when all these factors are taken into consideration, it is probable that the increase in availability of meat and fat, considerable though it was, could scarcely keep pace with the concurrent threefold growth in the human population. The national per capita consumption of these foods must therefore have stayed about the same at best and there may even have been a decrease.

The situation with respect to London suggests that the capital fared better than the country as a whole. The number of cattle sold at Smithfield Market rose about threefold between 1750 and 1850, from 71,000 to 227,000 and the sheep from just over 650,000 to over a million and a half.[34] The number of sheep more than doubled.[35] Here too the hundred-year increase in the amount of meat and fat available to the metropolis was probably greater than the changes in the number of animals would suggest. As already noted, the animals matured earlier and the individual mature weights of cattle and sheep tended to become greater. Also, some new meat markets opened up and furnished the capital with additional supplies. However, even when these factors are taken into consideration, it is unlikely that the increase in meat and fat supply could have reached the fivefold figure that defined the population increase of London between 1750 and 1850.[36] As was the case nationally, the per capita availability of animal foods in the metropolis would have remained at best unchanged and may even have declined slightly.

The overall figures that have been cited conceal wide per capita consumption differences within the populations of both London and the country as a whole. The skilled workman and the servant class usually ate adequately. However, the labourers and their families had little animal food. Their diets may even have worsened as the descendants of subsistence farmers became urbanized, and for many their meals consisted largely of bread and potatoes washed down with sugared tea.[37] Even these standards were affected adversely at times by rising prices or economic downturns. In contrast, the "upper middle class" could readily afford animal foods and maintain its disproportionately large share of the total available nationally.

Even with this advantage, however, the per capita meat and fat available for purchase by members of the upper middle class could not have become appreciably greater during the period under consideration and indeed may have fallen slightly. The quantity of animal products marketed, although increasing during the period under review, hardly kept pace with the approximately threefold rise in upper middle

[33] Holderness, op. cit., note 28 above, pp. 154–5, 166, 170.

[34] B R Mitchell, *British historical statistics*, Cambridge University Press, 1988, p. 708.

[35] Ibid., p. 708.

[36] Roy Porter, *London: a social history*, London, Hamish Hamilton, 1994, p. 131; Mitchell, op. cit., note 34 above, p. 19.

[37] B Seebohm Rowntree, *Poverty: a study of town life*, London, Macmillan, 1901, pp. 99–100, 115.

class numbers as suggested by comparing Joseph Massie's 1759 estimate[38] with that of W J Reader for 1881.[39] Similarly, B A Holderness concluded that per capita overall consumption of dairy products declined between 1750 and 1850.[40] Any market-imposed limitations aside, moreover, it is hard to conceive how in general any one person's intake of fat rich animal foods in a single meal could have exceeded the gargantuan amounts consumed individually by the affluent during the late eighteenth century. Restraints on greater consumption were if anything imposed by limits to the capacity of the human digestive system. In contrast to that of the eighteenth, the nineteenth-century increase in incidence of angina pectoris was not therefore associated with any evident increase in per capita intake of animal fats by the susceptible part of the population. Individually its members did not obviously eat more than their predecessors, but there were many more of them and on average they were older.

Turning to changes in other risk factors with origins in an earlier century, N Deerr documented a more than fourfold rise in sugar consumption during the nineteenth century, from 18.0 lbs annually per head in its first decade to 78.9 lbs in the last.[41] More recently, B R Mitchell published estimates that were not dissimilar; an average annual consumption of 19.6 lbs per head during the years 1799–1803, rising to 81.0 for 1894–98.[42] Sugar was used liberally by all sections of the population so that an increase in middle- and upper-class consumption probably reflected the national average, and sugar could therefore have contributed in some measure to a nineteenth-century rise in the incidence of angina pectoris. Coffee consumption in England was low at the beginning of the nineteenth century, possibly as a result of trade disruptions during the Napoleonic wars. It rose subsequently from an annual mean of 0.10 lbs per head during the years 1804–8 to a peak of 1.27 for the period 1854–58, after which there was a gradual decline to an average of 0.69 lbs per person during the 1894–98 quinquennium.[43] It would seem unlikely therefore that coffee contributed to any rising prevalence of angina pectoris in England during the Victorian era. The coming of the railways was unlikely to have made much impact on the general level of physical activity in view of the transformation in travelling patterns already effected by the improved speed and efficiency of horse-drawn transport (page 141). Some hardy souls who had been in the habit of riding long distances on horseback may have lowered their exercise tolerance as they took to the new means of transport. However, for most people there was no obvious change in physical activity as they changed from the stage coach to the train.

The only completely new risk factor to emerge in Victorian England was cigar smoking which became popular among the middle and upper classes and tended to replace other ways of using tobacco. Its medical significance has been shown in a recent cohort study of 17,774 men of between thirty to eighty-five years of age at

---

[38] Paul Langford, *A polite and commercial people: England 1727–1783*, Oxford University Press, 1992, p. 64.

[39] Reader, op. cit., note 8 above, p. 211.

[40] Holderness, op. cit, note 28 above, pp. 166–70.

[41] N Deerr, *The history of sugar*, 2 vols, London, Chapman and Hall, 1949–50, p. 532.

[42] Mitchell, op. cit., note 34 above, pp. 709–10.

[43] Ibid, pp. 709–10.

baseline and followed until either first hospitalization or death from cardiovascular disease or, if event-free, for twenty-four years. 14,682 had never smoked cigarettes and did not currently smoke a pipe. They were either non-smokers or had smoked a pipe in the past and constituted the control group. 1,546 had smoked cigars exclusively. The multivariate analysis included corrections for the cigar smokers being on average slightly older and having greater body mass indices, higher serum cholesterol levels, increased systolic and diastolic blood pressures, and diabetes more often. When compared with the controls, there was a modestly increased incidence of CHD among the cigar smokers with a relative risk of 1.27 (CL 1.12–1.45). It was somewhat greater among the men who smoked more than five cigars daily (RR 1.56, CL 1.21–2.01).[44] As the controls included some pipe smokers, the significance of the findings is increased, suggesting cigars could have made some small contribution to any nineteenth-century increase in coronary heart disease incidence.

In conclusion, there was probably some increase in the incidence of angina pectoris during the Victorian era, a time when populations were growing rapidly and becoming older. It remained for the most part a complaint of the middle and upper classes. In England there was little change in the pattern of lifestyle risk factors first established during the previous century, but as these lifestyles spread to other countries, angina pectoris ceased to be purely a "British disease".[45]

## Modern Times

The terms stable and unstable angina, myocardial infarction, sudden death and heart failure of ischaemic origin are currently used to describe the main clinical variations within the spectrum of coronary heart disease. Understanding of coronary heart disease during the 200 years following its 1768 recognition evolved with two contributions close in time laying the foundations for the modern classification of the clinical variants. In 1910 W P Obrastzow and K D Straschesko linked prolonged chest pain with myocardial infarction secondary to coronary arterial obstruction by thrombosis but compatible with short-term survival.[46] Two years later James B Herrick too delineated the distinctive clinical and pathological features of myocardial infarction, again with initial survival[47] and he subsequently established the electrocardiographic features that facilitated diagnosis in life.[48] However, the nature of coronary heart disease did not change during 200 years in anything but the absolute and relative incidence of its various manifestations. In the clinical descriptions by William Heberden[49] and contemporaries such as John Fothergill[50] it is possible

[44] C Iribarren *et al.*, 'Effect of cigar smoking on the risk of cardiovascular disease, chronic obstructive lung disease, and cancer in men', *N Engl J Med*, 1999, **340**: 1773–80, pp. 1775–6.

[45] Proudfit, op. cit., note 10 above, p. 209.

[46] W P Obrastzow and N D Straschesko, 'Zur Kenntnis der Thrombose der Koronarterien des Herzens', *Zschr Klin Med*, 1910, **71**: 116–32, pp. 118–21.

[47] James B Herrick, 'Clinical features of sudden obstruction of the coronary arteries', *JAMA*, 1912, **59**: 2015–20, pp. 2017–18.

[48] James B Herrick, 'Thrombosis of coronary arteries', *JAMA*, 1919, **72**: 387–90.

[49] William Heberden, 'Some account of a disorder of the breast', *Med Trans Coll Physns Lond*, 1772, **2**: 59–67, pp. 59–64.

[50] John Fothergill, 'Further account of the angina pectoris', *Medical Observations and Inquiries*, 1776, **5**: 252–8, p. 254.

to recognize all of the variants, including coronary thrombosis and myocardial infarction.

Coronary heart disease was not formulated in the International Classification of Disease (ICD) until as recently as 1931 and "myocardial degeneration", fatty or otherwise, was a term used until mid-century.[51] Once deaths attributable to coronary heart disease were tabulated as such, a dramatic twentieth-century rise in the number of deaths from this cause became clearly and unequivocally demonstrated in the official mortality figures of developed countries and with the evidence surviving six further *International list of causes of death* modifications. CHD ultimately became a leading cause of death in the western world, second only to cancer. Among white American males, it was by 1987 the leading cause of death at 161.7 per 100,000 per annum, with cancer deaths second at 158.4.[52] As a further example, United Kingdom government statistics indicated a one-third increase in a single twenty-year period that followed the introduction and subsequent unchanging use of the term "coronary heart disease" in the listings of causes of death. Between 1952–56 and 1972–76 male deaths rose from 168,077 to 248,077, female from 86,337 to 89,452.[53] The only departure from this trend was a transient drop in countries that suffered severe food deprivation during the Second World War. In Norway, for example, age-corrected annual mortality from circulatory diseases had fallen during the years 1943–45 to 78.7 per cent of the immediately pre-war level for men and 78.8 for woman. By the post-war period 1946–48 it had rebounded to 87.3 and 88.1 per cent respectively.[54]

In considering the reasons for this rise in CHD mortality, emphasis is being placed on circumstances prevailing in the United Kingdom although, in contrast to the late eighteenth-century situation, twentieth-century UK changes were paralleled by comparable developments in other parts of the western world. Also in contrast to the Georgian era, the extent and rapidity of the twentieth-century increase in coronary heart disease incidence are attributable in much greater measure to well documented demographic developments. During the first half of the century alone, the population of the United Kingdom grew in number by over one-third (Table XII.2)[55] and the increase was accompanied by an ever greater expectation of life. The improvement was due in large measure to a combination of improved housing, near complete eradication of deficiency diseases and, for the first time in history, a major impact of medical treatment, notably the introduction of immunotherapy for the prevention, and chemotherapy and antibiotics for the treatment of infectious diseases.[56] As a result there was a disproportionately large rise in the number of people reaching

[51] *Manual of the international list of causes of death: as adapted for use in England and Wales, Scotland and Northern Ireland; based on the fourth decennial revision by the International Commission, Paris, 1929*, London, HMSO, 1931, p. iii.

[52] National Center for Health Statistics, *Vital statistics of the United Stated 1983*, Vol 2, pt A DHHS pub no. (PHS) 87–1101, Washington, Government Printing Office, 1987, p. 12.

[53] Clive Osmond, 'Coronary heart disease mortality trends in England and Wales 1952–1991', *J Public Health Med*, 1995, **17**: 404–10, p. 410.

[54] Axel Strom and R Adelstein Jensen, 'Mortality from circulatory diseases in Norway 1940–45', *Lancet*, 1951, **i**: 126–9, p. 127.

[55] Mitchell, op. cit., note 34 above, pp. 13, 14.

[56] Porter, op. cit., note 19 above, pp. 578, 685.

Table XII.2
England and Wales population growth (thousands)

|  | Year | Male | Female | Total |
|---|---|---|---|---|
| All ages | 1901 | 15,769 | 16,843 | 32,612 |
|  | 1951 | 12,044 (33.5) | 22,771 (35.2) | 43,815 (34.4) |
| 50 + | 1901 | 2,205.3 | 2,584.7 | 4,790.0 |
|  | 1951 | 5,317.9 (141.1) | 6,897.4 (166.9) | 12,215.0 (155.0) |

Percentage increases in brackets.

Source: B R Mitchell, *British historical statistics*, Cambridge University, 1988, pp. 13, 14 (with permission).

middle and old age. Between 1901 and 1951 for example, the number of people in England and Wales aged fifty or over more than doubled.[57]

Some lifestyle risk factors that first became obvious during the eighteenth century increased in importance during the twentieth. The significance of others lessened. The need for salt diminished because with refrigeration it was no longer needed as a preservative. Sugar consumption in the United Kingdom rose, but to a limited extent, from a yearly average of 84.7 pounds per head during the decade 1900–9 to 106.0 pounds in 1970, a much slower rate of increase than during the nineteenth century.[58] Annual coffee consumption per head was static from the beginning of the twentieth century until the late 1930s at about 0.74 lbs per capita per year. It then rose fairly steadily to 4.4 lbs by 1970 probably because it was becoming a drink favoured by all sections of the population.[59] The incidence of coronary heart disease increased steadily both when average coffee consumption was static and when it was rising. There was a move from boiled to filtered and instant coffee[60] and the pattern of excessive and continuous consumption of black coffee by Georgian era coffee house patrons (see page 99) was not replicated in the twentieth century. Coffee can probably be exonerated as a recent risk factor.

In contrast, there is evidence to suggest that an increase in consumption of animal fats played as crucial a role in the twentieth century as it did in the eighteenth. Until mid-century, management of farm animals continued to have increase in weight and in fat content as the principle aims. In the United Kingdom as late as the beginning of the second half of the twentieth century, the sale values of animals were quoted as "fat stock prices". During the last part of the Victorian era steamships replaced sailing vessels and the turn of the century saw the introduction of refrigerator ships. This meant that cattle and sheep imports from the newly opened up and extensive grazing lands of Australasia and the Americas became available to augment home

[57] Mitchell, op. cit., note 34 above, pp. 13, 14.
[58] Ibid., pp. 710, 713.
[59] Ibid., pp. 710, 713.
[60] Michael J Klag *et al.*, 'Coffee intake and coronary heart disease', *Ann Epidemiol*, 1994, 4: 425–33, p. 431.

*Chapter XII*

*Table XII.3*

United Kingdom meat imports (thousands of cwt)

| 1885 | 6,712 | 1925 | 30,907 |
|------|-------|------|--------|
| 1895 | 12,098 | 1935 | 29,549 |
| 1905 | 18,680 | 1945 | 23,338 |
| 1915 | 25,432 | 1955 | 26,966 |

Source: B R Mitchell, *British historical statistics*, Cambridge University, 1988, p. 233 (with permission).

production in the more densely populated parts of the industrialized world and in the United Kingdom in particular. Meat imports to the UK rose fourfold between 1885 and 1915, although levelling off subsequently (Table XII.3).[61] Coronary heart disease in the first half of the twentieth century was still regarded as a "businessman's disease".[62] To a large extent the working classes had been "protected" by poverty from a disease associated with plenty. In 1901 B Seebohm Rowntree made a detailed survey of the state of the poor of York. He concluded that almost a half of the town's wage-earning class could not afford "sufficient for the maintenance of merely physical efficiency". His minimum diet for this allowed nine ounces of boiled bacon and the same weight of cheese as a week's intake.[63] However, with rising wages, low post-Second World War unemployment rates and new social supports, meat with its then high fat content became affordable by the working classes. Based on data from some ninety-seven surveys, Alison H Stephen and her colleagues calculated that, in the United Kingdom as a whole, fat as a percentage of total energy intake increased from 24.6 in the first ten years of the twentieth century to a peak of 40.3 in the decade 1970–79.[64] As a result, the consumption of foods high in saturated fatty acid content rose considerably. It was a re-enactment of changes in ancient Rome about which Lucretius commented, "At that time the lack of food consigned failing limbs at last to death. Now on the other hand abundance of things overwhelms them."[65] During the same period, obligatory physical activity declined considerably as towns became served by public transport networks, the car became generally available, and domestic appliances lightened domestic drudgery. Of particular significance for the working classes were the changes in farm, factory, building sites and docks as work became mechanized. Recreational exercise did not begin to compensate for the changes until the 1960s at earliest and became largely a pattern of middle- and upper- rather than working-class life.

In an important respect, developments during the past hundred years resembled those of the Georgian era. Two completely new risk factors first emerged at about the turn of the century. One was the introduction and subsequent increase in

[61] Mitchell, op. cit., note 34 above, p. 233.

[62] R G Wilkinson, *Unhealthy societies: the afflictions of inequality*, London, Routledge, 1996, p. 44.

[63] Rowntree, op. cit., note 37 above, pp. 99–100, 115.

[64] Alison H Stephen and G M Sieber, 'Trends in individual fat consumption in the United Kingdom 1900–1985', *Br J Nutr*, 1994, **71**: 775–88, p. 779.

[65] Titus Lucretius Carus, *De rerum natura Libro V*, vv 107–8, transl. R Gold (personal communication).

## The Aftermath

### Table XII.4
Cis- and trans-fatty acids as a percentage of A the fats in the diet and B the total diet*

|  |  |  | Margarine | | Butter |
|---|---|---|---|---|---|
|  |  |  | Soft (tub) | Hard (stick) |  |
| Unsaturated fatty acids | A | cis | 61.1 | 45.9 | 28.5 |
|  |  | trans | 7.4 | 20.1 | 1.5 |
|  | B | cis | 19.18 | 14.8 | 10.5 |
|  |  | trans | 3.30 | 6.72 | 1.25 |

* 35-day experimental diets; 30% fat; 20% of fat as margarine (soft or hard) or butter. 36 subjects.

Adapted from data published by A H Lichtenstein *et al.*, 'Effects of different forms of dietary hydrogenated fats on serum lipoprotein cholesterol levels', in *N Engl J Med*, 1999 **340**: 1933–40, p. 1935.

consumption of marine and vegetable oils that were artificially hydrogenated in the manufacture of margarine. Evidence was presented earlier (page 74) to indicate that during the last half of the twentieth century when vegetable and marine oils were partially hydrogenated in order to produce soft tub margarines, there was a coincident fall in coronary heart disease incidence. These soft margarines consist for the most part of cis-fatty acids with trans-fatty acids in relatively small amounts. Any theoretically harmful effects that the latter might have had were evidently outweighed by the benefits of replacing saturated by polyunsaturated fats in the diet, a change that resulted in significantly beneficial effects on the lipid profile (Table V.2)[66] and ultimately on CHD incidence and mortality (Table V.3).[67] In contrast, the hard stick margarines consumed extensively during the first half of the twentieth century were hydrogenated to a greater degree in order to make a product with the appearance and consistency of the more expensive butter with which they were competing. These hard margarines have a trans-fatty acid content two to three times that of soft margarines (Table XII.4).[68] Specifically the main constituent of hard margarines, the mono-unsaturated elaidic trans-fatty acid, has been found to affect the lipid profile adversely, producing a rise in total and LDL cholesterol and in the total-HDL cholesterol ratio (Table XII.5).[69] It must be noted too that in the early years of the twentieth century these hard margarines were not *substituted* for butter. For the poorer sections of the population they were an *addition* to a diet that had previously been very low in fats of any sort, including butter. The harmful effects of the hard margarines were not therefore countered by any concurrent beneficial dietary change. The Seven Countries study that involved 12,673 subjects in a 25-year follow-up showed location-to-location coronary heart disease mortality rates that were highly

[66] Jantine Brussaard *et al.*, 'Effects of amount and type of dietary fat on serum lipids, lipoproteins and apolipoproteins in man. A controlled 8-week trial', *Atherosclerosis*, 1980, **36**: 515–27, p. 522.

[67] Matti Miettinen *et al.*, 'Effect of cholesterol-lowering diet on mortality from coronary heart-disease and other causes. A twelve-year clinical trial in men and women', *Lancet*, 1972, **ii**: 835–8, p. 836.

[68] A H Lichtenstein *et al.*, 'Effects of different forms of dietary hydrogenated fats on serum lipoprotein cholesterol levels', *N Engl J Med*, 1999, **340**: 1933–40, p. 1935.

[69] Ibid., p. 1935.

*Table XII.5*
Effect of soft and hard margarines on the lipid profile (mg/dl)*

| Cholesterol | Margarine | | Butter |
|---|---|---|---|
| | Soft (tub) | Hard (stick) | |
| Total | 232 ± 28 | 243 ± 37 | 251 ± 36 |
| LDL | 159 ± 26 | 168 ± 30 | 177 ± 32 |
| HDL | 43 ± 9 | 42 ± 9 | 45 ± 10 |
| TC–HDL ratio | 5.65 ± 1.20 | 6.03 ± 1.27 | 5.85 ± 1.40 |

* 35-day experimental diets; 30% fat; 20% of fat as margarine (soft or hard) or butter. 36 subjects.

Adapted from data published by A H Lichtenstein *et al.*, 'Effects of different forms of dietary hydrogenated fats on serum lipoprotein cholesterol levels', in *N Engl J Med*, 1999, **340**: 1933–40, p. 1935.

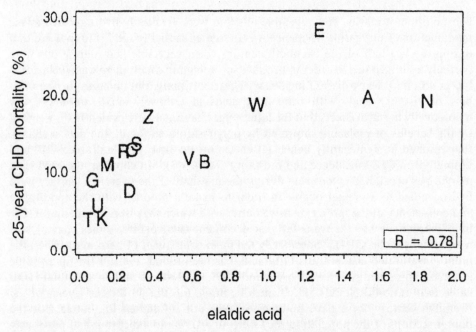

*Figure XII.1:* Association between average intake of trans-fatty (elaidic) acid and 25-year mortality rates from coronary heart disease (%) in the Seven Countries study. The letters refer to location (not listed). Source: Daan Kromhout *et al.*, 'Dietary saturated and trans-fatty acids and cholesterol and 25-year mortality from coronary heart disease. The Seven Countries Study', *Prev Med*, 1995, **24**: 308–15, p. 312. (With permission by Academic Press.)

and positively correlated with their differences in average per capita consumption of hard margarine (r = 0.78), a finding in keeping with this being a significant risk factor by reason of the trans-fatty acid content (Figure XII.1).[70]

[70] Daan Kromhout *et al.*, 'Dietary saturated and trans-fatty acids and cholesterol and 25-year mortality from coronary heart disease. The Seven Countries Study', *Prev Med*, 1995, **24**: 308–15, p. 312.

## The Aftermath

### Table XII.6

Cigarette tobacco consumption in the United Kingdom during the twentieth century (thousands of tons)

| Year | Males | Females | Total |
|------|-------|---------|-------|
| 1905 | 11.2  | —       | 11.2  |
| 1925 | 34.7  | 1.6     | 36.3  |
| 1940 | 61.6  | 11.5    | 73.1  |
| 1960 | 75.4  | 33.1    | 108.5 |

Source: *Compendium of health statistics*, 10th ed., London, Office of Health Economics, 1997, p. 21.

The second and very much more important factor was the introduction of manufacturing techniques for mass production of cheap cigarettes and their rapidly growing use by all classes during the first two-thirds of the past century, initially by men for the most part, but to an increasing extent latterly by women (Table XII.6).[71] Evidence was presented in an earlier chapter to suggest that pipe smoking with its beginnings in the seventeenth century and its increasing use in the eighteenth *may* have contributed in some small measure to the emergence of angina pectoris in the Georgian era, with secondary smoke possibly playing an additional part. However, in marked contrast, recent epidemiologic observations have established incontrovertibly a much greater and highly significant association between smoking cigarettes and ischaemic heart disease incidence, including a direct relationship between the amount smoked and the cardiac consequences.[72] It is very likely therefore that among men replacement of the pipe by cigarettes and their growing popularity among all classes from the end of the nineteenth century onwards has been a major factor contributing to the subsequent epidemic of ischaemic heart disease. The impact of cigarettes on women needs no similar qualification as with insignificant exceptions they had not smoked by any other method in preceding years.

In summary, the rising incidence of coronary heart disease, based on individual reports in the late eighteenth century and conjectural in the nineteenth, became unquestionable in the twentieth and explosive in extent as growing numbers and aging populations became exposed to the effects of two new risk factors, while at the same time adopting ever more widely most of the unhealthy dietary patterns that had their origins in Georgian England. In the United Kingdom there was increasing availability and affordability of fatty animal foods, hard margarines and cigarettes. During the same period obligatory physical activity declined greatly as work was mechanized, towns served by public transport networks and, most importantly, the car became generally available. Recreational exercise did not begin to compensate for this change until the 1960s at earliest. All of these changes were associated with a rapid rise in the incidence of coronary heart disease, greatest among male members of social classes IV and V and culminating during the 1960s

[71] *Compendium of health Statistics*, 10th ed, London, Office of Health Economics, 1997, p. 21.
[72] David Simpson, 'Trends in major risk factors. Cigarette smoking', *Postgrad Med J*, 1984, **60**: 20–5, p. 21.

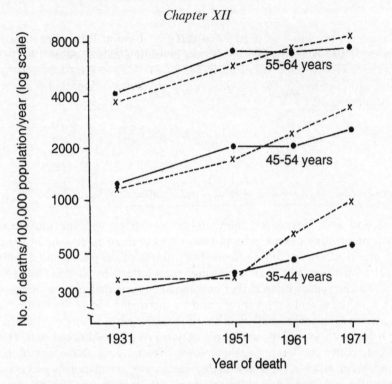

*Figure XII.2:* Non-valvular heart disease mortality in men, 1931–71, by age and social class. Solid circles indicate social classes I and II, crosses social classes IV and V. Source: M G Marmot *et al.*, 'Changing social-class distribution of heart disease', *Br Med J*, 1978, **ii**: 1109–12, p. 1110. (With permission from the BMJ Publishing Group.)

in an incidence exceeding that of social classes I and II (Figure XII.2).[73] Angina pectoris had become a complaint of the working man as well as the businessman. These changes followed in less developed countries as they caught up with the demographic and living patterns of Western Europe and North America, an example being the growing frequency of ischaemic heart disease in former Soviet satellite countries of Eastern Europe after they began to change to a market economy.[74]

The *natural* history of coronary heart disease, the record of which began for all practical purposes in 1768, drew towards its close almost exactly two centuries later when recognition of risk factors was followed by a start in their correction, achieved in part pharmacologically but also by lifestyle changes. Medical and surgical treatment of the established disease began to become effective at about the same time, but the beginnings of a fall in incidence followed increase in recreational physical activity,

[73] M G Marmot *et al.*, 'Changing social-class distribution of heart disease', *Br Med J*, 1978, **ii**: 1109–12, p. 1110.
[74] S Sans, H Kesteloot and D Kromhout on behalf of the task force, 'The burden of cardiovascular diseases mortality in Europe. Task force of the European Society of Cardiology on Cardiovascular Mortality and Morbidity Statistics in Europe', *Eur Heart J*, 1997, **18**: 1231–48, p. 1241.

fewer cigarettes smoked and changes in diet that have at least in part neutralized the impact of the Agricultural Revolution on eating habits. After 1968, with the USA in the lead and other countries including the United Kingdom and Australia following within a decade, the 200-year rise in incidence and mortality was replaced by the beginnings of a fall.[75]

---

[75] Lee Goldman and E Francis Cook, 'The decline in ischemic heart disease mortality rates. An analysis of the comparative effects of medical interventions and changes in lifestyle', *Ann Intern Med*, 1984, **101**: 825–36, pp. 825–31; Terry Dwyer and Basil S Hetzel, 'A comparison of trends of coronary heart disease mortality in Australia, USA, and England and Wales with reference to three major risk factors—hypertension, cigarette smoking and diet', *Int J Epidemiol*, 1980, **9**: 65–71, p. 66.

# XIII

# Rebuttals, Rejoinders and Refutations

"The lady doth protest too much, methinks"[1]

Before acceptance of the postulate that has been put forward, some possible concerns need to be addressed:

The conclusions are based in large measure on negative evidence, specifically the extreme paucity of documented references to chest pain on exertion before 1768.

A number of earlier clinical descriptions of what could be interpreted as angina pectoris are extant.

Coronary heart disease can occur in the absence of traditional risk factors.

Pathological evidence of coronary arterial and heart disease antedates Heberden's first description of angina pectoris.

There are causes of angina pectoris other than coronary arteriosclerosis, notably aortic valve stenosis and syphilitic narrowing of the coronary ostia.

## Negative Evidence

Negative evidence can have great significance on occasion and in widely differing circumstances. A striking example from the world of literature is to be found in Dostoyevsky's epic, *Crime and punishment* (1866). Raskolnikov, the student who murdered the old pawnbroker and her sister, committed the crime undetected and subsequently covered his tracks successfully. The suspicions of the St Petersburg police were aroused only because he was the one client of the murdered pawnbroker who did *not* reclaim the pledges that he had placed with her in pawn, an omission that led to his detection, conviction and exile to Siberia. As an example in real life, two Soviet physicists published a communication in *The Physical Review*, in June 1940, reporting that they had observed occasional spontaneous nuclear fission in samples of uranium. There was a complete lack of any American response to their publication and from 1940 onwards Russian scientists became aware of a sudden dearth of scientific publications by prominent American mathematicians, chemists, metallurgists and physicists. These negative observations convinced Soviet physicists, and secondarily the government of the USSR, that a large-scale secret atomic bomb project was underway in the United States.[2]

---

[1] William Shakespeare, *Hamlet*, III.ii.
[2] Richard Rhodes, *The making of the atomic bomb*, New York, Simon and Schuster, 1986, p. 327.

### Early Descriptions of Possible Angina Pectoris

Notwithstanding the conditions prevailing before the eighteenth century, there were undoubtedly some few individuals who had the potential for development of ischaemic heart disease. This can occur in the absence of exogenous risk factors for coronary arteriosclerosis, for example, in rare homozygous subjects with familial abnormalities of cholesterol metabolism.[3] Congenital coronary arterial anomalies can also very occasionally cause angina independently of arteriosclerotic disease.[4] Either of these could have accounted for Heberden's twelve-year-old patient with exertional chest pain. The present work does not therefore attempt to prove that angina pectoris was a totally new syndrome emerging in the mid-eighteenth century in the way, for example, that Acquired Immune Deficiency Syndrome (AIDS) first became manifest in the late 1970s. It *is* being suggested that before the mid-eighteenth century angina pectoris was too rare to have been recognisable as a distinct clinical entity by any one physician.

### Coronary Heart Disease Frequency in the Absence of Traditional Risk Factors

In mid-twentieth century studies, the frequency of symptomatic coronary heart disease occurring in the then apparent absence of risk factors may have been overestimated. When the association of lipid abnormalities with increased risk of coronary arterial disease was first recognized, "normality" of serum cholesterol was based on results of measurements that were made in apparently healthy subjects. Levels that were then accepted as normal would now be regarded as pathologically high and a consequence of the excessively fatty diets and possibly resulting obesity that has been all too common in western societies. As late as 1998, the CARE study, an investigation of the effect of pravastatin (a cholesterol lowering medication) on the incidence of coronary events among survivors of a first myocardial infarction was initiated because total serum cholesterol levels in the range of 5.2 to 6.2 mmol/L were then considered to be unproven as risk factors and therefore regarded as normal. Indeed the ethical decision to allow randomizing half the study population to placebo treatment was based on this premise. The term hypercholesterolaemia was reserved for levels above 6.2 mmol/L. The results of the CARE study itself showed that serum cholesterol concentrations earlier categorized as "average" should now be considered pathologically high, even 5.2 mmol/L being considered excessive.[5]

A measure of the incidence of overt coronary heart disease in populations with total serum cholesterol levels that are acceptable as normal by present standards

---

[3] Peter H Jones and Antonio M Gotto, 'Assessment of lipid abnormalities in the heart', in J Willis Hurst and Richard C Schlant (eds), *The heart, arteries and veins*, 7th ed., New York, McGraw Hill, 1990, p. 378.

[4] J Noble *et al.*, 'Myocardial bridging and milking effect of the left anterior coronary artery. Normal variant or obstruction?', *Am J Cardiol*, 1976, **37**: 993–9, p. 997.

[5] F M Sacks *et al.*, 'Relationship between plasma LDL concentrations during treatment with pravastatin and recurrent coronary events in the Cholesterol and Recurrent Events trial', *Circulation*, 1998, **15**: 1446–52, p. 1447.

can be derived from a number of epidemiologic studies. Among the most valuable is the MRFIT study which involved a six-year follow-up of over one-third of a million American males who were between thirty-five and fifty-seven years of age at entry and free of known coronary heart disease. The published results include reports of CHD death rates among a subgroup of men who did not smoke cigarettes and had low serum total cholesterol levels. This would have a direct bearing on circumstances that prevailed before the beginnings of the Agricultural Revolution when diets were perforce deficient in animal fats and cigarettes unknown. There were 45,353 such men in the MRFIT study who had initial total serum cholesterol levels below 4.68 mmol/L. Of these, 83 died as a result of coronary heart disease, a yearly rate of about 0.30 per thousand.[6] The United States findings have been paralleled by observations in China where Zhenming Chen and his colleagues studied 6,494 men and 2,857 women. They were observed for eight to thirteen years and their ages ranged from thirty-five to sixty-four years at recruitment. In a 2,162 subsection of these subjects the initial total serum cholesterol was below 3.53 mmol/L, their mean being 3.08. During the period of observation, there were four coronary heart disease deaths, which, assuming an average follow-up of about ten years, gives a death rate of roughly 0.18 per thousand per year.[7] Although smokers were not excluded from the study, this incidence is little more than half the rate observed in the USA investigation, the lower initial serum cholesterol level used to define the Chinese group possibly accounting for the difference. Both the MRFIT and the Chinese studies were initiated before treatment had made any appreciable impact on mortality. They both suggest therefore that a population living before the onset of the Agricultural Revolution and having perforce a low fat diet could well have been subject to comparable death rates from coronary heart disease, i.e. between 0.18 and 0.30 per thousand per year.

These low incidence rates suggest that when the serum total cholesterol levels are low, other recently recognised risk factors have little epidemiological significance (see page 74). As an example, Meir Stampfer and others conducted a *prospective* study of the relation of plasma homocysteine levels to risk of myocardial infarction. This amino acid is associated with premature arterial disease when present in excess. In what ultimately proved to be a low risk group generally, 14,916 male American physicians aged forty to eighty-four years at entry and with no prior infarction or stroke were followed for five years. Among patients with homocysteine levels in the 95th upper percentile or higher there were thirty-one cases, scarcely 0.2 per cent of the total population at risk.[8] Lp(a) also appears to be of doubtful importance as a risk factor when other lipid levels are low.[9] The same is true of coagulation and

[6] Jeremiah Stamler, Deborah Wentworth and James D Neaton, 'Is relationship between serum cholesterol and risk of premature death from coronary heart disease continuous and graded?', *JAMA*, 1986, **256**: 2823–8, p. 2825.

[7] Zhenming Chen *et al.*, 'Serum cholesterol and coronary heart disease in a population with low cholesterol concentrations', *Br Med J*, 1991, **303**: 276–82, p. 279.

[8] Meir Stampfer *et al.*, 'A prospective study of plasma homocyst(e)ine and risk of myocardial infarction in US physicians', *JAMA*, 1992, **268**: 877–81, p. 879.

[9] Bernard Cantin *et al.*, 'Is lipoprotein (a) an independent risk factor for ischemic heart disease in men? The Quebec cardiovascular study', *J Am Coll Cardiol*, 1998, **31**: 519–25, p. 521.

clotting functions. Thus G J Miller and co-workers found that when fat intake is low factor VII concentration is reduced[10] and in addition the impact of fibrinogen on CHD incidence has been found to be lower when serum LDL cholesterol levels are relatively low.[11]

If the 0.18 to 0.30 per thousand annual mortality reported in the Chinese and MRFIT studies is any indication, other manifestations of CHD such as angina pectoris could also be presumed to have been infrequent. A general physician would need to wait for years and see several thousand patients before finding a single case. This would have been the situation of the eighteenth-century doctor who was a general practitioner in the fullest sense, attending adults and children, men and women, young and old, victims of trauma, and patients with psychiatric as well as organic diseases. Recognition of a distinctive syndrome requires seeing, preferably not too far apart in time, some minimum number of patients with similar clinical features. Before 1768 Heberden saw patients with the typical chest pain on exertion with a frequency that averaged about once a year, and it was only after he had experience of a total of twenty that he could group these subjects together, showing as they did common features of a condition concerning which he "could find no satisfaction from books".[12] It is therefore understandable that a much greater rarity of angina pectoris in an earlier era could have precluded its recognition as a distinct condition by even the most observant of clinicians.

### Pathological Evidence of Coronary Arterial and Heart Disease before 1768

Arterial calcification has been described in Egyptian mummies, the earliest about thirty-five centuries old and the most notable that of the Pharaoh Menephtah. The incidence is of course unknown and observations were confined for the most part to the large arteries and to the aorta in particular.[13] Arteriosclerosis however is now known to be a diffuse process and the association of aortic with coronary arterial calcification is well recognized. Moreover, fibrous thickening of coronary arterial walls has been reported in a 3,000-year-old female mummy,[14] and "roughened" arteries were described in Bonet's *Sepulchretum* in 1679.[15] Twenty-nine years later "ossification" was observed in the coronary arteries by Thebesius, better known for the eponymously named veins and valves in the heart.[16] Coronary arterial

---

[10] G J Miller *et al.*, 'Fat consumption and factor VII coagulant activity in middle aged men. An association between a dietary and thrombogenic coronary risk factor', *Arteriosclerosis*, 1989, **78**: 19–24, p. 21.

[11] Jürgen Heinrich *et al.*, 'Fibrinogen and factor VII in the prediction of coronary risk. Results from the PROCAM study in healthy men', *Arterioscler Thromb*, 1994, **14**: 54–9, p. 56.

[12] William Heberden, 'Some account of a disorder in the breast', *Med Trans Coll Physns Lond*, 1772, **2**: 59–67, pp. 59–64, 62.

[13] H T Blumenthal (ed.), *Cowdry's arteriosclerosis: a survey of the problem*, 2nd ed., Springfield, ILL, Thomas, 1967, p. 6.

[14] Allen R Long, 'Cardiovascular renal disease. Report of a case three thousand years ago', *Arch Pathol*, 1931, **12**: 92–4.

[15] T Bonet, *Sepulchretum sive anatomia practica ex cadaveribus morbo denatis*, Geneva, Chouët, 1679, p. 387.

[16] J O Leibowitz, *The history of coronary heart disease*, London, Wellcome Institute of the History of Medicine, 1970, p. 74.

"encrustations" were described in 1740 by Johann Crell,[17] and W Cowper, who lived from 1669 to 1709, speculated that coronary arterial blood flow could become impeded.[18] The seventeenth- and early eighteenth-century pathological descriptions have been summarized by J O Leibowitz.[19]

These early descriptions of what was apparently coronary arterial calcification and sclerosis might be considered indicative of coronary heart disease having existed before the mid-eighteenth century, even if of unknown prevalence and the consequences unrecognized clinically. There is, however, recent evidence to show that calcification in coronary arterial walls is not necessarily indicative of luminal stenosis or obstruction sufficient to cause symptomatic myocardial ischaemia. Calcification has been found at autopsy to extend over about 8 per cent of the aorta and the coronary arteries of black Jamaicans thus examined and in a similar percentage of both Guatemalan Indians and Durban Bantu, yet in all of these groups clinically overt coronary arterial disease is virtually unknown.[20] J N Morris reviewed London Hospital autopsy records of the early years of the twentieth century and found that coronary arteriosclerosis was then extensive.[21] It was a period when symptomatic coronary heart disease was very rare among the deprived social classes living in the catchment area of the hospital. Sclerotic coronary arterial changes and the chest pain of myocardial ischaemia were apparently dissociated.

The strongest evidence suggesting that coronary arterial anatomic changes and frequency of overt clinical coronary arterial disease can be disparate is provided by recent studies showing the effect of serum cholesterol reduction on pathological coronary arterial anatomy on the one hand and the incidence of symptomatic ischaemic heart disease on the other. In a Dutch study it was found that following successful lowering of serum cholesterol any changes in coronary arterial lumen diameter at the point of narrowing by plaque were measured in as little as hundredths of a millimetre, but the number of cardiac events was almost halved.[22] The results of twelve similar trials were reviewed by Gilbert Thompson. Following lipid-lowering therapy quantitative serial angiography showed that evidence of coronary arterial plaques persisted and may even have worsened, albeit less in treated than untreated patients. However, epidemiologic studies of the same patients demonstrated a dramatic reduction in the incidence of symptomatic coronary arterial disease that became evident within months.[23] D Sutton and R G Grainger observed that "radiologically visible coronary artery calcification in persons over 40" plays no significant

[17] Johann F Crell, 'Dissertatio de arteria coronaria instar ossis indurata observatio 1740', in A Haller, *Disputationes ad morborum historiam et curationem facientes. Vol II, Ad morbos pectoris*, Lausanne, M M Bousquet, 1757, p. 565.

[18] Leibowitz, op. cit., note 16 above, p. 113.

[19] Ibid., pp. 70–1.

[20] Jeremiah Stamler, 'Epidemiology of coronary heart disease', *Med Clin N Am*, 1973, **57**: 5–46, p. 14.

[21] J N Morris, 'Recent history of coronary disease', *Lancet*, 1951, **i**: 69–73, p. 71.

[22] J Wouter Jukema *et al.*, 'Effects of lipid lowering by pravastatin on progression and regression of coronary artery disease in symptomatic men with normal to moderately elevated serum cholesterol levels', *Circulation*, 1995, **91**: 2528–40, p. 2534.

[23] Gilbert R Thompson, 'Angiographic trials of lipid-lowering therapy: end of an era?', *Br Heart J*, 1995, **74**: 343–7, p. 345.

part in the diagnosis of coronary heart disease.[24] Richard Frink and his colleagues found that at autopsy moderate degrees of calcification were often present in absence of significant stenosis.[25] Giuseppi Sangiorgi and his colleagues quantified coronary artery calcium at autopsy by contact microradiography while morphologic coronary artery integrity was maintained by perfusion at physiological pressures. They too found that throughout the entire range there was very poor correlation between the extent of calcification and the amount of reduction in luminal diameter.[26]

Two reasons for the discrepancy between the presence of coronary calcification and the absence of symptomatic coronary heart disease have been postulated. Firstly, degenerative changes in the arterial wall are often associated with weakening and consequent dilatation of the vessel, so that the calcified plaques project outwardly rather than into the lumen which consequently retains its size. Secondly, lipids are absorbed from cholesterol-rich and unstable plaques when serum lipid levels are reduced, whether by diet restriction, medication or both. Whilst calcific changes persist, fat-laden plaques become fibrous with stabilization of the previously fragile overlying cap. These developments, which have been observed directly in animal studies, minimize the successive risk of plaque fracture, extrusion of lipid into the lumen of the coronary artery, clot formation with blockage, and organization with subsequent increasing narrowing of the vessel, should the patient survive the episode. Persistent calcification is not therefore necessarily indicative of either flow-limiting arterial stenoses or potential for blood vessel occlusion by clot.[27]

Leibowitz has reviewed the pathological descriptions prior to the mid-eighteenth century that have been interpreted as evidence of myocardial infarction, but in many of these the evidence is inconclusive. Seventeenth- and eighteenth-century pathological descriptions, when available, are often difficult to recognize as myocardial infarction, examples being references to polyps, ulcers or "tubercles".[28] Solid substances found in the left ventricular cavity were probably clots. However, the distinction between antemortem and postmortem thrombi had not been recognized by the eighteenth century and clots in the left ventricular cavity can be associated with conditions other than myocardial infarction. More suggestive of an infarct are descriptions of cardiac rupture as cited by William Harvey in a letter to Professor Riolan of Paris and in accounts by Giovanni Battista Morgagni and S F Morand. Certainly in Harvey's patient and that of Morgagni, the rupture could have complicated a

[24] D Sutton (ed.), *A textbook of radiology and imaging*, 3rd ed., London, Churchill Livingstone, 1980, p. 491.

[25] Richard J Frink *et al.*, 'Significance of calcification of the coronary arteries', *Am J Cardiol*, 1970, **26**: 241–7, p. 244.

[26] Giuseppi Sangiorgi *et al.*, 'Arterial calcification and not lumen stenosis is highly correlated with atherosclerotic plaque burden in humans: a histologic study of 723 coronary artery segments using non-decalcifying methodology', *J Am Coll Cardiol*, 1998, **31**: 126–33, p. 130.

[27] B Greg Brown *et al.*, 'Lipid lowering and plaque regression. New insights into prevention of plaque disruption and clinical events in coronary disease', *Circulation*, 1993, **87**: 1781–9, p. 1782.

[28] Leibowitz, op. cit., note 16 above, pp. 77ff.

myocardial infarction.[29] However, cardiac rupture as described in the eighteenth century must sometimes have been an entity different from the current one. Of the mere half dozen cases documented by Leibowitz, two involved the *right* ventricle, one incidentally resulting in the sudden demise of King George II.[30] In an era in which rheumatic heart disease was prevalent, infections common and bacterial endocarditis incurable, myocardial abscesses were a possible cause of cardiac rupture. Morgagni did describe a single case in which a tendinous left ventricular wall suggested presence of scarring as a sequel of myocardial infarction and his finding of a left ventricular aneurysm in another autopsy could imply a similar cause.[31] In both of these instances the victims must have survived the episode by months, if not years. An autopsy reported by Crell stands alone in describing an intracoronary soft yellow-white body which could be extruded. It had a worm-like form and the part of the heart through which this artery passed was withered and pulpy.[32] The description is compatible with either a thrombosis or with extruded contents of a ruptured soft atheromatous lesion, but it stands alone. Although most of these pathological reports were preceded by short clinical descriptions, none made reference to chest pain on effort.

In conclusion, thousands of pathological reports concerning the heart were extant from the period under consideration, notably, but not exclusively, in the writings of Bonet, Crell and Morgagni. The findings reviewed suggest that among them there were just seven autopsy descriptions that might be ascribed to myocardial infarction and that antedated Heberden's 1768 description of angina. Among the multitude of clinical descriptions accompanying the autopsy reports there were but two mentions of pain recognizable as angina pectoris having been a feature of the preceding illness, both by Morgagni and described in Chapter III. It must be noted too that in an era in which valvular disease of the heart and its infective complications were both probably much more prevalent than today, emboli, either sterile or infected, could have been the cause of myocardial infarction (although not angina of effort) with far greater relative frequency than is currently the case. Of the handful of pathological descriptions compatible with myocardial infarction that were recorded before 1768, none is necessarily secondary to coronary arterial disease.

### Aortic and Coronary Ostial Stenoses

Aortic valve stenosis can cause angina pectoris in the absence of coronary arterial disease, but is very much rarer than coronary arteriosclerosis. It was probably less common still before the mid-eighteenth century. Arthur Boon and his colleagues and William Roberts found that risk factors for aortic stenosis included both raised

[29] William Harvey, *Exercitatio anatomica, de motu cordis et sanguinis in animalibus*, Rotterdam, Arnold Leers, 1648, pp. 99–102, 82; Giovanni Battista Morgagni, *The seats and causes of diseases*, transl. Benjamin Alexander, 3 vols, London, A Miller and T Cadell, 1769, vol. 1, Letter xxvii, p. 846; S F Morand, 'Sur quelques accidents remarquables dans les organes de la circulation du sang', *Mémoires de l'Académie Royale des Sciences*, 1732, p. 428–34.
[30] Leibowitz, op. cit., note 16 above, p. 82.
[31] Morgagni, op. cit., note 29 above, p. 846.
[32] Crell, op. cit., note 17 above, p. 565.

total serum cholesterol and hypertension.[33] Reasons for considering both of these to have been rare prior to the Georgian era have been discussed in Chapters V and VII.

It is uncommon for coronary ostial stenosis to occur as an isolated manifestation of syphilitic cardiovascular disease. There is almost invariably an accompanying aortic aneurysm, aortic incompetence or both. Aortic incompetence could lower exercise tolerance and thereby reduce susceptibility to effort induced pain, whilst the continuous pain of aortic aneurysm would tend to mask any chest discomfort induced by exertion. Syphilis was common among the poor but angina pectoris rare. William Osler became a professor of medicine in 1874. By 1889, after fifteen years in practice at the Montreal General and Philadelphia University Hospitals, he reported having seen only one patient with angina in his hospital clinics, although syphilis had been widespread in the working population from which his hospital practice was drawn. He could not comment on his experience at the Johns Hopkins Hospital, as records of fee and non-fee paying patients were not kept separately.[34]

As in the western world generally, sexual relations with multiple partners is common in the United States where some 40 million people do not have access to medical care. There is a large immigrant population that came to the USA from countries where preventive medicine is virtually non-existent. Despite this, exertional chest pain as a manifestation of cardiovascular syphilis is so rare that in 1998 a patient with classical angina of effort and angiographically proven syphilitic coronary ostial stenosis was deemed unusual enough to warrant selection for a *New England Journal of Medicine* weekly pathological exercise.[35] It would appear probable that both prior and subsequent to 1768 syphilitic coronary ostial narrowing was not associated with angina pectoris with a frequency sufficient to result in its recognition as a distinct clinical entity.

[33] Arthur Boon *et al.*, 'Cardiac valve calcification: characteristics of patients with calcification of the mitral annulus or aortic valve', *Heart*, 1997, **78**: 472–4, p. 473; William C Roberts, 'The senile cardiac calcification syndrome', *Am J Cardiol*, 1986, **58**: 572–4.

[34] William Osler, 'The Lumleian lectures on angina pectoris, Lecture I', *Lancet*, 1910, **i**: 697–702, p. 698.

[35] 'Case records of the Massachusetts General Hospital. Case 10–1998. A 46-year-old man with chest pain and coronary ostial stenosis', *N Engl J Med*, 1998, **338**: 897–903, p. 899.

# XIV

# Conclusion

It may be now asked, to what purpose tends all this labourious buzzling and groping?[1]

William Heberden's 1768 description of angina pectoris and his subsequent writings on the subject have been reviewed. Rare earlier descriptions of what might be understood as the pain of myocardial ischaemia were critically examined. Historical reasons have been given for considering angina pectoris to have been a symptom complex of exceeding rarity prior to Heberden's lifetime rather than a common but unrecognized affliction. Causes for its sudden emergence were sought, together with possible bases for a subsequent rapid increase in prevalence. As angina pectoris was initially a complaint confined almost exclusively to upper- and middle-class Englishmen, reasons for this were sought in the changes in all aspects of life that were taking place in Georgian England and the extent to which they differed from developments or lack of them in other countries. Finally, the subsequent 200-year relationship of coronary heart disease incidence to changes in demographic and lifestyle risk factors, old and new, was reviewed.

There is known to have been a modest growth in the total population of England during the early and middle years of the Georgian era and, particularly among the prosperous, some increase in the numbers of people who lived to middle and old age. These changes accelerated towards the end of the century, with a resulting growth in the number of individuals who reached an age at which they would have been susceptible to symptomatic coronary heart disease. These demographic changes, however, were deemed insufficient by themselves and too late in time to account alone for the sudden emergence and late-eighteenth-century documented prevalence of angina pectoris among the English upper and middle classes. Other possible causes were therefore sought.

During the eighteenth century there were revolutionary changes in agricultural practice in England and, as a result, a dramatic increase in both the availability and the fat content of animal foods. These included veal and beef, lamb and mutton, game, bacon, poultry, eggs and dairy products. There was in consequence a very great increase in the consumption of animal fats, notably by the members of society for whom these foods were readily affordable. Twentieth-century studies suggest that the changes in animal husbandry introduced during the Georgian era would have resulted in the fats becoming increasingly saturated, with an accompanying reduction in their polyunsaturated fatty acid content. These developments are thought to constitute the principle cause for the initial appearance and the subsequent increase

---

[1] John Graunt (1620–74), *Natural and political observations made upon the Bills of Mortality*, ed. Jacob H Hollander, Baltimore, Johns Hopkins Press, 1939, p. 77.

in prevalence of angina pectoris among the more prosperous sections of English society during the late eighteenth century.

During the Georgian era the changing diet of the well-to-do was also characterized by greater consumption of salt, sugar and coffee, reduction in fibre and possibly some lessening of fish and vegetable intake. Reasons have been adduced for considering these changes to be relevant ancillary risk factors for development of coronary heart disease, although less certain in their effects than the changes in fat consumption. Obesity was common, with people tending to gain weight as they grew older. High consumption of saturated fats, low fibre intake, very liberal coffee consumption, rising salt intake and obesity have all been implicated since as contributors to increase in blood pressure. This raises the possibility, although incapable of proof, that hypertension with its complications became increasingly prevalent during the course of the Georgian era.

The eighteenth century was the first in which tobacco consumption was at a high level, although caution is needed in ascribing significance to this because cigarettes were then unknown. People smoked pipes exclusively and tobacco was often chewed or taken as snuff, and the role of these as risk factors for development of coronary heart disease is unproven. Increasing secondary exposure to smoke, a known hazard, may have been important. Recruits to the growing business and professional classes became less active physically as they became able to afford servants. There is also evidence to suggest that improvements in horse-drawn vehicles resulted in middle- and upper-class people travelling in carriages more and walking or riding on horseback less as the century progressed. These changes had a possible impact on levels of physical activity comparable to those which resulted from rising car ownership during the twentieth century. Finally there were some increasing pressures unique to the rising middle classes, notably stresses associated with upward mobility, the need to remain subservient to those possessed of "ancienne richesse" and the growing anxieties that accompanied financial insecurity. These causes for worry could be considered significant in light of the currently recognized association of mental stress with predisposition to development of coronary heart disease. Each risk factor was initially considered separately, but two or more would frequently have coexisted in individuals or groups of people and interacted in ways now known to have not only additive but multiplicative effects on coronary heart disease incidence.

Heberden's case reports and those of later eighteenth-century physicians included not only the typical and stable pain that occurs with exertion and is relieved by rest, but also its onset at rest, unstable angina, prolonged episodes of pain with collapse, congestive changes and in some instances death. It would appear, therefore, that not only angina of effort but coronary heart disease in most if not all of its clinical variations became manifest and then increasingly prevalent during the late eighteenth century. The risk factors that have been considered could therefore be deemed contributory to the emergence of coronary heart disease in all of its clinical presentations.

By the early nineteenth century angina pectoris had been recognized throughout the western world and it probably became somewhat more prevalent during the

Victorian era when demographic factors played a more important role than formerly, with rapid growth of populations and their aging as expectation of life lengthened. The dietary risk factors that were first embraced in eighteenth-century England retained their importance in the nineteenth and became characteristic of other countries as they began to apply the farming practices developed in England during the earlier Agricultural Revolution. During the twentieth century there was an undoubted great increase in the prevalence of angina pectoris as a manifestation of coronary heart disease. Populations rose in numbers and aged as expectation of life lengthened. By mid-century, improving economic conditions in the developed world resulted in high risk diets becoming affordable by members of all social classes, whilst arrival of the car and mechanization in the workplace contributed to their ever more sedentary lifestyles. As in the eighteenth century, the impact of completely new risk factors became felt. In the Victorian era it was the cigar, and in the early twentieth century the introduction of hardened margarines with their high trans-fatty acid content and, above all in importance, the cheap cigarette. With all these developments angina pectoris became for the first time a complaint widespread amongst all the social classes of developed countries. By the 200th anniversary of Heberden's presentation to the Royal College of Physicians of London, angina pectoris had become a marker of the coronary heart disease that had become the leading cause of death throughout the developed world. This anniversary, however, marked the beginnings of effective lifestyle and medical interventions that were followed by a decline in incidence and mortality. The "natural" history of angina pectoris had come to an end.

England had led the way in the agricultural and social changes that have been described, and Georgian England was characterized by a degree of inventiveness and innovation greater than in all the centuries of recorded human endeavour that had preceded it. The Agricultural Revolution resulted in greater prosperity, diminution of want and hunger, ability to feed a growing and productive urban population. It was accompanied by a better distribution system and a consequent reduction in the impact of famine. It contributed in no small measure to better health among the general population, a rising expectation of life and an improvement in its quality. These formidable advances must be weighed in the balance when considering any untoward consequences, one of which has been the theme of this work. At the same time, the events of the eighteenth century carry a warning for the future. The evidence presented in Chapters IV and V suggests that the chemical differences between the fats of farmed animals on the one hand and those of marine mammals and fish on the other are not endogenous, but the result of changes in the land animals as a result of the human intervention in their feeding patterns. As marine mammals become threatened and killing them either restricted or abolished, their availability for human consumption becomes less. As the seas, rivers and lakes are vacuumed clean and traditional ways of fishing replaced by farming of fish, their fat content is being increased and its composition altered by artificial feeding.[2] The

---

[2] R George and R Bhopal, 'Fat composition of free living and farmed sea species: implications for human diet and sea-farming technique', *Br Food J*, 1995, **97**: 19–22.

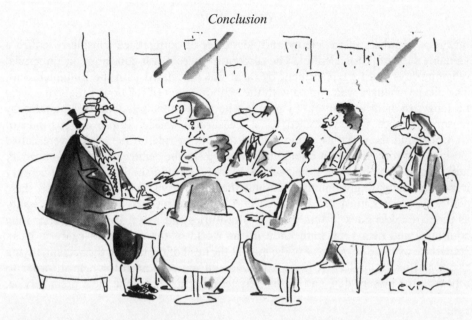

*Illustration 11:* 'Okay, will somebody please bring me up to date?' (Arnie Levin, cartoonist). (Reproduced from the *New Yorker* collection, 29 January 1996. From cartoon bank with permission.)

eighteenth-century changes in land animal feeding practices are now being replicated in the waters. Whether this will prove deleterious to human health is indeterminate at present but the possibility exists. The cloud may be no smaller than a man's hand, but a cloud it is.

In a sense, the reader has been throughout in the position of a person going through a door marked "pull" when everyone else is moving in the opposite direction and following instructions to "push". We are now living in a world which passes judgement on major lifestyles in ways that are almost Orwellian in their simplicity. Animal fats, excess calorie intake, sugar, salt and coffee are bad; fish, vegetables and fibre are good. Tobacco consumption and inactivity are bad; exercise is good. In the preceding chapters the reader was projected into a world that was almost exactly the reverse. In England, the eighteenth century was an era in which animal fats were used in increasing amounts in order to prepare dishes for which gourmet cooks and fashionable hostesses were esteemed. Obesity was seen as an indication of success and "roast beef was the Englishman's sacramental meal".[3] It was a time when sugar was enjoyed and welcomed as a product of an expanding empire of which people were proud, and with the prosperity of which they identified themselves. High fibre foods were deemed nutritionally undesirable and eating white bread was a symbol of refinement. Vegetables were held in low esteem whilst salt was welcomed as a condiment and valued as a preservative. The atmosphere in which men drank coffee was convivial, often intellectually stimulating and valuable for the transaction of

[3] Roy Porter, *English society in the eighteenth century*, Harmondsworth, Penguin, 1990, p. 21.

business. Members of the clergy and advocates of temperance considered coffee a valuable substitute for alcohol. The discontinuance of fish consumption on special religious days and its replacement by meat was associated with the Enlightenment. The dietary changes were linked with the abandonment of religious rituals that were no longer thought meaningful by people who prided themselves on being guided by reason. Tobacco was welcomed as a pleasurable solace. Improved methods of transport and the resulting reduced need to walk or ride on horseback were hailed as signs of progress and an unqualified blessing. In the eighteenth century coronary heart disease involved the privileged exclusively. During the late twentieth century it became increasingly common among the underprivileged. Because of all these contrasts, readers must be able to effect a complete reversal in attitude, necessary as they are taken back in time some two centuries and more. Personally, after long continued and near total immersion in the world of the eighteenth century, I can empathize with the *cri du coeur* of the man at the head of the table in the accompanying cartoon (Illustration 11). It is an expression of my own need for help in order to return to the present day, and in this respect the artist has done me a great service.

# Bibliography

Acierno, L J (1994). *The history of cardiology*, Carnforth, Lancs, Parthenon.

Adshead, S A M (1992), *Salt and civilization*, New York, St Martin's Press.

Ahola, I, Jauhiainen, M, and Aro, A (1991), 'The hypercholesterolaemic factor in boiled coffee is retained by a paper filter', *J Intern Med*, **230**: 293–7.

Albert, William (1972), *The turnpike road system in England 1663–1830*, Cambridge University Press.

Allbutt, Clifford (1915), *Diseases of the arteries including angina pectoris*, London, Macmillan.

Anonymous (1785), 'A letter to Dr. Heberden, concerning the angina pectoris; and an account of the dissection of one, who had been troubled with that disorder', *Med Trans Coll Physns Lond*, **3**: 1–11.

Antar, M A, Little, J A, Lucas, C, Buckley, G C, and Csima, A (1970), 'Inter-relationship between the kinds of dietary carbohydrate and fat in hyper-lipoproteinemic patients, Part 3: Synergistic effect of sucrose and animal fat on serum lipids', *Atherosclerosis*, **11**: 191–201.

Appel, L J, Moore, T J, Obarzanek, E, Vollmer, W M, Svetkey, L P, Sacks, F M, Bray, G E, Vogt, T J, Cutler, J A, Windhauser, M M, *et al.* (1997), 'A clinical trial of the effects of dietary patterns on blood pressure', *N Engl J Med*, **336**: 1117–24.

Armstrong, W A, Huzel, J P (1989), 'Food, shelter and self help', in G E Mingay (ed.), *The agrarian history of England and Wales, Volume VI: 1750–1850*, Cambridge University Press.

Aronow, W S (1978), 'Effect of passive smoking on angina pectoris patients', *N Engl J Med*, **299**: 21–4.

Ascherio, A, Rimm, E B, Stampfer, M J, Giovanucci, E L, and Willett, W C (1995), 'Dietary intake of marine n-3 fatty acids, fish intake and the risk of coronary heart disease among men', *N Engl J Med*, **332**: 977–82.

Assmann, G and Schulte, J H (1992), 'Relation of high-density lipoprotein cholesterol and triglycerides to incidence of atherosclerotic coronary artery disease (the PROCAM experience)', *Am J Cardiol*, **70**: 733–7.

Aurelianus, C (1950), *On acute diseases and On chronic diseases*, transl. I E Drabkin, University of Chicago Press.

Austin, M A (1991), 'Plasma triglyceride and coronary artery disease', *Arterioscler Thromb*, **11**: 2–14.

Bair, C W, and Marion, W M (1978), 'Yolk cholesterol in eggs from various species', *Poult Sci*, **57**: 1260–5.

Baker, W J (1988), *Sports in the western world*, Urbana and Chicago, University of Illinois Press.

Balarajan, R, Bulusu, L, Adelstein, A M, and Shukla, V (1984), 'Patterns of mortality among migrants to England from the Indian subcontinent', *Br Med J*, **289**: 1185–7.

*Bibliography*

Balfour, G W (1876), *Clinical lectures on diseases of the heart and aorta*, London, Churchill.

Bang, H O, and Dyerberg, J (1951), 'Mortality from circulatory disease in Norway 1927–48', *Lancet*, **i**: 126–9.

Barker, D J P, and Osmond, C (1986), 'Infant mortality, childhood nutrition and ischaemic heart disease in England and Wales', *Lancet*, **i**: 1077–81.

Baugh, D A (ed.) (1975), *Aristocratic government and society in England*, New York, Francis Watts.

Beamish, R E, Singal, P, and Dhalla, N S (eds) (1985, *Stress and heart disease*, Boston, Martinus Nijhoff Publishing.

Ben-Shlomo, Y, Smith, G D, Shipley, M J, and Marmot, M G (1994), 'What determines mortality risk in male former cigarette smokers?', *Am J Public Health*, **84**: 1235–42.

Berlin, J A, and Colditz, G A (1990), 'A meta-analysis of physical activity in the prevention of coronary heart disease', *Am J Epidemiol*, **132**: 612–28.

Black, S (1795), 'Case of angina pectoris with remarks', *Memoirs of the Medical Society of London*, **4**: 261–79.

Black, S (1819), *Clinical and pathological reports*, Newry, Alexander Wilkinson.

Blomquist, C G, and Salton, B (1983), 'Cardiovascular adaptations to physical training', *Ann Rev Physiol*, **45**: 169–89.

Blumenthal, H T (ed.) (1967), *Cowdry's arteriosclerosis: a survey of the problem*, 2nd ed., Springfield, ILL, Thomas.

Bogart, H (1813), *An inaugural dissertation on angina pectoris*, New York, C S Van Winkle.

Bonet, T (1679), *Sepulchretum sive anatomia practica ex cadaveribus morbo denatis*, Geneva, Chouët.

Boon, A, Cheriex, E, Lodder, J, and Kessels, F (1997), 'Cardiac valve calcification: characteristics of patients with calcification of the mitral annulus or aortic valve', *Heart*, **78**: 472–4.

Bosma, H, Marmot, M G, Hemingway, H, Nicholson, A C, Brunner, E, and Stansfeld, S A (1997), 'Low job control and risk of coronary heart disease in Whitehall II (prospective cohort) study', *Br Med J*, **314**: 558–65.

Boston Collaborative Drug Surveillance Program report, Jick, H, Miettinen, O S, Neff, R K, Shapiro, S S, Heinonen, O P, and Slone, D (1972), 'Coffee drinking and acute myocardial infarction', *Lancet*, **ii**: 1278–81.

Boswell, J (1989), *The London journal 1762–1763*, ed. F A Pottle, M K Danziger, and F Brady, London, McGraw-Hill.

Bowden, P W (1985), 'Agricultural prices, wages, farm profits and rents', in Thirsk, J (ed.), *The agrarian history of England and Wales, Volume V: 1640–1750. II. Agrarian change*, Cambridge University Press.

Boyd, W (1970), *A textbook of pathology*, 8th ed., Philadelphia, Lea and Febiger.

Braudel, F (1995), *The Mediterranean and the Mediterranean world in the age of Philip II*, transl. S Reynolds, 2 vols, Berkeley, University of California Press.

Breckon, B, and Parker, J (1991), *Tracing the history of houses*, Newbury, Countryside Books.

# Bibliography

Broder, S, Memgan, T C Jr, and Bolognesi, D (1994), *Textbook of AIDS medicine*, London, Williams and Wilkins.

Brown, B G, Zhao, X Q, Sacco, D E, and Albers J J (1993), 'Lipid lowering and plaque regression. New insights into prevention of plaque disruption and clinical events in coronary disease', *Circulation*, **87**: 1781–9.

Brown, J and Beecham, H A (1989), 'Farming practices', in G E Mingay (ed.), *The agrarian history of England and Wales, Volume VI: 1750–1850*, Cambridge University Press.

Brunner, E, Davey Smith, G, Marmot, M, Canner, R, Beksinska, M, and O'Brien, J (1996), 'Childhood social circumstances and psychosocial behavioural factors as determinants of plasma fibrinogen', *Lancet*, **347**: 1008–13.

Brussaard, J H, Dallinga-Thie, G, Groot, P H, and Katan, M B (1980), 'Effects of amount and type of dietary fat on serum lipids, lipoproteins and apolipoproteins in man. A controlled 8-week trial', *Atherosclerosis*, **36**: 515–27.

Burch, G E, and Colcolough, H L (1970), 'Postcardiotomy and postinfarction syndromes—a theory', *Am Heart J*, **80**: 290–1.

Burns, A (1809), *Observations on some of the most frequent and important diseases of the heart*, Edinburgh, T Bryce.

Burr, M L, Fehily, A M, Rogers, S, Welsby, E, King, S, and Sandham, S (1989), 'Effect of changes in fat, fish and fibre intakes on death and myocardial reinfarction: diet and reinfarction trial', *Lancet*, **ii**: 757–61.

Bush, M L (ed.) (1992), *Social orders and social classes in Europe since 1500*, London, Longman.

Campbell, J (1774), *Political survey of Great Britain*, London, printed by the author.

Cannon, J, and Griffiths, R (1989), *The Oxford illustrated history of the British monarchy*, Oxford University Press.

Cantin, B, Gagnon, F, Moorjani, S, Depres, J P, Lamarche, B, Lupien, P J, and Dageneus, G R (1998), 'Is lipoprotein (a) an independent risk factor for ischemic heart disease in men? The Quebec cardiovascular study', *J Am Coll Cardiol*, **31**: 519–25.

Carvalho, A C A, Colman, R W, and Lees, R S (1974), 'Platelet function in hyperlipoproteinemia', *N Engl J Med*, **290**: 434–8.

'Case records of the Massachusetts General Hospital Case 10–1998. A 46-year-old man with chest pain and coronary ostial stenosis' (1998), *N Engl J Med*, **13**: 897–903.

Chartres, J A (1985), 'The marketing of agricultural produce', in Thirsk, J (ed.), *The agrarian history of England and Wales, Volume V: 1640–1750. II. Agrarian change*, Cambridge University Press.

Chen, W J L, and Anderson, J W (1986), 'Hypocholesterolemic effects of soluble fibres', in Vahouny, G V, and Kritchevsky, D (eds.), *Washington symposium on dietary fibre*, New York, Plenum Press.

Chen, Z, Peto, R, Collins, R, MacMahon, S, Lu, J, and Li, W (1991), 'Serum cholesterol and coronary heart disease in a population with low cholesterol concentration', *Br Med J*, **303**: 276–82.

Cheyne, G (1733), *The English malady; or, A treatise of nervous diseases of all kinds, as spleen, vapours, lowness of spirits, hypochondriacal and hysterical distempers*, Dublin, S Powell.

Christensen, W N, and Hinkle, L E Jr (1961), 'Differences in illness and prognostic signs in two groups of young men', *JAMA*, **177**: 247–53.

Clay, C (1985), 'Landlords and estate management in England', in Thirsk, J (ed.), *The agrarian history of England and Wales, Volume V: 1640–1750. II. Agrarian change*, Cambridge University Press.

Cockerell, H A L, and Green, E (1976), *The British insurance business, 1547–1970*, London, Heinemann Educational Books.

Collins, E J T (1989), 'Introduction' to 'The agricultural servicing and processing industries', in Mingay, G E (ed.) *The agrarian history of England and Wales, Volume VI: 1750–1850*, Cambridge University Press.

*Compendium of health statistics*, (1997), 10th ed., London, Office of Health Economics.

Corvisart, J N (1818), *Essaie sur les maladies et les lésions organiques du coeur et des gros vaisseaux*, Paris, Méquignon-Marvis.

*Cowdry's Arteriosclerosis and Thrombosis* (1967), Blumenthal, H T (ed.), 2nd ed., Springfield, Illinois, Thomas.

Crawford, M A (1968), 'Fatty acid ratios in free-living and domestic animals. Possible implications for atheroma', *Lancet*, **i**: 1329–33.

Crawford, M A (ed.) (1968), *Comparative nutrition of wild animals: the proceedings of a symposium held at the Zoological Society of London held on 10 and 11 November 1966*, London, published for the Zoological Society of London by Academic Press.

Crawford, M A, Gale, M M, Woodford, M H, and Casperd, N M (1970), 'Comparative studies on fatty acid composition of wild and domestic meats', *Int J Biochem*, **1**: 295–305.

Crell, J F (1757), 'Dissertatio de arteria coronaria instar ossis indurata observatio 1740', in Haller, A, *Disputationes ad morborum historiam et curationem facientes*, Vol. 2, *Ad morbos pectoris*, Lausanne, M M Bousquet.

*The Critical Review or Annals of literature* (1772).

Daviglus, M L, Stamler, J, Orencia, A J, Dyer, A R, Liu, K, Greenland, P, Walsh, M K, Morris, D, and Shekelle, R B (1997), 'Fish consumption and the 30-year risk of fatal myocardial infarction', *N Engl J Med*, **336**: 1046–53.

Dawber, T R (1980), *The Framingham study: the epidemiology of atherosclerotic disease*, Cambridge, MA, Harvard University Press.

Dawber, T R, Kannel, W B, and Gordon, T (1974), 'Coffee and cardiovascular disease, observations from the Framingham study', *N Engl J Med*, **291**: 871–4.

De Groot, A P, Luyken, R, and Pikaar, N A (1963), 'Cholesterol lowering effect of rolled oats' (letter), *Lancet*, **ii**: 303–4.

Deerr, N (1949–50), *History of sugar*, 2 vols, London, Chapman and Hall.

Desportes, E H (1811), *Traité de l'angine de poitrine, ou nouvelles recherches sur une maladie de la poitrine, que l'on a presque toujours confondue avec l'asthme, les maladies du coeur, etc.*, Paris, Méquignon.

Després, J P, Lamarche, B, Mauriege, P, Cantin, B, Dagenais, G R, Moorjani, S, and Lupien, P J (1996), 'Hyperinsulinemia as an independent risk factor for ischemic heart disease', *N Engl J Med*, **334**: 952–7.

Dhawan, J, Bray, C L, Warburton, R, Ghambhir, D S, and Morris, J (1994), 'Insulin resistance, high prevalence of diabetes and cardiovascular risk in immigrant Asians. Genetic or environmental effect?', *Br Heart J*, **72**: 413–21.

Diamond, J (1997), *Guns, germs and steel: the fates of human societies*, W W Norton.

Dobson, J F (1927), 'Erasistratus', *Proc Royal Soc Med*, **20** (2): 825–32.

Dobson, M J (1997), *Contours of death and disease in early modern England*, Cambridge University Press.

Dressler, W J (1956), 'A post-myocardial-infarction syndrome', *JAMA*, **160**: 1379–83.

Drewnowski, A (1992), 'Sensory properties of fats and fat replacements', *Nutr Rev*, **50** (4, Part 2): 17–20.

Drummond, J C, and Wilbraham, A (1959), *The Englishman's food*, London, Readers Union and Jonathan Cape.

Ducimetiere, P, Eschwege, E, Papoz, L, Richard, J L, Claude, J R, and Rosselin, G (1980), 'Relationship of plasma insulin levels to the incidence of myocardial infarction and coronary heart disease mortality in a middle-aged population', *Diabetologia*, **19**: 205–10.

Dwyer, T, and Hetzel, B S (1980), 'A comparison of trends of coronary heart disease mortality in Australia, USA and England and Wales with reference to three major risk factors—hypertension, cigarette smoking and diet', *Int J Epidemiol*, **9**: 65–71.

Eckles, C H (1956), *Dairy cattle and milk production*, 5th ed. revised by E L Anthony, New York, Macmillan.

Elton, G R (1974), *England under the Tudors*, 2nd ed., London, Methuen.

Emmett, P M, and Heaton, K W (1995), 'Is extrinsic sugar a vehicle for dietary fat?', *Lancet*, **345**: 1537–40.

Ernle, Lord (1925), *The land and its people: chapters in rural life and history*, London, Hutchinson.

Ernle, Lord (1888), *The pioneers and progress of English farming*, London, Longmans, Green.

Ernst, E, and Resch, K L (1993), 'Fibrinogen as a cardiovascular risk factor: meta-analysis and review of the literature', *Ann Intern Med*, **118**: 956–63.

Faure, L, and Cazeilles, M (1953), 'Pericardite arguë récidivante et infarctus du myocarde', *Journal de Médecine de Bordeaux et du Sud Ouest*, **130**: 489–92.

Fisher, H A L (1946), *A history of Europe*, London, Edward Arnold.

Fishman, A P and Richards, D W (eds) (1964), *Circulation of the blood: men and ideas*, New York, Oxford University Press.

Floud, R, Gregory, A, and Wachter, K (1990), *Height, health and history: nutritional status in the United Kingdom 1750–1980*, Cambridge University Press.

Forsdahl, A (1977), 'Are poor living conditions in childhood and adolescence an important risk factor for atherosclerotic heart disease?', *Br J Prev Soc Med*, **31**: 91–5.

Fothergill, J (1776), 'Case of an angina pectoris with remarks', *Medical Observations and Inquiries*, **5**: 233–51.

Fothergill, J (1776), 'Further account of the angina pectoris', *Medical Observations and Inquiries*, **5**: 252–8.

Frink, R J, Achor, R W P, Brown, A L Jr, Kincaid, O W, and Brandenburg, R O

(1970), 'Significance of calcification of the coronary arteries', *Am J Cardiol*, **26**: 241–7.

Fussell, G E (1929), 'The size of English cattle in the eighteenth century', *Agric Hist*, **3**: 160–81.

Fussell, G E, and Goodman, C (1930), 'Eighteenth century estimates of British sheep and wool production', *Agric Hist*, **4**: 131–51.

Galton, F (1884), 'The weights of British noblemen during the last three generations', *Nature*, **29**: 266–8.

Garrett, L (1994), *The coming plague*, New York, Farrar, Straus and Giroux.

George, D M (1965), *London life in the eighteenth century*, New York, Harper and Row.

George, R, and Bhopal, R (1995), 'Fat composition of free living and farmed sea species: implications for human diet and sea-farming technique', *Br Food J*, **97**: 19–22.

Gibson, J P (1989), 'Altering milk composition through genetic selection', *J Dairy Sci*, **72**: 2815–25.

Glasse, H (1971), *The art of cookery made plain and easy*, facsmile reprint of 1796 ed., Hamden, CT, Archon Books.

Gleibermann, L (1973), 'Blood pressure and dietary salt in human populations', *Ecol Food Nutr*, **2**: 143–56.

Gold, K V, and Davidson, D M (1988), 'Oat bran as a cholesterol-reducing dietary adjunct in a young, healthy population', *West J Med*, **148**: 299–302.

Goldie, M, and Locke, J (1993), 'Jonas Proast and religious toleration 1688–92', in Walsh, J, Haydon, C, and Taylor, S (eds.), *The Church of England* c. *1689–*c. *1833: from toleration to tractarianism*, Cambridge University Press.

Goldman, L, and Cook, E F (1984), 'The decline in ischemic heart disease mortality rates. An analysis of the comparative effects of medical interventions and changes in lifestyle', *Ann Intern Med*, **101**: 825–36.

Goodman, J (1993), *Tobacco in history*, London, Routledge.

Goodman, L S and Gilman, A (1996) *Goodman & Gilman's The pharmacological basis of therapeutics*, 9th ed., ed. J G Hardman, and L E Limbird, New York, McGraw-Hill.

Grant, K I, Marais, M P, and Dhansay, M A (1994), 'Sucrose in a lipid-rich meal amplifies the postprandial excursion of serum and lipoprotein triglyceride and cholesterol concentrations by decreasing triglyceride clearance', *Am J Clin Nutr*, **59**: 853–60.

Grant, M (1991), 'Ancient writers bibliography', in *idem, The founders of the western world: a history of Greece and Rome*, New York, Charles Scribner and Sons.

Grant, M (1978), *History of Rome*, New York, Charles Scribner and Sons.

Grant, W (1779), *Some observations on the origins, progress, and method of treating the atrabilious temperament and gout*, London, T Cadell.

Graunt, J (1939), *Natural and political observations made upon the Bills of Mortality*, ed. J H Hollander, Baltimore, Johns Hopkins University Press.

Gray, S, and Wykott, V J (1940–41), 'Tobacco trade in the eighteenth century', *Southern Econ J*, **7**: 1–26.

Grigg, D (1992), *The transformation of agriculture in the west*, Oxford, Blackwell.

Grobbee, D E, Rimm, E B, Giovanucci, E, Colditz, G, Stampfer, M, and Willett, W (1990), 'Coffee, caffeine, and cardiovascular disease in men', *N Engl J Med*, **323**: 1026–32.

Habbakuk, H J (1975), 'England's nobility', in Daniel A Baugh (ed.), *Aristocratic government and society in England*, New York, Francis Watts.

Hall, A P (1965), 'Correlations among hyperuricemia, hypercholesterolemia, coronary disease and hypertension', *Arthritis Rheum*, **8**: 846–64.

Haller, A (1757), *Disputationes ad morborum historiam et curationem facientes*, Vol. 2, *Ad morbos pectoris*, Lausanne, M M Bousquet.

Hammond, E C (1966), 'Smoking in relation to death rates of one million men and women', *Nat Cancer Inst Monogr*, **19**: 127–204.

Hargis, P S (1988), 'Modifying egg yolk cholesterol in the domestic fowl', *World Poult Sci J*, **44**: 17–29.

Hargreaves, A D, Logan, R L, Elton, R A, Buchanan, K D, Oliver, M F, and Riemersma, R A (1992), 'Glucose tolerance, plasma insulin, HDL cholesterol and obesity: 12-year follow-up and development of coronary heart disease in Edinburgh men', *Atherosclerosis*, **94**: 61–9.

Harley, D (1993), 'The beginnings of the tobacco controversy: puritanism, James I and the royal physicians', *Bull Hist Med*, **67**: 28–50.

Hart, D (1985), 'Gout and non-gout through the ages', *Br J Clin Pract*, **39**: 91–2.

Harvey, W (1648), *Exercitatio anatomica, de motu cordis et sanguinis in animalibus*, Rotterdam, Arnold Leers.

Harvey, W (1848), 'A second disquisition to John Riolan', in *The works of William Harvey MD*, London, Sydenham Society.

Haskell, W L, Brachfield, N, Bruce, R A, Davis, P O, Dennis, C A, and Fox, S M (1989), 'Task force II: Determination of occupational working capacity in patients with ischemic heart disease', *J Am Coll Cardiol*, **14**: 1025–34.

Hayes, C J, Baldwin, M W and Cole, C W (1956), *History of Europe*, 2 vols, New York, Macmillan.

Heberden, E (1989), *William Heberden: physician of the age of reason*, London, Royal Society of Medicine Services.

Heberden, W, Case notes, *Index historiae morborum*, Royal College of Physicians of London, manuscript 342.

Heberden, W (1802), *Commentaries on the history and cure of diseases*, 2nd ed., London, T Payne.

Heberden, W (1818), *Commentaries on the history and cure of diseases*, from the last London ed., Boston, Wells and Lilly.

Heberden, W (1772), 'Some account of a disorder in the breast', *Med Trans Coll Physns Lond*, **2**: 59–67.

Hechter, H H, and Borhani, N O (1965), 'Mortality and geographic distribution of arteriosclerotic heart disease', *Public Health Rep*, **80**: 11–24.

Heckers, H, Göbel, V, and Kleppel, U (1994), 'End of the coffee mystery: diterpene alcohols raise serum low-density lipoprotein cholesterol and triglyceride levels' (letter), *J Intern Med*, **235**: 192–3.

Heinrich, J, Ballersen, L, Schulte, H, Assmann, G, and van de Loo, J (1994), 'Fibrinogen and factor VII in the prediction of coronary risk. Results from the PROCAM study in healthy men', *Arterioscler Thromb*, **14**: 54–9.

Herrick, J B (1912), 'Clinical features of sudden obstruction of the coronary arteries', *JAMA*, **59**: 2015–20.

Herrick, J B (1919), 'Thrombosis of coronary arteries', *JAMA*, **72**: 387–90.

Heyden, S, Tyroler, H A, Heiss, G, Hames, C G, and Bartel, A (1978), 'Coffee consumption and mortality. Total mortality, stroke mortality, and coronary heart disease mortality', *Arch Intern Med*, **138**: 1472–5.

Hickey, N, Mulcahy, R, Daly, L, Graham, I, O'Donoghue, S, and Kennedy, C (1983), 'Cigar and pipe smoking related to four year survival of coronary patients', *Br Heart J*, **49**: 423–6.

Hinkle, L E Jr, Whitney, L H, Lehman, E W, Dunn, J, Benjamin, B, King, R, Plakun, A, and Flehinger, B (1968), 'Occupation, education and coronary heart disease. Risk is influenced more by education and background than by occupational experiences, in the Bell System', *Science*, **161**: 238–46.

Hoffman, C J, Miller, R H, Hultin, M B (1992), 'Correlation of factor VII activity and antigen with cholesterol and triglycerides in healthy young adults', *Arterioscler Thromb*, **12**: 267–70.

Hoffmann, F (1748), 'Consultationes medicae: casus lxxxiii', in original Latin in Bogart, H, (1813) *An inaugural dissertation on angina pectoris*, New York, C S Van Winkle.

Holderness, B A (1989), 'Prices, production and output', in Mingay, G E (ed.), *The agrarian history of England and Wales, Volume VI: 1750–1850*, Cambridge University Press.

Hollingsworth, T H (1964), *Demography of the British peerage, Population Studies*, **18**: Supplement No. 2, London, Population Investigation Committee, London School of Economics.

Home, E (1794), 'A short account of the author's life', in Hunter, J, *A treatise on the blood, inflammation and gunshot wounds*, London, John Richardson.

Hooper, J (1792), 'A case of angina pectoris', *Memoirs of the Medical Society of London*, **1**: 238–43.

Hopkins, D R (1983), *Princes and peasants: smallpox in history*, University of Chicago Press.

Hopkins, P N, and Williams, R R (1981), 'A survey of 246 reputed coronary risk factors', *Atherosclerosis*, **40**: 1–52.

Houston, R A (1992), *Population history of Britain and Ireland, 1500–1750*, London, Macmillan Education.

Howe, G M (1970), *National atlas of disease mortality in the United Kingdom*, London, Butler and Tanner.

Howell, T H (1969), 'George Cheyne's essay on health and long life', *Gerontology*, **9**: 226–8.

Hubert, H H, Feinleib, M, McNamara, P M, and Castelli, W P (1983), 'Obesity as an independent risk factor for cardiovascular disease. A 26-year follow-up of participants in the Framingham heart study', *Circulation*, **67**: 968–70.

Huchard, H (1889), *Maladies du coeur et des vaisseaux*, Paris, Octave Doin.

Hughes, E (1934), *Studies in administration and finance 1558–1825*, Philadelphia, Porcupine Press.

Hunton, P (1995), 'The broiler industry. Thirty-four years of progress', *Poultry International*, **34**: 28–30.

Hurst, J W and Schlant, R C (eds) (1990), *The heart, arteries and veins*, 7th ed., New York, McGraw-Hill.

Iacono, J M, Marshall, M W, Dougherty, R M, and Wheeler, M A (1975), 'Reduction in blood pressure associated with high polyunsaturated fat diets that reduce blood cholesterol in man', *Prev Med*, **4**: 426–43.

Interstate Cooperative Research Group (1988), 'Intersalt: an international study of electrolyte excretion and blood pressure. Results for 24-hour urinary sodium and potassium excretion', *Br Med J*, **297**: 319–28.

Iribarren, C, Tekawa, I S, Sidney, S, and Friedman, G D (1999), 'Effect of cigar smoking on the risk of cardiovascular disease, chronic obstructive lung disease, and cancer in men', *New Engl J Med*, **340**: 1773–80.

Izzo, J L Jr, Ghosal, A, Kwong, T, Freeman, R B, and Jaenike, J R (1983), 'Age and prior caffeine use alter the cardiovascular and adrenomedullary responses to oral caffeine', *Am J Cardiol*, **52**: 769–73.

Jackson, R, and Beaglehole, R (1987). 'Trends in dietary fat and cigarette smoking and the decline in coronary heart disease in New Zealand', *Int J Epidemiol*, **16**: 377–82.

Jacobsen, B K, Bjelke, E, Kvale, G, and Heuch, I (1986), 'Coffee drinking, mortality, and cancer incidence: results from a Norwegian prospective study', *J Nat Cancer Inst*, **76**: 823–31.

Jick, H J, Miettinen, O S, Neff, R K, Shapiro, S, Heinonen, O P, and Slone, D (1973), 'Coffee and myocardial infarction. A report from the Boston Collaborative Surveillance Program', *N Engl J Med*, **289**: 63–7.

Jones, P H, and Gotto, A M (1990), 'Assessment of lipid abnormalities in the heart', in Hurst, J W and Schlant, R C (eds), *The heart, arteries and veins*, 7th ed., New York, McGraw-Hill.

Joyce, J (1967), *The story of passenger transport in Britain*, London, I Allan.

Judd, P A, and Truswell, A S (1981), 'The effect of rolled oats on blood lipids and fecal steroid excretion in man', *Am J Clin Nutr*, **34**: 2061–7.

Jukema, J W, Bruschke, A V, van Boven, A J, Reiber, J H, Ball, E T, Zwinderman, A H, Jansen, H, Boerma, G J, van Rappard, F M, Lie, K I, *et al.* (1995), 'Effects of lipid lowering by pravastatin on progression and regression of coronary artery disease in symptomatic men with normal to moderately elevated serum cholesterol levels. The Regression Growth Evaluation Study (REGRESS)', *Circulation*, **91**: 2528–40.

Kaijser, L, and Berglund, B (1985), 'Effect of nicotine on coronary blood flow in man', *Clin Physiol*, **5**: 541–52.

Kannel, W (1975), 'Role of blood pressure in cardiovascular disease: the Framingham study', *Angiology*, **26**: 1–14.

Kannel, W B, and Thom, T J, 'Statistical data of clinical importance, incidence, prevalence and mortality of cardiovascular disease', in Hurst, J W, and Schlant, R C (eds) (1990), *The heart, arteries and veins*, 7th ed., New York, McGraw-Hill.

Kaplan, G A, and Salonen, J T (1990), 'Socioeconomic conditions in childhood and ischaemic heart disease during middle age', *Br Med J*, **301**: 1121–3.

Katan, M B (1995), 'Fish and heart disease', *N Engl J Med*, **332**: 1024–5.

Kato, H, Tillotson, J, Nichaman, M Z, Rhoads, G G, and Hamilton, H B (1973), 'Epidemiological studies of coronary heart disease and stroke in Japanese men living in Japan, Hawaii and California. Serum lipids and diet', *Am J Epidemiol*, **97**: 372–85.

Kawachi, I, Colditz, G A, Speizer, F E, Manson, J E, Stampfer, M J, Willett, W C, and Hennekens, C H (1997), 'A prospective study of passive smoking and coronary heart disease', *Circulation*, **95**: 2374–9.

Kawachi, I, Colditz, G A, and Stone, C B (1994), 'Does coffee drinking increase the risk of coronary heart disease? Results from a meta-analysis', *Br Heart J*, **72**: 269–75.

Keys, A (1980), *Seven countries: a multivariate analysis of death and coronary heart disease*, Cambridge, MA, and London, Harvard University Press.

Keys, A (1971), 'Sucrose in the diet and coronary heart disease', *Atherosclerosis*, **14**: 193–202.

Khaw, K-T, Wareham, N, Luben, R, Bingham, S, Oakes, S, Welch, A, and Day, N (2001), 'Glycated haemoglobin, diabetes, and mortality in men in Norfolk cohort of European Prospective Investigation of Cancer and Nutrition (EPIC-Norfolk)', *Br Med J*, **322**: 15–18.

King, G (1936), *Natural and political observations and conclusions upon the state and condition of England 1696*, ed. G E Barnett, Baltimore, Johns Hopkins Press.

King, L S (1958), *The medical world of the eighteenth century*, University of Chicago Press.

Kirby, R W, Anderson, J W, Sieling, B, Rees, E D, Chen, W-J L, Miller, R E, and Kay, R M (1981), 'Oat-bran intake selectively lowers serum low-density lipoprotein cholesterol concentrations of hypercholesterolemic men', *Am J Clin Nutr*, **34**: 824–9.

Klag, M J, Mead, L A, LaCroix, A Z, Wang, N Y, Coresh, J, Liang, K Y, Pearson, T A, and Levine, D M (1994), 'Coffee intake and coronary heart disease', *Ann Epidemiol*, **4**: 425–33.

Klatsky, A L, Armstrong, M A, and Friedman, G D (1990), 'Risk of cardiovascular mortality in alcohol drinkers, ex-drinkers and non-drinkers', *Am J Cardiol*, **66**: 1237–42.

Kligfield, P, and Filutowski, K (1995), '"Dr. Anonymous" unmasked: resolution of an eighteenth century mystery in the history of coronary artery disease', *Am J Cardiol*, **75**: 1166–9.

Knapp, V J (1996), 'The coming of vegetables, fruits and key nutrients to the European diet', *Nutr Health*, **10**: 313–21.

Kromhout, D, Bosschieter, E B, and Coulander, C de L (1982), 'Dietary fibre and 10-year mortality from coronary heart disease, cancer and all causes. The Zutphen study', *Lancet*, **ii**: 518–22.

Kromhout, D, Bosschieter, E B, and Coulander, C de L (1985), 'The inverse relation between fish consumption and 20-year mortality from coronary heart disease', *N Engl J Med*, **312**: 1205–9.

Kromhout, D, Menotti, A, Bloemberg, B, Araranis, C, Blackburn, H, Buzina, R, Dontas, A S, Fidanza, F, Giampaoli, and Jansen A (1995), 'Dietary saturated and trans-fatty acids and cholesterol and 25-year mortality from coronary heart disease. The Seven Countries Study', *Prev Med*, **24**: 308–15.

Krüger, Ø, Aase, A, and Steinar, W (1995), 'Ischaemic heart disease mortality among men in Norway: reversal of urban–rural difference between 1966 and 1989', *J Epidemiol Community Health*, **49**: 271–6.

Kushi, L H, Lew, R A, Stare, F J, Ellison, L R, Eclozy, M, Bourke, G, Daly, L, Graham, I, Hickey, N, Mulcahy, R *et al.* (1985), 'Diet and 20-year mortality from coronary heart disease. The Ireland–Boston diet-heart study', *N Engl J Med*, **312**: 811–18.

LaCroix, A Z, Mead, L A, Liang, K Y, Thomas, C B, and Pearson, T A (1986), 'Coffee consumption and the incidence of coronary heart disease', *N Engl J Med*, **315**: 977–82.

Lancisi, G M (1971), *De subitaneis mortibus*, transl. P D White and A V Boursy, New York, St John's University Press.

Landers, J (1993), *Death and the metropolis: studies in the demographic history of London 1670–1830*, Cambridge University Press.

Lane, J (1984), 'The medical practitioners of provincial England in 1783', *Med Hist*, **28**: 353–71.

Langford, P (1992), *A polite and commercial people: England 1727–1783*, Oxford University Press.

Larson, C S (1995), 'Biological changes in human populations with agriculture', *Annu Rev Anthropol*, **24**: 185–213.

Latham, P M (1876), *Collected works*, vol. 1, *Diseases of the heart*, London, New Sydenham Society.

Lawes, J B, and Gilbert, J H (1859), 'Experimental inquiry into the composition of some of the animals fed and slaughtered as human food', *Philos Trans Roy Soc*, London, **149**: 493–680.

Lawrence, M, Neil, A, Mant, D and Fowler, G (eds) (1996), *Prevention of cardiovascular disease: an evidence-based approach*, Oxford General Practice series No. 33, Oxford University Press.

Ledger, H P (1968), 'Body composition as a basis for comparative study of some East African mammals', in M A Crawford (ed.), *Comparative nutrition of wild animals: the proceedings of a symposium held at the Zoological Society of London held on 10 and 11 November 1966*, London, published for the Zoological Society of London by Academic Press.

LeGrady, D, Dyer, A R, Shekelle, R B, Stamler, J, Liu, K, Paul, O, Lepper, M, and Shryock, A M (1987), 'Coffee consumption and mortality in the Chicago Western Electric Company study', *Am J Epidemiol*, **126**: 803–12.

Leibowitz, J O (1970), *The history of coronary heart disease*, London, Wellcome Institute of the History of Medicine.

Lerman, A, Webster, M W, Chesebro, J H, Edwards, W D, Wei, C M, Fuster, V, and Burnett, J C Jr (1993), 'Circulating and tissue endothelin immunoreactivity in hypercholesterolaemic pigs', *Circulation*, **88**: 2923–8.

Lichtenstein, A H, Jauhiainen, M, McGladdery, S, Ausman, L M, Jalbert, S M, Vilella-Bach, S M, Ehnholm, C, Frohlich, J, and Schaefer, E J (1999), 'Effects of different forms of dietary hydrogenated fats on serum lipoprotein cholesterol levels', *N Eng J Med*, **340**: 1933–40.

Lichtstein, E, Chapman, I, and Gupta, P K (1976), 'Diagonal ear-lobe crease and coronary artery sclerosis', (letter) *Ann Intern Med*, **85**: 337–8.

Lillywhite, B (1963), *London coffee houses*, London, George Allen and Unwin.

Long, A R (1931), 'Cardiovascular renal disease. Report of a case three thousand years ago', *Arch Pathol*, **12**: 92–4.

Lyon, T P, Yankley, A, Gofman, J W, and Strisower, B (1956), 'Lipoproteins and diet in coronary heart disease; a five-year study', *Calif Med*, **84**: 325–8.

Lyons, A S, and Petricelli, R J, II (1978), *Medicine: an illustrated history*, New York, Harry N Abrams.

Macdonell, W R (1913), 'On the expectation of life in ancient Rome and in the provinces of Hispania, Lusitania and Africa', *Biometrika*, **9**: 366–80.

McDonough, P, Duncan, G J, Williams, D, and House, J (1997), 'Income dynamics and adult mortality in the United States, 1972 through 1989', *Am J Publ Health*, **87**: 1476–83.

McDougall, J I, and Michaels, L (1972), 'Cardiovascular causes of sudden death in "De subitaneis mortibus" by Giovanni Maria Lancisi', *Bull Hist Med*, **45**: 486–94.

McElroy, C L, Gissen, S A, and Fishbein, M C (1978), 'Exercise-induced reduction in myocardial infarct size after coronary artery occlusion in the rat', *Circulation*, **57**: 958–62.

McKeigue, P M, and Marmot, J G M (1988), 'Mortality from coronary artery disease in Asian communities in London', *Br Med J*, **297**: 903.

McKeigue, P M, Marmot, M G, Adelstein, A M, Hunt, S P, Shipley, M J, Butler, S M, Riemersma, R A, and Turner P R (1985), 'Diet and risk factors for coronary heart disease in Asians in northwest London', *Lancet*, **ii**: 1086–90.

McKeown, T (1976), *The modern rise of population*, London, Edward Arnold.

MacMahon, S, Peto, R, Cutler, J, Collins, R, Sorlie, P, Neaton, J, Abbott, R, Godwin, J, Dyer, A, and Stamler, J (1990), 'Blood pressure, stroke, and coronary heart disease. Part I, Prolonged differences in blood pressure: prospective observational studies corrected for the regression dilution bias', *Lancet*, **335**: 765–74.

*Manual of the international list of causes of death: as adapted for use in England and Wales, Scotland and Northern Ireland; based on the fourth decennial revision by the International Commission, Paris, 1929* (1931), London, HMSO.

Markowe, H L, Marmot, M G, Shipley, M J, Bulpitt, C J, Meade, T W, Stirling, Y, Vickers, M V, and Semmence, A (1985), 'Fibrinogen: a possible link between social class and coronary heart disease', *Br Med J*, **291**: 1312–14.

Marmot, M G, Adelstein, A M, Robinson, N, and Rose, G A (1978), 'Changing social-class distribution of heart disease', *Br Med J*, **ii**: 1109–12.

Marmot, M G, Bosma, H, Hemingway, H, Brunner, E, and Stansfeld, S (1997), 'Contribution of job control and other risk factors to social variations in coronary heart disease incidence', *Lancet*, **350**: 235–9.

Marmot, M G, Shipley, M J, and Rose, G (1994), 'Inequalities in death-specific explanations of a general problem', *Lancet*, **i**: 1003–6.

Marmot, M G, and Smith, G D (1989), 'Why are the Japanese living longer', *Br Med J*, **299**: 1547–51.

Martin, J M, Hulley, S B, Browner, W S, Kuller, L H, and Wentworth, D (1986), 'Serum cholesterol, blood pressure, and mortality: implications from a cohort of 361,662 men', *Lancet*, **ii**: 933–9.

Mathias, P. (1979), *The transformation of England: essays in the economic and social history of England in the eighteenth century*, New York, Columbia University Press.

Mayr-Harting, H, and Harris, P (1986), 'St. Etheldreda and the death of Gervase', *Int J Cardiol*, **12**: 369–71.

Michaels, L (1966), 'Aetiology of coronary heart disease: an historical approach', *Br Heart J*, **28**: 258–64.

Miettinen, M, Turpeinen, O, Karvonen, M J, Elosuo, R, and Paavilainen, E (1972), 'Effect of cholesterol-lowering diet on mortality from coronary heart-disease and other causes. A twelve-year clinical trial in men and women', *Lancet*, **ii**: 835–8.

Miller, G J, Cruikshank, J K, Ellis, L J, Thompson, R L, Wilkes, H C, Stirling, Y, Metropolous, K A, Allison, J V, Fox, T E, and Walker, A O (1989), 'Fat consumption and factor VII coagulant activity in middle aged men. An association between a dietary and thrombogenic coronary risk factor', *Arteriosclerosis*, **78**: 19–24.

Miller, M, Seidler, A, Moalemi, A, and Pearson, T A (1998), 'Normal triglyceride levels in coronary heart disease events: the Baltimore coronary observational long-term study', *J Am Coll Cardiol*, **31**: 1252–7.

Mingay, G E (ed.) (1989), *The agrarian history of England and Wales, Volume VI: 1750–1850*, Cambridge University Press.

Mitchell, B R (1988), *British historical statistics*, Cambridge University Press.

Mitchell, B R, and Deane, P (1971), *Abstract of British historical statistics*, Cambridge University Press.

Morand, S F (1732), 'Sur quelques accidents remarquables dans les organes de la circulation du sang', *Mémoires de l'Académie Royale des Sciences.*

Morgagni, G B (1769), *The seats and causes of diseases*, transl. B Alexander, 3 vols, London, A Miller and T Cadell.

Morgan, A D (1968), 'Some forms of undiagnosed coronary disease in nineteenth-century England', *Med Hist*, **12**: 344–58.

Morison, S E (1965), *The Oxford history of the American people*, New York, Oxford University Press.

Morris, J N (1951), 'Recent history of coronary disease', *Lancet*, **i**: 69–73.

Morris, J N, Chave, S P, Adam, C, Sirey, C, Epstein, L, and Sheehan, D J (1973), 'Vigorous exercise in leisure-time and incidence of coronary heart-disease', *Lancet*, **i**: 333–9.

Morris, J N, Kagan, A, Pattison, D C, and Gardner, M J (1966), 'Incidence and prediction of ischaemic heart-disease in London busmen', *Lancet*, **ii**: 553–9.

Morris, J N, Marr, J W, and Clayton, D G (1977), 'Diet and heart: a postscript', *Br Med J*, **ii**: 1307–14.

Morris, N, and Rothman, D J (eds) (1996), *The Oxford history of the prison: the practice of punishment in western society*, Oxford University Press.

Muir, J, and Mant, D (1996), 'Multiple risk', in Lawrence, M, Neil, A, Mant, D and Fowler, G (eds), *Prevention of cardiovascular disease: an evidence-based approach*, Oxford University Press.

Muntzel, M, and Drüeke, T (1992), 'A comprehensive review of the salt and blood pressure relationship', *Am J Hypertens*, Suppl 4, 1S-42S.

Murphy-Chutorian, D R, Wexman, M P, Greco, A J, Heininger, J A, Glassman, E, Gaull, G E, Ng, S K, Feit, F, Wexman, K, and Fox, A C (1985), 'Methionine intolerance: a possible risk factor for coronary artery disease', *J Am Coll Cardiol*, **6**: 725–30.

Murray, S S, Bjelke, E, Gibson, R W, and Schuman, L M (1981), 'Coffee consumption and mortality from ischemic heart disease and other causes: results from the Lutheran Brotherhood study 1966–1978', *Am J Epidemiol*, **113**: 661–7.

Myers, M G, and Basinski, A (1992), 'Coffee and coronary heart disease', *Arch Intern Med*, **152**: 1767–72.

Naismith, D J, Akenyanju, P A, Szanto, S, and Yudkin, J (1970), 'The effect, in volunteers, of coffee and decaffeinated coffee on blood glucose, insulin, plasma lipids and some factors involved in blood clotting', *Nutr Metab*, **12**: 144–51.

National Centre for Health Statistics (1987), *Vital statistics of the United States 1983*, DHHS pub no. (PHS) 87–1101, Washington, Government Printing Office.

Noble, J, Bourassa, M G, Petitclerc, R, and Dyrda, I (1976), 'Myocardial bridging and milking effect of the left anterior descending coronary artery. Normal variant or obstruction?', *Am J Cardiol*, **37**: 993–9.

Nygård, O, Vollset, S E, Refsum, H, Stensvold, I, Tverdal, A, Nordrehang, J E, Ueland, M, and Kvale, C (1995), 'Total plasma homocysteine and cardiovascular risk profile. The Hordaland homocysteine study', *JAMA*, **274**: 1526–33.

Oberman, A (1985), 'Exercise and the primary prevention of cardiovascular disease', *Am J Cardiol*, **55**: 10d–20d.

Obrastzow, W P, and Straschesko, N D (1910), 'Zur Kenntnis der Thrombose der Koronarterien des Herzens', *Zschrf Klin Med*, **71**: 116–32.

O'Dea, K, Traianedes, K, Chisholm, K, Leyden, H, and Sinclair, A J (1990), 'Cholesterol-lowering effect of a low-fat diet containing lean beef is reversed by the addition of beef fat', *Am J Clin Nutr*, **52**: 491–4.

O'Gorman, F (1997), *The long eighteenth century: British political and social history 1688–1832*, London, Arnold.

Osler, W (1910), 'The Lumleian lectures on angina pectoris, Lecture I', *Lancet*, **i**: 697–702.

Osler, W (1901), *The principles and practice of medicine*, 4th ed., Edinburgh and London, Y J Pentland.

Osmond, C (1995), 'Coronary heart disease trends in England and Wales 1952–1991', *J Public Health Med*, **17**: 404–10.

Overton, M (1996), *Agricultural revolution in England: the transformation of the agrarian economy 1500–1850*, Cambridge University Press.

Page, L B, Damon, A, and Moellering R C Jr (1974), 'Antecedents of cardiovascular disease in six Solomon Islands societies', *Circulation*, **49**: 1132–46.

Parker, R A C (1955–6), 'Coke of Norfolk and the agrarian revolution', *Econ Hist Rev*, 2nd series, **8**: 156–66.

Parkinson, J (1973), 'An essay on the shaking palsy 1817', reprinted in Wilkins, R H and Brady, I A, *Neurological classics*, New York, Johnson Reprint Corporation, pp. 88–92.

Parry, C H (1799), *An inquiry into the symptoms and causes of the syncope anginosa, commonly called angina pectoris*, Bath, R Cruttwell.

Paston-Williams, S (1993), *The art of dining: a history of cooking and eating*, London, National Trust.

Pepys, S (1970–83), *The diary of Samuel Pepys*, ed. R C Latham, and W Matthews, 11 vols, University of California Press.

Picard, L (2000), *Dr. Johnson's London*, London, Weidenfeld and Nicolson.

Pickering, G (1964), 'Systemic arterial hypertension', in Fishman, A P and Richards, D W (eds), *Circulation of the blood: men and ideas*, New York, Oxford University Press.

Pietinen, P, Vartiainen, E, Seppanen, R, Aro, A and Puska, P (1996), 'Changes in diet in Finland from 1972 to 1992: impact on coronary heart disease risk', *Prev Med*, **25**: 243–50.

Pietinen, P, Vartiainen, E, Seppanen, R, Aro, A, Puska, P and Huttunen J K (1987), 'Dietary fat and blood pressure—a review', *Eur Heart J*, **8**: Suppl B, 9–17.

Pinsky, C, and Bose, R (1988), 'Pyridine and other coal tar constituents as free radical-generating environmental neurotoxicants', *Mol Cell Biochem*, **84**: 217–22.

Pliny the Elder (1942), *Natural history*, transl. H Rackham, 10 vols, Cambridge, MA, Harvard University Press.

The Pooling Project Research Group (1978), 'Relationship of blood pressure, serum cholesterol, smoking habit, relative weight and ECG abnormalities to incidence of major chronic events: final report of the pooling project', *J Chron Dis*, **31**: 201.

Porter, R (1990), *English society in the eighteenth century*, Harmondsworth, Penguin Books.

Porter, R (1997), *The greatest benefit to mankind: a medical history of humanity from antiquity to the present*, London, HarperCollins.

Porter, R (1994), *London: a social history*, London, Hamish Hamilton.

Porter, R, and Rousseau, G S (1998), *Gout: the patrician malady*, New Haven and London, Yale University Press.

Price, F W (ed.) (1946), *A textbook of the practice of medicine*, London, Oxford University Press.

Prothero, R E (1888), *The pioneers and progress of English farming*, London, Longmans, Green.

Proudfit, W L (1983), 'Origin of concept of ischaemic heart disease', *Br Heart J*, **50**: 209–12.

Przyklenk, K (1994), 'Nicotine exacerbates postischemic contractile dysfunction of "stunned" myocardium in the canine model: possible role of free radicals', *Circulation*, **89**: 1272–81.

Pyörälä, K (1979), 'Relationship of glucose tolerance and plasma insulin to the incidence of coronary heart disease: results from two population studies in Finland', *Diabetes Care*, **2**: 131–41.

Ramazzini, B (1964), *Diseases of workers*, transl. from the Latin text, *De morbis artificum*, of 1713, by W C Wright, London, Hafner.

Ramsay, G D (1952), 'The smugglers' trade, a neglected aspect of English commercial development', *Royal Hist Soc Trans*, 5th series, **2**: 131–57.

Razzell, P E (1965), 'Population change in eighteenth-century England: a re-interpretation', *Econ Hist Rev*, 2nd series, **18**: 312–32.

Razzell, P E (1993), 'The growth of population in eighteenth century England. A critical reappraisal', *J Econ Hist*, **53**: 743–71.

Reader, W J (1966), *Professional men: the rise of the professional classes in nineteenth-century England*, London, Weidenfeld and Nicolson.

Reaven, G M (1979), 'Effects of differences in amount and kind of dietary carbohydrate on plasma glucose and insulin responses in man', *Am J Clin Nutr*, **32**: 2568–78.

Reaven, G M, Lithell, H, and Landsberg, L (1996), 'Hypertension and associated metabolic abnormalities—the role of insulin resistance and the sympathoadrenal system', *N Engl J Med*, **334**: 374–81.

Reed, W (1866), *The history of sugar and sugar yielding plants*, London, Longmans, Green.

Registrar-General (1885), *Supplement to 45th annual report of the registrar-general of births, deaths and marriages in England and Wales*, London, Eyre and Spottiswood.

Reiser, S, Hallfrisch, J, Michaelis, O E IV, Lazar, F L, Martin, R E, and Prather, E S (1979), 'Isocaloric exchange of dietary starch and sucrose in humans. Effects on levels of fasting blood lipids', *Am J Clin Nutr*, **32**: 1659–69.

Reisin, E, Abel, R, Modan, M, Silverberg, D S, Eliahou, H E, and Modan, B (1978), 'Effect of weight loss without salt restriction on the reduction of blood pressure in overweight hypertensive patients', *N Engl J Med*, **298**: 1–6.

Rhodes, R (1986), *The making of the atomic bomb*, New York, Simon and Schuster.

Roberts, W C (1986), 'The senile cardiac calcification syndrome', *Am J Cardiol*, **58**: 572–4.

Robertson, W (1896), *History of the reign of Charles the Fifth*, 3 vols, London, George Routledge and Sons.

Robinson, E (1972), *The early English coffee house*, 2nd ed., Christchurch, Dolphin Press.

Rogers, J E T (1909), *Six centuries of work and wages: a history of English labour*, London, Swan Sonneschein.

Rose, F C (1995), *The history of migraine from Mesopotamia to medieval times*, *Cephalalgia*, Supplement 15.

Rosengren, A, and Wilhelmsen, L (1991), 'Coffee, coronary heart disease and mortality in middle-aged Swedish men: findings from the Primary Prevention Study', *J Intern Med*, **230**: 67–71.

Rosenman, R H, Friedman, M, Straus, R, Wurm, M, Kositchek, R, Hahn, W, and Werthessen, N T (1964), 'A predictive study of coronary heart disease', *JAMA*, **189**: 15–22.

Rosenthal, J, Simone, P G, and Silbergleit, A (1974), 'Effects of prostaglandin deficiency natriuresis, diuresis and blood pressure', *Prostaglandins*, **5**: 435–40.

Rowntree, B S (1901), *Poverty: a study of town life*, London, Macmillan.

Russell, G (1979), 'Bulimia nervosa: an ominous variant of anorexia nervosa', *Psychol Med*, **9**: 429–48.

Ryle, J A, and Russell, W T (1949), 'The natural history of coronary heart disease', *Br Heart J*, **11**: 370–89.

Sacks, F M, Moye, L A, Davis, B R, Cole, T G, Rouleau, J L, Nash, D T, Pfeffer, M A, and Braunwald, E (1998), 'Relationship between plasma LDL concentrations during treatment with pravastatin and recurrent coronary events in the Cholesterol and Recurrent Events trial', *Circulation*, **15**: 1446–52.

Sandler, D P, Comstock, G W, Helsing, K J, and Shore, D L (1989), 'Deaths from all causes in non-smokers who lived with smokers', *Am J Public Health*, **79**: 163–7.

Sangiorgi, G, Rumberger, J A, Severson, A, Edwards, W D, Gregoire, J, Fitzpatrick, L A, and Schwartz, R S (1998), 'Arterial calcification and not lumen stenosis is highly correlated with atherosclerotic plaque burden in humans: a histological study of 723 coronary artery segments using non-decalcifying methodology', *J Am Coll Cardiol*, **31**: 126–33.

Sans, S, Kesteloot, H, and Kromhout, D, on behalf of the task force (1997), 'The burden of cardiovascular diseases mortality in Europe. Task force of the European Society of Cardiology on Cardiovascular Mortality and Morbidity Statistics in Europe', *Euro Heart J*, **18**: 1231–48.

Santow, G (1995), '*Coitus interruptus* and the control of natural fertility', *Popul Stud*, **49**: 19–43.

Savage, P J, and Saad, M F (1993), 'Insulin and atherosclerosis: villain, accomplice, or innocent bystander?', *Br Heart J*, **69**: 473–5.

Schaeffer, G B (1787), *De angina pectoris vulgo se dicta. Dissertatio inauguralis medica*, Gottingen, H M Grape.

Schaible, T F, and Scheuer, J (1985), 'Cardiac adaptations to chronic exercise', *Prog Cardiovasc Dis*, **27**: 297–324.

Schama, S (8 April 1996), 'Mad cows and Englishmen', *New Yorker*.

Schofield, R S (1972–3), 'Dimensions of illiteracy 1750–1850', *Explorations in Economic History*, **10**: 437–54.

Schroeder, H A (1958), 'Degenerative cardiovascular disease in the Orient. II Hypertension', *J Chron Dis*, **8**: 312–33.

Schumpeter, E (1960), *English overseas trade statistics, 1697–1808*, Oxford, Clarendon Press.

Scott, S, and Duncan, C J (1999), 'Nutrition, fertility and steady-state population dynamics in a pre-industrial community in Penrith, northern England', *J Biosoc Sci*, **31**: 505–23.

Seed, J (1992), 'From "middling sort" to middle class in late eighteenth- and early nineteenth-century England' in Bush, M L (ed.), *Social orders and social classes in Europe since 1500*, London, Longman.

Sharpe, J A (1988), *Early modern England: a social history 1550–1760*, London, Edward Arnold.

Shaukat, N, de Bono, D P, and Jones, D R (1995), 'Like father like son? Sons of patients of European or Indian origin with coronary artery disease reflect their parents' risk factor patterns', *Br Heart J*, **74**: 318–23.

Shell, E R (2001), 'New World Syndrome', *Atlantic Monthly*, **287**: 50–3.

Sigfusson, N, Sigvalduson, H, Steingrimsdottir, L, Gudmundsdottir, I, Stefansdottir, I, Thorsteinsson, T, and Sigurdsson, G (1991), 'Decline in ischaemic heart disease in Iceland and changes in risk factor levels', *Br Med J*, **302**: 1371–5.

Simpson, D (1984), 'Trends in major risk factors. Cigarette smoking', *Postgrad Med J*, **60**: 20–5.

Sinclair, A J, and O'Dea, K J (1987), 'The lipid levels and fatty composition of the lean portions of pork, chicken and rabbit meats', *Food Techol*, Australia, **39**: 232–3.

Sinclair, A J, Slattery, W J, and O'Dea, K J (1982), 'The analysis of polyunsaturated fatty acids in meat by capillary gas-liquid chromatography', *J Sci Food Agric*, **33**: 771–6.

Slicher van Bath, B H (1965), *The agrarian history of western Europe A.D. 500–1800*, transl. O Ordish, London, Edward Arnold.

Smith, S (1857), 'On the evidence of the prolongation of life during the eighteenth century', *Transactions of the National Association for the Promotion of the Social Sciences*.

Spiller, R C (1996), 'Cholesterol, fibre and bile acids', *Lancet*, **347**: 415–16.

Sprague, H B (1966), 'Environment in relation to coronary heart disease', *Arch Environ Health*, **13**: 4–12.

Stamler, J (1973), 'Epidemiology of coronary heart disease', *Med Clin N Am*, **57**: 5–46.

Stamler, J, Stamler, R, and Pullman, T N (eds) (1967), *The epidemiology of hypertension: proceedings of an international symposium ... Chicago, Illinois*, London, Grune and Stratton.

Stamler, J, Wentworth, D, and Nealon, J D (1986), 'Is relationship between serum cholesterol and risk of premature death from coronary heart disease continuous and graded?', *JAMA*, **256**: 2823–8.

Stampfer, M J, Krauss, R M, Ma, J, Blanche, P J, Holl, L G, Sacks, F M, and Hennekens, C H (1996), 'A prospective study of triglyceride level, low-density lipoprotein particle diameter, and risk of myocardial infarction', *JAMA*, **276**: 882–8.

Stampfer, M J, Malinow, M R, Willett, W C, Newcomer, L M, Upston, B, Ullmann, D, Tishler, P V, and Hennekens, C H (1992), 'A prospective study of plasma homocyst(e)ine and risk of myocardial infarction in US physicians', *JAMA*, **268**: 877–81.

Stensvold, I, Tverdal, A, and Jacobsen, B K (1996), 'Cohort study of coffee intake and death from coronary heart disease over 12 years', *Br Med J*, **312**: 544–5.

Stephen, A H, and Sieber, G M (1994), 'Trends in individual fat consumption in the United Kingdom 1900–1985', *Br J Nutr*, **71**: 775–88.

Storch, K, Anderson, J W, and Young, V R (1984), 'Oat bran muffins lower serum cholesterol of healthy young people', *Clin Res*, **32**: 740A (abstr).

Strom, A and Jensen, R A (1951), 'Mortality from circulatory diseases in Norway 1940–45', *Lancet*, **i**: 126–9.

Suetonius Tranquillus, G (2000), *Lives of the Caesars*, transl. C Edwards, New York, Oxford University Press.

Sutton, D (ed.) (1980), *A textbook of radiology and imaging*, 3rd ed., Edinburgh, Churchill Livingstone.

Sutton, D, and Grainger, R G (1969), *Textbook of radiology*, 1st ed, Edinburgh and London, E & S Livingstone.

Sutton, J D (1989), 'Altering milk composition by feeding', *J Dairy Sci*, **72**: 2801–14.

Sydenham, T (1710), *Compleat method of curing almost all diseases*, 4th ed., London, T Home and R Parker.

*Syndrome X*, American Heart Association Internet posting, http://www.americanheart.org/

Sytkowski, P A, Kannel, W B, and D'Agostino, R B (1990), 'Changes in risk factors and the decline in mortality from cardiovascular disease. The Framingham Heart Study', *N Engl J Med*, **322**: 1635–41.

Tann, J (1989), 'Corn milling', in G E Mingay (ed.), *The agrarian history of England and Wales, Volume VI: 1750–1850*, Cambridge University Press.

Thelle, D S, Heyden, S, and Fodor, J G (1987), 'Coffee and cholesterol in epidemiological and experimental studies', *Atherosclerosis*, **67**: 97–103.

Thirsk, J (1985), 'Agricultural policy: public debate and legislation', in J Thirsk (ed.), *The agrarian history of England and Wales, Volume V: 1640–1750. II, Agrarian change*, Cambridge University Press.

Thirsk, J (ed.) (1967–91), *The agrarian history of England and Wales*, 8 vols, Cambridge University Press.

Thompson, G R (1995), 'Angiographic trials of lipid-lowering therapy: end of an era?' *Br Heart J*, **74**: 343–7,

Treasure, C B, Klein, J L, Weintraub, W S, Talley, J D, Stillabower, M E, Kosinski, A S, Zhang, J, Boccuzzi, S J, Cedarholm, J D, and Alexander R W (1995), 'Beneficial effects of cholesterol-lowering therapy on the coronary endothelium in patients with coronary artery disease', *N Engl J Med*, **332**: 481–7.

Trevelyan, G M (1947), *English social history*, 3rd ed., London, Longmans, Green.

Trevelyan, G M (1978), *English social history*, illustrated edition, London, Longman.

Trevelyan, G M (1947), *History of England*, London, Longmans, Green.

Turberville, A S (ed.) (1952), *Johnson's England*, 2 vols, Oxford, Clarendon Press.

Tverdal, A, Stensvold, I, Solvoll, K, Foss, O P, Lund-Larsen, P, and Bjartveit, K (1990), 'Coffee consumption and death from coronary heart disease in middle aged Norwegian men and women', *Br Med J*, **300**: 566–9.

Tyroler, H A, and Cassel, J (1964), 'Health consequences of culture change, II. The effect of urbanization on coronary heart mortality in rural residents', *J Chronic Dis*, **17**: 167–77.

Urgert, R, Meyboom, S, Kuilman, M, Rexwinkel, H, Visser, M N, Klerk, M, and Katan, M B (1996), 'Comparison of the effect of cafetière and filtered coffee on serum concentrations of liver aminotransferases and lipids: six month randomised controlled trial', *Br Med J*, **313**: 1362–5.

Urgert, R, Van der Weg, G, Kosmeyer-Schuil, T G, van de Bovenkamp, P, Hovenier, R, and Katan, M B (1995), 'Levels of the cholesterol elevating diterpenes cafestol and kahweol in various coffee brews', *J Agric Food Chem*, **43**: 2167–72.

Van Boven, A J, Jukema, J W, Zwinderman, A H, Crijns, A J, Liek, I, and Brusche, A V (1996), 'Reduction of transient myocardial ischemia with pravastatin in addition to the conventional treatment in patients with angina pectoris. REGRESS Study Group', *Circulation*, **94**: 1503–5.

Van Horn, L V, Liu, K, Parker, D, Emidy, L, Liao, Y L, Pan, W G, Guinette, D, Hewitt, J, and Stamler, J (1986), 'Serum lipid response to oat product intake with a fat modified diet', *J Am Diet Assoc*, **86**: 759–64.

Vekshtein, V I, Young, A C, Vita, J A, Nabel, E G, Fish, R D, Bird, J, Selwyn, A P, and Ganz, P (1989), 'Fish oil improves endothelial dependent relaxation in patients with coronary arterial disease', *Circulation*, Suppl II, Abstr 1727.

Von Schacky, C, and Weber, P C (1985), 'Metabolism and effects on platelet function of the purified eicosapentaenoic and docosahexaenoic acids in humans', *J Clin Invest*, **76**: 2446–50.

Wall, J (1776), 'Letter to Heberden', *Medical Observations and Inquiries by a Society of Physicians in London*, **5**: 233–51, in Proudfit, W L (1983), 'Origin of concept of ischemic heart disease', *Br Heart J*, **50**: 209–12.

Walsh, J, Haydon, C, and Taylor, S (eds.) (1993), *The Church of England c. 1689–c. 1833: from toleration to tractarianism*, Cambridge University Press.

Walsh, J, and Taylor, S (1993), 'The Church and Anglicanism in the "long" eighteenth century', in Walsh, J, Haydon, C, and Taylor, S (eds), *The Church of England c.1689–c. 1833: from toleration to tractarianism*, Cambridge University Press.

Wang, I Y, and Fraser, I S (1994), 'Reproductive function and contraception in the postpartum period', *Obstet Gynecol Surv*, **49**: 56–63.

Ward, J, and Yell, J (eds. and transl.) (1993), *The medical casebook of William Brownrigg, M.D., F.R.S. (1712–1800) of the Town of Whitehaven in Cumberland*, *Medical History*, Supplement No. 13, London, Wellcome Institute for the History of Medicine.

Warren, J (1812), 'Remarks on angina pectoris', *N Engl J Med Surg*, **1**: 1–11.

Welborn, T A, and Wearne, K (1979), 'Coronary heart disease incidence and cardiovascular mortality in Busselton with reference to glucose and insulin concentrations', *Diabetes Care*, **2**: 154–60.

Welin, L, Eriksson, H, Larsson, B, Ohlson, L O, Svardsudd, K, and Tillin, G (1992), 'Hyperinsulinemia is not a major coronary risk factor in elderly men. The study of men born in 1913', *Diabetologia*, **35**: 766–70.

Wells, A J (1994), 'Passive smoking as a cause of heart disease', *J Am Coll Cardiol*, **24**: 546–54.

Whitsett, T L, Manion, C V, and Christensen, H D (1984), 'Cardiovascular effects of coffee and caffeine', *Am J Cardiol*, **53**: 918–22.

Wilkinson, R G (1996), *Unhealthy societies: the afflictions of inequality*, London and New York, Routledge.

Wiseman, J (1986), *A history of the British pig*, London, Duckworth.

Withering, W (1785), *An account of the foxglove, and some of its medical uses: with practical remarks on dropsy, and other diseases*, Birmingham, M Swinney.

Wolf, S G (1985), 'History of the study of stress and heart disease', in Beamish, R E, Singal, P, and Dhalla, N S (eds), *Stress and heart disease*, Boston, Martinus Nijhoff Publishing.

Wood, G B (1852), *A treatise on the practice of medicine*, Philadelphia, Lippincott, Grambo.

Woodforde, J (1927), *The diary of a country parson 1788–1792*, ed. J Beresford, 3 vols, Oxford University Press.

Wright, A, Burstyn, P G, and Gibney, M J (1979), 'Dietary fibre and blood pressure', *Br Med J*, **ii**: 1541–3.

Wrigley, E A (1985), 'Urban growth and agricultural change: England and the continent in the early modern period', *J Interdis Hist*, **15**: 683–728.

Wrigley, E A, Davies, R S, Oeppen, J E, and Schofield, R S (1997), *English population history from family reconstitution 1580–1837*, Cambridge University Press.

Wrigley, E A, and Schofield, R S (1981), *The population history of England 1541–1871: a reconstruction*, Cambridge, MA, Harvard University Press.

Yano, K, Reed, D M, and MacLean, J M (1987), 'Coffee consumption and incidence of coronary heart disease' (letter), *N Engl J Med*, **316**: 946.

Young, A (1770), *The farmers' tour through the north of England or the northern tour*, 4 vols, London, W Strahan.

Young, G M (ed.) (1934), *Early Victorian England*, 2 vols, London, Oxford University Press.

Yudkin, J (1957), 'Diet and coronary thrombosis: hypothesis and fact', *Lancet*, **ii**: 155–62.

Yudkin, J (1964), 'Dietary fat and dietary sugar in relation to ischaemic heart disease and diabetes', *Lancet*, **ii**: 4–5.

Yudkin, J and Roddy, J (1964), 'Levels of dietary sucrose in patients with occlusive atherosclerotic disease', *Lancet*, **ii**: 6–8.

Zeiher, A M, Drexler, H, Saurbier, B, and Just, H (1993), 'Endothelium mediated

coronary flow modulation in humans: effects of age, atherosclerosis, hypercholesterolemia and hypertension', *J Clin Invest*, **92**: 652–62.
Zock, P L, Katan, M B, Merkus, M P, van Dusseldorp, M, and Hanyvan, J L
(1990), 'Effect of a lipid-rich fraction from boiled coffee on serum cholesterol',
*Lancet*, **335**: 1235–7.

# Index

# Index

217